The Multiple Pregnancy Sourcebook

Pregnancy and the First Days with Twins, Triplets, and More

• • •

Nancy A. Bowers, R.N., B.S.N.

CB

CONTEMPORARY BOOKS

Chicago   New York   San Francisco   Lisbon   Madrid   Mexico City   Milan
New Delhi   San Juan   Seoul   Singapore   Sydney   Toronto

Library of Congress Cataloging-in-Publication Data

Bowers, Nancy A.
   The multiple pregnancy soucebook / Nancy A. Bowers.
     p. cm.
   Includes bibliographical references and index.
   ISBN 0-7373-0306-9
   1. Multiple pregnancy.   2. Multiple pregnancy—Economic aspects.
    I. Title.
RG567.B684 2001
618.2'5—dc21   00-065999
                                                          CIP

Published by Contemporary Books
A division of The McGraw-Hill Companies
4255 West Touhy Avenue, Lincolnwood, Illinois 60712, U.S.A.

2 3 4 5 6 7 8 9 10 DOC/DOC 0 9 8 7 6 5 4 3 2

International Standard Book Number: 0-7373-0306-9

Printed and bound by R. R. Donnelley & Sons Co.

McGraw-Hill books are available at special quantity discounts to use as premiums and sales promotions, or for use in corporate training programs. For more information, please write to the Director of Special Sales, Professional Publishing, McGraw-Hill, Two Penn Plaza, New York, NY 10121-2298. Or contact your local bookstore.

The purpose of this book is to educate. It is sold with the understanding that the publisher and author shall have neither liability nor responsibility for any injury caused or alleged to be caused directly or indirectly by the information contained in this book. While every effort has been made to ensure its accuracy, the book's contents should not be construed as medical advice. Each person's health needs are unique. To obtain recommendations appropriate to your particular situation, please consult a qualified health care provider.

Contents

Acknowledgments   xi

PART I
The Joys and Challenges of Multiple Pregnancy   1

    A Book for Mothers   2
    How the Book Was Written   2
    Words and Meanings   4

Chapter One
Welcome to the World of Multiples   7

    How Multiples Come About   10
    Placentas in Multiple Pregnancy   13
    Identical or Fraternal?   15
    Diagnosis of Multiple Pregnancy   16
    Surprise Multiples   17

Chapter Two
Multiple Pregnancy After Infertility   19

    Understanding Infertility Technology
        Before You Get Pregnant   19
    Preventing Higher-Order Multiples   22
    Concerns About Multiple Pregnancy After Infertility   24
    Future Children   29

Chapter Three

Emotions in Multiple Pregnancy   31

Common Concerns   32
Dads Have Emotions and Worries, Too   33
Out-of-Control Worries   34
Balancing Your Concerns   35
Finding Support   37

Chapter Four

Multiple Pregnancy Nutrition: Eating for Everyone   39

What Are You Eating Now?   39
Nutritional Recommendations for
    Multiple Pregnancy   40
Supplementing Your Diet   50
Fluids   52
Vegetarians   53
Diabetes   53
Eating Disorders   54
Food Additives   54
Food-Borne Illnesses   55
How Are You Eating?   56
Weight Gain   57

Chapter Five

Your Changing Body   61

Your Amazing Uterus   62
Outfitting Your Fast-Growing Body   62
Digestion in Early Pregnancy   64
Digestion in Later Pregnancy   66
Urination   66
Shortness of Breath   67
Fatigue   67
Insomnia   68
Aches and Pains   70
Blood Vessel Changes   72
Diastasis Recti   72
Itching   73
Circulation   74
Skin Changes   75

Chapter Six
Adapting Your Lifestyle with a Multiple Pregnancy   77

Working Outside the Home   77
Homemakers and Caring for Children   80
Exercise   82
Social Activities   85
Intimacy and Sexual Relations   86
Travel   87
Lifestyle Hazards   88
What Is Really Important?   90

Chapter Seven
Prenatal Care for You and Your Babies   91

Choosing a Care Provider   91
Perinatologist   93
Your First Prenatal Appointment   95
Prenatal Care   97
Prenatal Education   102

Chapter Eight
Fetal Growth and Development   105

The Beginning of Pregnancy   105
Single Fetal Development   106
Multiple Fetal Development   108
Intrauterine Behavior   109

Chapter Nine
Prenatal Diagnosis and Testing in Multiple Pregnancy   113

Ultrasound   114
Alpha Fetoprotein   117
Chorionic Villus Sampling   118
Amniocentesis   119
Nonstress Test   120
Biophysical Profile   121
Doppler Flow Ultrasound   122
Fetal Movement   122
Decision Making   123

PART II

The Joys and Challenges of Being High-Risk   125

The Facts   126
Facing the Facts   127

Chapter Ten

Preterm Labor and Birth   131

What Is Preterm for Multiples?   131
Why Is Preterm Birth a Concern?   132
Causes of Preterm Labor   134
Signs of Preterm Labor   135
Premature Rupture of Membranes   139
Predicting Preterm Labor   141
Treating Preterm Labor with Medications   145
Other Ways to Manage Preterm Labor   149
Reducing the Chances of Preterm Labor—
    What Can You Do?   155

Chapter Eleven

Other Complications in Multiple Pregnancy   157

High Blood Pressure   157
Intrauterine Growth Restriction   162
Gestational Diabetes   165
Amniotic Fluid Problems   166
Placental Problems   169
Umbilical Cord Problems   174
Fetal Loss—When Multiples Die During Pregnancy   175

Chapter Twelve

Bed Rest   181

Problems of Bed Rest   182
How to Cope with Bed Rest   183

Chapter Thirteen

Multifetal Pregnancy Reduction   191

    Who Is a Candidate?   192
    The Procedure   193
    Risks and Complications   194
    Decision Making   194

PART III

The Joys and Challenges of Giving Birth to Multiples   197

Chapter Fourteen

Planning for the Birth of Your Babies   199

    What to Bring to the Hospital   199
    Support in Labor and Delivery   201
    Comfort in Labor and Birth   205
    Delivery Decisions   211

Chapter Fifteen

Labor and Vaginal Birth of Multiples   219

    Signs of Labor   219
    Hospital Admission   221
    Procedures for the Birth of Multiples   222
    Labor   227
    Labor Induction   235
    What About Vaginal Birth After Cesarean?   236
    Cord Blood Banking   237

Chapter Sixteen

Cesarean Birth of Multiples   239

    Preparing for a Cesarean Delivery   240
    In the Operating Room   241

Chapter Seventeen

Your Recovery and Postpartum Care   245

The First Hours of Recovery   246
Your Care in the Hospital   247
Managing Pain After Birth   248
Other Discomforts   249
Your Body Isn't Pregnant Anymore   250
Postpartum Blues and Depression   254
Birth Control   257
Tips for Coping   257

PART IV

The Joys and Challenges of Multiple Babies   259

Chapter Eighteen

Well-Baby Care in the Hospital   261

The First Hours for Your Babies   261
Newborn Appearance and Characteristics   262
Newborn Procedures and Treatments   265
Initial Newborn Care   266

Chapter Nineteen

Your Babies in Intensive Care   271

Who Will Care for Your Babies?   272
Health and Survival of Premature Babies   273
Physical Needs of Premature Babies   275
Common Health Problems of Premature Babies   279

Chapter Twenty

Specialized Care for Babies   283

Developmental Care   283
Kangaroo Care   289
Co-Bedding of Multiples   291
Being Your Babies' Advocate   294
Your Emotions When Your Babies Are in the NICU   295

Chapter Twenty-One

Getting to Know Your Babies 299

Time with Your Babies in the Hospital—
Rooming-In 299
Bonding 300
Tips for Bonding in the Hospital 304

Chapter Twenty-Two

Feeding Multiple Babies—Creative Dining 307

Breastfeeding 307
Benefits of Breastfeeding 308
Bottle Feeding Multiples 326

Chapter Twenty-Three

Surviving the First Days at Home 329

The Nursery—Your Babies' Room 329
Essential Equipment 331
Baby Showers for Multiples 337
Getting Help 338

Epilogue 341

Appendix A 343

Declaration of Rights and Statement of Needs of Twins
and Higher Order Multiples

Appendix B 349

Sample Menus

Appendix C 353

Birth Plan for Multiples

Glossary 357

Selected Bibliography 369

Resources 377

Index 405

Acknowledgments

So many individuals have shared their expertise in the development of this book. I am extremely indebted to all of them for this project and for their dedication to the care of multiple birth families.

I am especially grateful to my husband, my son, and twins, for their ongoing encouragement and support of my efforts.

My thanks and gratitude go to: John P. Elliott, M.D., Phoenix Perinatal Associates, for his painstaking reviews of the book content, and for his zeal and expertise in improving the care of women with multiple pregnancies; Washington C. Hill, M.D., F.A.C.O.G., Sarasota Perinatal Center, for his support and content review, and for his leadership within the professional perinatal community; Janet Bleyl, executive director of The Triplet Connection, for her review and her effective work in supporting families of higher-order multiples; Maureen Boyle, executive director of MOST, for her review and her years of dedication to higher-order multiple birth families; Lisa Cranwell Bruce, R.N.C., M.S., F.N.P.C., for her continuous support, terrific suggestions, and experience as a nurse, mother of twins, and Marvelous Multiples® educator; Cheryl Griffin, R.D., L.D., for her experience with expectant mothers of multiples, her nutrition knowledge, and the creation of the wonderful menus for the book; Karen Kerkhoff Gromada, M.S.N., R.N., I.B.C.L.C., director of the Breastfeeding Answer Center and author of *Mothering Multiples*, for her friendship and encouragement and her detailed reviews of the information on bonding and breastfeeding; Candace Hurley of Sidelines, for her contributions to the chapter on bed rest and her commitment to women with high-risk pregnancies; Linda G. Leonard, R.N., M.S.N., associate professor and twin-triplet specialist in the School of Nursing, University of British Columbia, for her knowledgeable reviews of the emotional and psychosocial aspects of multiple pregnancy; Linda M. Lutes, M.Ed., infant development specialist and NIDCAP trainer, for her detailed input to the chapter on developmental care and her pioneering work with co-bedding; Joyce Martin of the National Center for Health Statistics, for her dedication to compiling and reporting all the mind-boggling national multiple birth statistics; Mary Slaman-Forsyth, executive director of the Twin to Twin Transfusion Syndrome Foundation, for her contributions to the information on twin-to-twin transfusion and her ongoing support of families experiencing this problem; Amy Spangler, M.N., R.N., I.B.C.L.C., former president of the International Lactation Consultant Association, and author of *Breastfeeding, A Parent's Guide,* for the use of her well-researched benefits of breastfeeding; Martha Strange, M.D., neonatologist, Brookwood Medical Center, for her review of the chapters on the NICU and her tireless dedication to sick babies and their families.

Finally, I am deeply indebted to the many mothers of multiples whose experiences, feelings, and thoughts are reflected in the quotations in this book.

• • •

PART I

The Joys and Challenges of Multiple Pregnancy

Congratulations, you're going to have twins or triplets—or more! Are you still dazed from hearing those words? Have all your thoughts suddenly turned to mountains of diapers, limousine strollers, and stereo babies? You aren't alone. More women than ever before are finding out that they have multiple pregnancies and and the beginning of a very special experience.

The experiences of multiple pregnancy, birth, and parenting are unique—shared by about 3 percent of all families—making you and your babies very special. Having multiples brings countless joys; all the blessings of one baby are literally multiplied. But whether your multiple pregnancy is a *precious* gift after many months of infertility or a total surprise, you now have an important responsibility. Many challenges lie ahead for you and your babies during the next few months. Pregnancy and birth with twins, triplets, and higher multiples are prone to complications and problems, placing all of you at increased risk. Fortunately, many of these difficulties are manageable, and some are preventable. With the help of your health care providers, you can do a lot to take care of yourself, prevent problems, and have healthy babies.

A BOOK FOR MOTHERS

The Multiple Pregnancy Sourcebook is written directly to you, the
expectant mother of multiples. As your babies' mother, you are ultimately their keeper and nurturer, and the one who brings them
into the world. This book can take you through each step of your
multiple pregnancy—from diagnosis until your first days with your
new babies. Expectant fathers, grandparents, other family members, friends, or professionals reading this book: Put yourselves in
the mother's place as you read. She has a tremendous responsibility, carrying and birthing several babies at once. When you understand this experience from her perspective, you'll be better
equipped to relate to her feelings and help her face the pressures
and obligations ahead.

HOW THE BOOK WAS WRITTEN

The Multiple Pregnancy Sourcebook is a comprehensive resource
for multiple pregnancy and birth. Along with current medical literature and methods of clinical care, the anecdotes and accounts of
many parents and professionals were used in its development.
Mothers of multiples shared many words of wisdom ("I wish I had
known about. . .")—and these are highlighted throughout the
book. Health professionals offered advice about vital aspects of
multiple pregnancy care; and as a mother of twins, a perinatal
nurse, and multiple birth educator, I have personal and professional experience that brought unique insights. All these resources
were united under several basic principles:

- Multiple pregnancy is high-risk. That is, the chances for
  problems and complications are greater than with single

pregnancy. While being high-risk is neither a prophecy of doom nor a sentence to a difficult pregnancy, it is a fact that cannot be changed or sugar-coated.

- Women *do* have control over some risks in pregnancy. By changing their actions and behaviors, women can minimize or eliminate certain risks.
- As with any pregnancy, multiple pregnancy can have some complications that are beyond anyone's control and happen despite anything that the mother or healthcare provider does.
- By learning about complications, warning signs, and symptoms, women are more likely to get earlier treatment and improve their babies' chances for a healthier outcome.
- Parents and health care providers form a team. Mutual respect and cooperation are essential for the most effective care for mother and babies.

Using these principles, *The Multiple Pregnancy Sourcebook* is designed to help you through your pregnancy and the birth of your babies. You'll find answers to the most common questions parents have when they learn they are having multiples, and information about important topics you need to know—things you may not anticipate right now. Each chapter has information about the changes and challenges you might face in the coming weeks and months, as well as detailed explanations with easy-to-understand definitions of medical terms. You'll discover tools to help you make informed choices and interact with your care providers so that you can have the healthiest pregnancy possible. And you'll find clear discussions of medical procedures and treatments. Throughout the book are quotes from others who have "been there"—who have had experiences you may share. All this, even the unpleasant parts, is written to motivate you to take good care of yourself and your babies.

WORDS AND MEANINGS

You have probably heard many words and expressions that relate to having more than one baby: *twins, multiples, supertwins,* and *higher-order multiples,* just to name a few. It is confusing when several different terms mean the same thing. Here is a brief list of terms related to multiples and how they are used in this book:

- *Multiple pregnancy:* Pregnancy with more than one baby.
- *Twinning:* The process of two or more babies being formed at the same time.
- *Multiples:* Two or more babies carried in a multiple pregnancy.
- *Twins:* Two babies carried in the same pregnancy.
- *Triplets:* Three babies carried in the same pregnancy
- *Higher-order multiples:* More than two babies, usually refers to triplets and quadruplets.
- *Very high multiples:* More than triplets, usually refers to four, five, six, and more.
- *Singleton:* One baby in a single pregnancy.

Many different health care providers are involved in the care of a woman with a multiple pregnancy. Doctors, nurse midwives, nurse practitioners, and nurses work with other professionals to care for you and your babies. As you read, write down questions to ask at your prenatal visits. Your care providers may be delighted that you are so knowledgeable, and it can help them answer specific questions about your pregnancy. Remember that the information in this book does not take the place of medical care or the advice of your health care providers. Nor does all of the information apply to every pregnancy, because each situation is unique.

Throughout the book, you are likely to find related topics that spark your interest. At the end of the book is a list of resources that includes books, organizations, and Web sites current at the time this book was written. A glossary of terms and an index are also included.

Enjoy this book. Use it along with other resources to discover all you can about multiple pregnancy. Share what you learn with your doctor and health care providers. Together, you can develop a plan of care that is best for you and your babies.

Chapter One

Welcome to the World of Multiples

In the past, having multiples was fairly uncommon, and many mothers felt alone and isolated in their multiple birth experiences. But today, it seems that everywhere you look there are twins, triplets, and higher-order multiples—in doctors' offices, malls, schools, on TV—and nearly everyone today has a friend or relative with multiples. It's not your imagination; the birth rates for multiples have skyrocketed in the past couple of decades as illustrated in Figure 1.1. In the early 1970s, about 1 in 55 live births was a twin, triplets were extremely unusual, and very high multiples were a rare phenomenon. Today the rate of twins is 1 in 36 live births. Triplets now occur at a rate of one in five hundred, and quadruplets are much more common. In 1998, there were 118,295 babies born in multiple births in the United States, including 104,137 twins, 6,919 triplets, 627 quadruplets, and 79 quintuplets and higher. Just since 1980, the number of twins has risen 62 percent, and the number of higher-order multiples has increased over 470 percent. In 1998, births of the first surviving septuplets (seven) and octuplets (eight) made news across the world.

In the United States as well as many other countries, multiple birth rates continue to rise while the birth rate for single babies has started to fall. There are several explanations for such an

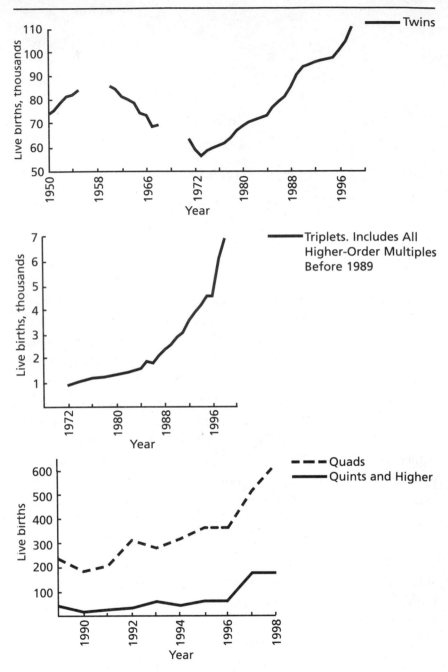

Source: National Center for Health Statistics, Hyattsville, Maryland.

Figure 1.1

incredible increase in multiple births. The last twenty years has witnessed a trend in women waiting until later in their lives to have children. Women over the age of forty-five are ten times more likely to have twins than women under the age of twenty. A natural mechanism for twinning increases with a woman's age until about her late thirties. This can cause more than one egg to develop in a monthly cycle, and multiples often result.

Another reason multiple births are more common in older women is just the opposite of this natural twinning ability. Delaying pregnancy until after age thirty is often associated with *infertility*, which is the inability to conceive or carry a baby. Conditions that cause infertility, such as endometriosis, can worsen with time; and women are more likely to have ovulation problems as they get older. Medications and procedures for treating infertility can promote the development of more than one baby. Over half of twins and nearly all higher-order multiples result from some type of infertility treatment. Chapter Two gives more details on infertility treatments and multiple pregnancy.

Other factors also increase the chances of having more than one baby. Race makes a difference. African American women have the highest rate of twinning of all races, and Asian women have the lowest rate. Although fraternal multiples—those developed from separate fertilized eggs—do seem to run in families, the exact mechanism of inheritance is not clear. Most researchers believe that twinning passes through the mother's line. And the more children a woman already has, the greater her chances of having multiples, especially if she has had multiples before.

> At our first ultrasound, the technicians started giggling and asked if we knew we were having twins. I nearly fell off the table. With four children already, twins never even crossed my mind.

HOW MULTIPLES COME ABOUT

Twinning has always had a magical aura and has been the source of fascination throughout history. It is indeed remarkable to see babies, children, and adults who look exactly the same. Of course, one of the first things expectant parents want to find out is if their babies are identical or fraternal.

Identical Multiples

About one-third of all multiple birth children are identical. Identical multiples occur when one egg is fertilized by one sperm. This fertilized egg (called a *zygote,* or early *embryo*) divides and forms two, three, or more identical zygotes. These identical twins, triplets, or more are *monozygotic,* because they form from one zygote. See Figure 1.2. Each multiple in a monozygotic set has the same chromosome makeup, and a set is always the same sex, either all boys or all girls. However, many people do not understand this concept. No wonder parents are amused when asked if boy/girl twins are identical.

> The general public is pretty ignorant about twins. When people would ask if my boy/girl twins were identical, I would look at them deadpan and say, "Well no, not if you look in their diapers." This usually got the message across!

Some babies may look so much alike that their own parents cannot easily tell them apart. Although identical multiples have the same genes, they are not the same people. Despite appearances, each identical multiple is an individual with a unique personality and identity, right down to individual fingerprints. About 25 percent of identical twins are opposite, or mirror images, of each other, with one being right-handed and the other left-handed or having birthmarks on opposite sides.

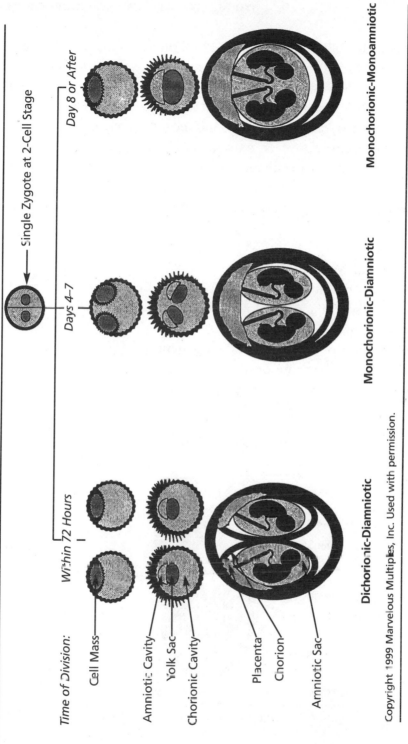

Figure 1.2   Identical Twins

Copyright 1999 Marvelous Multiples, Inc. Used with permission.

Identical twinning occurs at a fairly constant rate, approximately 1 in 250 births. Although reproductive technologies have helped explain how monozygotic twinning occurs, *why* it happens remains a mystery. Monozygotic twinning is not related to the mother's age, race, or heredity, and most researchers believe it is a random event. However, more and more monozygotic multiples are occurring in pregnancies from infertility treatments. It is thought that infertility medications and technologies can alter the structure of the egg or the zygote, making it more susceptible to division.

Fraternal Multiples

Fraternal multiples occur when two or more eggs are fertilized by separate sperm and develop at the same time. These zygotes are called *dizygotic* if there are two, *trizygotic* if there are three, and so on. Each of these zygotes is a genetically different individual, and may be the same or different sexes. See Figure 1.3. These multiples are siblings who are carried together in the same preg-

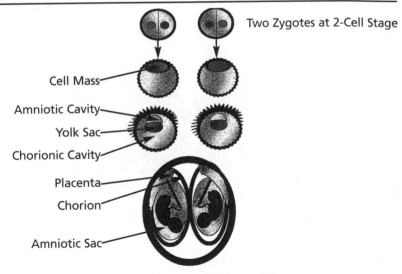

Two Zygotes at 2-Cell Stage

Cell Mass
Amniotic Cavity
Yolk Sac
Chorionic Cavity
Placenta
Chorion
Amniotic Sac

Copyright 1999 Marvelous Multiples, Inc. Used with permission.

Figure 1.3   Fraternal Twins (Dichorionic-Diamniotic)

nancy. The rate of fraternal twinning is influenced by factors including infertility treatments, heredity, race, and the mother's age.

Higher-Order Multiples
Most higher-order multiples are fraternal. However, identical multiples are increasingly more common with *assisted reproductive technology (ART)* such as in vitro fertilization. (Chapter Two has more information on how this happens.) Spontaneous triplets often have a set of identical twins and a separate fraternal multiple. Or they can all be identical, forming from one zygote that divided three times. See Figure 1.4.

PLACENTAS IN MULTIPLE PREGNANCY

The placenta is a disc-shaped organ that develops in the early part of your pregnancy and attaches to your blood supply through the inner walls of your uterus. The umbilical cord connects the baby

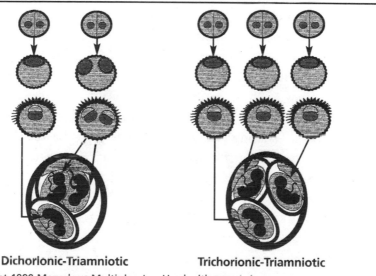

Dichorionic-Triamniotic   Trichorionic-Triamniotic

Copyright 1999 Marvelous Multiples, Inc. Used with permission.

Figure 1.4   Triplets

to the placenta as the lifeline for nutrition and oxygen. Two membranes, or layers of tissue, develop with the placenta and surround the baby. The outer membrane layer is the *chorion*. An inner membrane called the *amnion* forms a sac filled with fluid, often called the *amniotic sac* or bag. The *amniotic sac* and the *amniotic fluid* provide a safe, nurturing place for the baby to grow.

In a single pregnancy, one baby has one placenta, one chorion, and one amnion. Multiple birth babies can have several combinations of these placental structures. The number of placentas and whether they are separate or shared can help determine whether multiples are fraternal or identical. How these placental structures are configured is important in your babies' health during pregnancy and is called the *chorionicity*.

Each fraternal multiple has a placenta, a chorion, and an amnion, just as with a singleton. Each fraternal placental structure functions independently of the others. Occasionally, these separate placentas may be located so close to each other that they grow or fuse together, giving the appearance of one large placenta.

Identical multiples often share some of these placental structures. How much they share depends on when the zygote divides. This division timeline is illustrated in Figure 1.2. If division occurs in the first few days after fertilization, each baby can develop totally separate placental structures, just as fraternal multiples do. Two babies would have a chorionicity called *dichorionic-diamniotic*, three would have *trichorionic-triamniotic*, and so on. Later division can result in babies sharing one placenta. When two babies share one placenta with one chorion but have separate amniotic sacs, they have a *monochorionic-diamniotic* chorionicity. The thin amniotic membrane separating the babies is often visible on early ultrasound. About two-thirds of identical twins are dichorionic-diamniotic, and one-third are monochorionic-diamniotic.

When division occurs after about eight days, the babies may have a *monochorionic-monoamniotic* chorionicity, with both babies in the same amniotic sac. This occurs in only about 1 to 5 percent of identical multiples. Very late division, about thirteen to fifteen days after fertilization, is how conjoined (*Siamese*) twins form. Not only do these babies share placentas and membranes, they also share parts of their bodies and organs. Conjoined twins are extremely rare, occurring in about 1 in 100,000 births. Most of these are identified by ultrasound very early, and they often die during pregnancy. Those who survive may have a chance for surgical separation, depending on how much they share.

IDENTICAL OR FRATERNAL?

Most expectant parents are eager to find out whether their babies are identical or fraternal. This is also important for your babies' health, as babies with shared placentas can have more difficulties in pregnancy. About 15 percent of babies with a shared placenta develop *twin-to-twin transfusion syndrome* (*TTTS*). This occurs when blood passes from one baby to the other through connecting blood vessels within the placenta. See Chapter Eleven for more information on TTTS and how it is diagnosed and treated. There are also great dangers for babies that share the same amniotic sac because of umbilical cord entanglement. Early diagnosis of these conditions is essential.

Determining whether babies are identical or fraternal is also important after birth, as identical multiples are at greater risk for birth defects. And identical multiples have similar health risks throughout life: if one develops a disease such as diabetes or heart disease, the identical siblings are likely to develop the disease as well.

So, how do you find out if your babies are identical or fraternal? There are several very accurate ways to determine zygosity. Babies who share one chorion or amnion in pregnancy are always identical. First trimester ultrasound is very accurate in identifying these structures and can detect the thin membrane layers between babies. Ultrasound can show a triangle-shaped area of the placenta called the *lambda* or *twin peak sign* that indicates a dichorionic placenta. With triplets, doctors look for the *ipsilon zone*, a y-shaped area formed by 3 different membranes. If babies are different sexes, they are, without a doubt, fraternal. Having different blood types also means they are fraternal. When babies of the same sex look very different (hair, eye color), they are probably fraternal.

However, when babies are the same sex, look very much alike, yet have separate placentas, determining if they are identical becomes a bit more difficult. As you learned earlier, babies can be identical even with separate placentas. Microscopic examination of the placentas after birth may provide some answers. However, *DNA* (*deoxyribonucleic acid*) testing is the most accurate option, as DNA is the chemical material that makes up genes. Identical twins have the same genes and the same DNA patterns. Your obstetrician or pediatrician can help you locate a lab that performs DNA testing, sometimes called DNA fingerprinting, which can be performed before birth on amniotic fluid obtained in an amniocentesis. Once the babies are born, the test is as simple as using sampling swab on the inside of each child's cheek. You may decide that there is enough physical evidence that your babies are or are not identical, without doing further testing. But testing is always an option, and something that your children may elect to do when they are adults.

DIAGNOSIS OF MULTIPLE PREGNANCY

As few as twenty years ago, twins and other multiples were often a surprise at delivery to the parents as well as to the doctor. Although women often sensed that they were carrying more than one baby because of an increased appetite or a larger-than-usual abdomen, doctors could rely only on hearing a second fetal heartbeat or an x-ray to confirm that twins were on the way. Today's widespread use of *ultrasound* has made the early diagnosis of multiple pregnancy very simple and accurate, using sound waves to create an image of internal structures. A vaginal ultrasound is used in early pregnancy because it can show tiny structures very accurately; abdominal ultrasound is used later because it gives a larger, more panoramic view.

Ultrasound can detect a *gestational sac* (the fluid-filled structure that contains the developing baby) as early as three weeks after conception. By seven weeks after your last menstrual period, your babies' heartbeats can be seen on ultrasound as tiny flashes of light. When more than one baby is seen, you may have additional ultrasounds throughout the rest of your pregnancy.

> At my first OB appointment at ten weeks, I was already wearing maternity clothes. The OB told me that either my dates were wrong, or I was having twins. I never took the "twins" possibility seriously because there is no history of twins anywhere in my family. I wasn't on fertility drugs either. Also, I have endometriosis, and I was told that I would probably never be able to have kids—Ha! I was scheduled for an ultrasound at fourteen weeks. As the technician was moving the wand around, I got excited and gasped, "Look, there's the baby." In a very calm voice the tech said, "There's two." We could not believe it. It was the most unexpected thing that has ever happed to me. By the time I was dressed, my husband was already showing the ultrasound pictures to everybody in the waiting room. I can't explain the mixed emotions we had—fear, excitement, happiness, all kind of rolled into one.

SURPRISE MULTIPLES

The first ultrasound might not detect all the babies. Early embryonic structures can be difficult to interpret and might be incorrectly identified. Identical twins with a single placenta can be overlooked in very early pregnancy because the sacs are so close together that they appear as one. Also, it is possible to miss a multiple with a gestational sac located far apart from the others. In pregnancies resulting from infertility procedures, surprise multiples sometimes appear on follow-up ultrasounds.

> There were twins on the first ultrasound when I was just six weeks. The next week there was only one. I was heartbroken. But at eight weeks we saw three strong heartbeats! I was almost afraid to go back for the next ultrasound.

It is important to learn as much as possible about the type of multiple pregnancy you have and its chorionicity. Early diagnosis helps your care providers monitor your pregnancy and gives you and your babies the best chances for a healthy outcome.

Chapter Two

Multiple Pregnancy After Infertility

Hearing the words "You're pregnant" is the dream of over six million infertile couples in the United States. One couple in six struggles month after month with doctor's appointments, medications, timed intercourse, and invasive procedures in their quest for a baby. The cost of this is great, both financially and emotionally, so it's no wonder that many couples see having several babies at once as a bonus. For older couples whose childbearing years are limited, the prospect of multiples is a special gift. Although multiple pregnancy is indeed a blessing, it is not an easy path. More than one baby can make a much-wanted pregnancy a big challenge, beginning as early as the first trimester.

UNDERSTANDING INFERTILITY TECHNOLOGY BEFORE YOU GET PREGNANT

If you are currently trying to get pregnant with infertility treatments, you are more likely to have multiples than are women who are able to conceive without this help. It is important to receive counseling and education *before* any treatments or medications are started. This counseling should include discussions of the risks and benefits of each infertility medication and procedure as well as other treatment alternatives. Ask to see statistics for twins, triplets, and other multiples for your infertility doctor or clinic, so you can compare this information with national data. It is also important to discuss the potential for conceiving very high multiples and how to minimize the chances of that happening.

The chance of conceiving multiples is increased with the use of *ovulation-stimulating drugs*. These drugs help a woman's ovaries produce more than one egg, sometimes called *superovulation*. Multiple births can occur when several eggs are produced, released, and fertilized.

Clomiphene citrate (Clomid or Serophene) works by helping the pituitary gland (located at the base of the brain) produce more follicular stimulating hormone (FSH) and luteinizing hormone (LH). These hormones then stimulate the ovary to ripen a follicle (egg sac) and to release an egg. Clomiphene has a twinning rate of about 5 to 10 percent. Although triplets and other higher-order multiples are much less common with clomiphene, there are reports of quadruplets, quintuplets, and even a sextuplet conception.

> I didn't think much of my doctor's warning about the chance of multiples with Clomid. I recall thinking to myself, "That would never happen to me!" The amazement and disbelief must have shown on my face when I first saw those two little heartbeats. My second pregnancy was a singleton, also with Clomid, but it ended with miscarriage. My third pregnancy was once again the result of Clomid, and with my husband by my side, we watched as the ultrasound revealed what we now knew was possible—another set of twins!

Other infertility drugs are synthetic or natural preparations of FSH and/or LH. These drugs also stimulate the development of many eggs and often result in multiples because there is no way to predict how many eggs will fertilize. With drugs such as Gonal F, Follistim, Repronex, and Puregon, the incidence of multiple births is about 15 to 20 percent. About three-fourths of these are twins, and about one-fourth are higher-order multiples.

Naturally occurring hormones excreted in the urine of post-menopausal women are found in fertility drugs such as Pergonal and Humegon (which contain human menopausal gonadotropins), as well as Metrodin and Fertinex (which contain FSH). The incidence of multiple births with these drugs is higher, about 20 to 40 percent. As with other drugs, most of the multiple births are twins, but higher-order multiples frequently occur.

Some troubling side effects of ovulation-stimulating medications can be more likely in multiple pregnancies. One complication, *ovarian hyperstimulation syndrome (OHSS)*, occurs in about 1 to 5 percent of treatment cycles. In OHSS, the ovaries enlarge with many cysts and often look like clusters of grapes on an ultrasound exam. Women with mild OHSS have bloating and pelvic pain due to enlarged ovaries and fluid in the pelvic cavity. Severe OHSS can lead to extreme swelling, electrolyte imbalances, blood clots, kidney damage, twisting of the ovaries, and fluid build-up in the chest and abdomen. Hospitalization is often required, and sometimes fluid must be drawn out of the woman's chest or abdominal cavity.

Multiple births also occur with the use of *assisted reproductive technologies (ART)*. These highly technical procedures include *in vitro fertilization (IVF)*, *gamete intrafallopian transfer (GIFT)*, *and intracytoplasmic sperm injection (ICSI)*, among others. ART procedures involve removing eggs from the woman's ovaries and placing them with sperm. With most ART procedures, fertilization occurs in the laboratory, and then the embryos are placed in the woman's fallopian tube or uterus. Although superovulation drugs are used to stimulate the development of many eggs, ART allows more control. Couples make decisions about the number of eggs to fertilize as well as the number of embryos to transfer to the woman's uterus. About 37 percent of births from ART are multiples. Twin pregnancies are most common, but higher-order multiples occur about 6 to 7 percent of the time, especially if large numbers of embryos are transferred.

Although most multiples are fraternal, identical twinning can occur with infertility treatments. Ovulation-stimulating drugs and manipulation of the eggs and embryos in ART procedures appear to cause one embryo to divide into two or more identical embryos. Although the chance of identical twins following ART is small, about 3 percent, two embryos could become triplets, three embryos could turn into quadruplets, and so on.

It is important for doctors to thoroughly discuss the potential problems of multiple pregnancies with infertile couples *before* treatments begin. However, most doctors and infertility counselors are frustrated in their efforts, and often say they feel like they are talking to a brick wall. Desperate couples hear the information and mentally comprehend what is said but are often unable or unwilling to apply the risks to themselves. "It won't happen to me," or "I don't have much time, I want to have twins" are frequent responses. The births of septuplets and octuplets in the past few years have led many women to believe that they, too, would be able to carry so many babies successfully. In reality, nearly all women pregnant with very high multiples lose all their babies or have devastating outcomes after preterm birth.

PREVENTING HIGHER-ORDER MULTIPLES

What can be done to help couples become pregnant without risking the problems of higher-order multiple pregnancies? When many follicles (egg sacs) develop with ovulation-stimulating medication, one alternative is to withhold medication until some of the follicles stop growing and hormone levels drop. Then the cycle can be restarted with fewer numbers of follicles and fewer eggs released. Some infertility clinics use a long series of low-doses of medication, which stimulates only a very small number of follicles to develop.

Another recommendation has been to limit the number of embryos that are transferred in an IVF cycle. The American Society for Reproductive Medicine (ASRM) recommends that in women with the most favorable prognosis, no more than two high-quality embryos should be transferred during IVF. The number of embryos recommended for transfer increases based on the patient's age and infertility difficulty. Many centers now grow embryos in a special culture material that allows the embryos to develop one to two days longer into the *blastocyst* stage (a later stage of embryo development). By waiting, doctors can tell which embryos appear best developed and use only those for embryo transfer. The chance of pregnancy is greater and the risk for higher-order multiples lower when fewer of these "good" embryos are transferred.

Some clinics use a technique called *immature oocyte retrieval*. Instead of using drugs to stimulate eggs to grow, immature oocytes (eggs) are retrieved from the ovaries and allowed to mature in the lab. The best eggs are fertilized, and the embryos are returned to the woman's uterus. Of course, the success of any procedure depends on the woman and the experience of the care providers. So be sure to talk with your doctor about what is best for your individual case.

If you would like some ideas about what is involved in being the parents of two, three, or more babies, it might be helpful to contact a parents of multiples club, or ask your doctor and nurses for the names of multiple birth parents. Going to a twins club meeting, spending a day with a family, or watching a video about multiples can help you understand some of the joys and challenges. Sharing this with your family is important as well.

CONCERNS WITH MULTIPLE PREGNANCY AFTER INFERTILITY

Little compares to the thrill of a positive pregnancy test after many failed attempts. For many couples, the relief of getting pregnant is quickly replaced by the worry that something might go wrong, and it's natural to have mixed feelings when the ultrasound shows two or more babies. Like couples who naturally conceive multiples, you might have many questions about what lies ahead and how you will manage. Because of your previous infertility, you can also face some unique challenges with your multiple pregnancy.

> After several minutes of reading the ultrasound screen, the technicians looked at us poker-faced and asked, "How many children did you want?" I knew then that we were three for three! All the embryos we transferred had "taken." I was ecstatic—my husband's face was ashen.

Nosy Questions

Most parents of multiples are often asked questions that seem personal and intrusive. "Did you take fertility drugs?" is one of the most common questions. If your answer is yes, whether you share this depends on how open you are about your infertility experience. Be prepared for a variety of opinions, both helpful and hurtful. Some people are just nosy, while others ask because they are having a hard time getting pregnant themselves and need the encouragement of your success. A good answer to such questions is, "Is there a reason you are asking?" This puts nosy people in their place and allows those who are truly interested to open up to you. Of course, you can always smile and tell people "They are a blessing," which is true!

Premium Pregnancies

Many couples and health care providers consider pregnancy after infertility a "premium" pregnancy. Conceiving these babies comes about at a great price, both literally and figuratively. With so much at stake, it isn't unusual for infertile couples to expect to be treated as extraordinary. However, many are rudely awakened to find they are "just another patient" when they enter the obstetrical care system. Although this pregnancy is very special to you, your care provider may not treat you as "more special" than others. Obviously, multiple pregnancy involves a more intensive plan of care, but every woman and her pregnancy is special, and care providers should be equally committed to each. Your doctor and others, including nurse-midwives, nurses, and ultrasound technicians, understand your situation, but you should not have unrealistic expectations about your care. Be patient as you learn the new office and personnel. It is easier to handle the changes ahead when you understand how the system works. Communicating your needs to your care providers goes a long way toward making you feel better.

Prenatal Care

Finding the right care provider for your multiple pregnancy after infertility is an important task. Someone who has experience and the credentials necessary to care for women with multiple pregnancies often has insights into your unique emotional and physical needs. Chapter Seven has more information on choosing a multiple pregnancy care provider.

Once you have chosen a doctor, recognize that some aspects of your care will be different than they were during infertility. One of the biggest changes is the frequency of your visits. You may have had several appointments a month while you were trying to get pregnant. And right after your pregnancy is confirmed, you will probably have regular blood tests and ultrasounds, which can be very reassuring. Most women expect this level of care to continue and are shocked when they call to make their first appointment with their obstetrician and find it is not scheduled for four to six weeks, and the next appointment is a month after that! Feelings of panic and abandonment are common without those frequent, reassuring visits. If you feel this way, ask for an appointment earlier in your pregnancy. You can begin to see your obstetrician even if you have not been "released" from infertility care.

Your infertility doctor usually writes a referral letter to the obstetrician that outlines your history and how you became pregnant. There may be details of your infertility experience that you do not want discussed in your referral letter, such as use of a sperm or egg donor or a pregnancy reduction. However, unless you plaster a big sign across your chest that says "Formerly Infertile" or discuss your experience openly with staff or in the waiting room, no one but your care providers will know your medical history. Although this information is confidential and should be discussed with you privately, many aspects of your infertility care can have an impact on your pregnancy and need to be discussed among the care providers.

You also might be expecting to have the same close relationships with your obstetric care providers as you did with the infertility clinic staff. Unfortunately, obstetric offices, especially large ones, tend to be busy, and staff members have less time to develop personal connections with patients. But in time, the new relationships with your obstetric care providers may become just as close as they were with the infertility staff.

Difficulties After Infertility

Since the infertility road to pregnancy was so difficult, some women expect the pregnancy itself to be easier. After all you had to do get these babies, don't you deserve a break? Unfortunately, this isn't always so. Pregnancies after infertility can have more difficulties than naturally occurring pregnancies. This is also true in singleton pregnancies after infertility. The reasons for this are not fully understood, but it may be linked to hormonal factors. The type of treatment used to conceive also seems to play a role. Pregnancies following ART and superovulation drugs tend to be more complicated than less intensive treatments. Although many pregnancies after infertility are uneventful, they can have complications, making special care more likely. Don't become discouraged by this. Instead, let it inspire you to become more knowledgeable and alert to the needs of your multiple pregnancy.

> After the ultrasound, our obstetrician said that there could be a problem with one of our babies because of an abnormal umbilical cord. Our thoughts immediately turned to questioning our decisions, wondering if we were being handed a terrible fate because we decided to pursue a donor embryo pregnancy, or because we chose to pursue treatment with the help of infertility doctors. This experience was something that felt far more dramatic to us, having "fresh scars" from our infertility, than I believe it otherwise would have. No doubt that this situation is difficult for anyone, but with recent memories of infertility and weakened emotional strength from the years of losses, we felt particularly vulnerable.

Many women feel like they are walking on eggshells throughout pregnancy. It's natural to be fearful of losing babies you wanted so desperately. Some women are so afraid of loss that they are reluctant to get attached to their babies during pregnancy. Some barely prepare a nursery or delay this task until the last minute, for fear that taking such a step might somehow curse their luck. If you find yourself with these fears to the point that you can't connect with your unborn babies, talk with others who have been infertile or speak to your doctor, nurses, or a counselor.

> We have been skeptical of things going right, and fearful that something may go wrong. I really believe that if we hadn't been infertile, we could have relaxed a bit more and left this situation behind us more than we've been able to.

Another aspect of the infertility experience that many people overlook is the financial impact of months or years of expensive treatments. The average cost of an IVF cycle in the United States is nearly $8,000, and many couples must go through more than one cycle before getting pregnant. Only a handful of states currently have laws requiring insurers to cover some form of infertility diagnosis and treatment. Not surprisingly, these states often have higher multiple-birth rates than states where insurance is not mandated.

> Your financial resources are so stretched because of the infertility, that once you become pregnant, especially with multiples, finances can be a real stressor. Not that they aren't for any couple having a child, or multiples, but when you have to spend literally tens of thousands of dollars just to get pregnant, money can be a real problem.

Your infertility experience can actually be valuable in a number of ways. A long history of infertility can strengthen your resolve to make it through a difficult pregnancy. Having been through the treatments and invasive procedures of infertility can help you feel less afraid of the medical interventions of a high-risk pregnancy. Your experience with the medical care "system" often helps you know how and what to ask for. Many women are so excited about being pregnant that they find it easier to cope with the inconveniences and stresses. Some see the problems of multiple pregnancy as merely a part of the experience and not as something to be dreaded. For many, the worst days with a complicated multiple pregnancy are better than the best days of infertility.

Parenting

Parenting multiples is a challenge to anyone, but parenting after infertility has its own unique difficulties. After birth, some parents become overanxious and overprotective of their children and may have guilt feelings about discipline. They might set extremely high expectations of themselves and feel unworthy when they don't meet those expectations. Others resent having the less-than-perfect picture of parenting that they imagined. In addition, some parents feel they are unable to complain about the normal strains of parenting because, "After all, this is what we wanted." They feel pressured by friends or family who expect them to be happy regardless of the difficulties or they can feel let down by people "who should have known." Parents can also feel misled—they either weren't told or didn't get the message that parenting two, three, four, or more babies isn't easy. Some parents feel they are "second class" because they had to use fertility treatments to conceive.

These are common feelings, and realizing that others have had similar experiences is the first step in dealing with them. Resources such as parents of multiples clubs and other formerly infertile parents can help you learn that you aren't alone.

FUTURE CHILDREN

Although many parents who are blessed with multiples feel their family is complete, some do want to have more children. But, they worry that they may have to go through another long, involved infertility process to conceive. Because of this, many couples think they don't need to use birth control. After all, look what they had to do to get pregnant the first time! Surprisingly, pregnancy seems to somehow "fix" the problem of infertility for some women. Imagine their astonishment when they find they are pregnant "on their own." Even more of a shock is that this can occur right on the heels of having multiples. For those who do need infertility treatment to conceive, there is the additional worry that they might have multiples again.

Talk candidly with your care providers about your plans for future children. Moreover, do discuss birth control options. It can be very hard on your body as well as your emotions to become pregnant very quickly after a birth, and that pregnancy can be at greater risk for problems. Also, your babies will need your full attention in the first few years.

Chapter Three

Emotions in Multiple Pregnancy

For parents expecting just one baby, pregnancy and birth are normal, everyday events. But these experiences may seem overwhelming when you are having multiples. Multiple pregnancy is a unique experience, both physically and emotionally. The hormonal and physical changes of pregnancy bring about a whole roller coaster of emotions and moods. You feel excited, confused, and anxious all at the same time.

If you are like most parents, the idea of carrying and giving birth to several babies makes you feel a bit panicky. You may start wondering and worrying about what might happen. Is multiple pregnancy difficult? Will my babies be okay? How much weight should I gain? How long can I continue to work? What happens if I have to be on bed rest or in the hospital? What about finances? Who will care for our other children? Is labor with twins twice as long or twice as painful? Will I need a cesarean delivery? Does every multiple pregnancy result in tiny premature babies? Will I have enough love to go around? There are endless things to consider! As you go through the next weeks and months, it helps to know that these questions, emotions, and anxieties are normal.

COMMON CONCERNS

At first, you might feel hesitant about having more than one baby, especially if your multiples are a surprise or you are having higher-order multiples. You might be especially anxious if you had a difficult pregnancy or a loss in the past. And it takes a while to get over your initial shock, even if you were prepared for the possibility of multiples. Although it can take time, you get used to the idea of having all these babies. Even then, you have days when you find it hard to believe it's happening. Some days you feel overwhelmed with joy, and some days you feel just overwhelmed.

> After already having four children, this was an unwanted pregnancy. We had tried to have my tubes tied, but because of scheduling and hospital mix-ups, it never happened. When others offered congratulations I could only say thank you through gritted teeth for about six months. But now, my babies are a tremendous joy and blessed addiction that I wish for everyone.

> I had three miscarriages before conceiving my twins, and at first I was not too convinced that my pregnancy would last. The joys and concerns of having twins didn't come about until my second trimester.

As the weeks of pregnancy go by, you begin to see and feel remarkable changes in your body. It's a little scary to watch your body grow so quickly, and you wonder if your skin can stretch enough or if there's enough room for your babies. New sensations, aches, and pains begin. As you start sensing your babies' movements, it can be a strange feeling. But these are marvelous confirmations of becoming a mother. Most women recognize individual baby movements and personalities before their babies are born! A mom of quints relates, "It was amazing to watch my body grow . . . my belly grew 3½ inches in one week!"

Mixed with all the physical changes are the emotions that come with a high-risk pregnancy. It's natural to feel vulnerable or on edge when things aren't in your control. Although you may not have complications, you could find yourself on a different path from what you had imagined. Being on bed rest or in the hospital probably isn't in your plans. Waiting for results of tests and procedures can be emotionally exhausting, too. Some medications used to treat complications can make you more anxious or depressed. You may also feel afraid for your babies, not knowing what lies ahead. It isn't unusual to feel disappointed and helpless when the course of your pregnancy doesn't match what you had planned or hoped.

When the time gets closer to the birth of your babies, you start worrying about the actual process of birth. Many women are concerned about how a vaginal birth occurs with multiples and whether cesarean delivery is needed. As the reality of becoming a parent to several babies begins to sink in, you wonder what it will be like to care for your babies and how you will manage at home.

DADS HAVE EMOTIONS AND WORRIES, TOO

Men experience many emotions during pregnancy as they try to adjust to their new role as expectant father. Most expectant fathers want to be involved in the pregnancy experience and are eager to attend prenatal visits. Some have pregnancy symptoms along with the mother, such as nausea or weight gain.

Multiple pregnancy can add pressures for expectant fathers. Along with their normal concerns about the health of mother and babies, men worry about possible complications. Fathers often feel a special protectiveness and want to shield the mother from bad news or problems at home. They also have finances on their minds, especially if the family is dependent on the mother's income. Men often have to become the cook, housekeeper, and child care provider when mothers are unable to carry through with these roles. They also begin to think about how their lives will change and worry that there may be little room for them after the babies are born. Expectant fathers often feel great pressure to be strong and supportive of the mother and other family members, even though they are afraid. Many men have difficulty expressing such worries and feelings. They need opportunities to talk with other expectant fathers as well as men who have "survived" multiple pregnancy and who are managing parenthood.

OUT-OF-CONTROL WORRIES

Having worries is natural, especially about something you've never been through before. However, it can be positive when these worries motivate you to take good care of yourself. Being anxious about the health of your babies is why you seek prenatal care, eat properly, and avoid dangers to yourself and your unborn babies. Having concern encourages you to learn about the potential problems of your pregnancy. A little fear can make you more attentive to your body's signals and motivate you to take action if you suspect a problem.

Although some worry is normal, extreme anxiety or stress has negative effects. Stress not only affects your relationships with your family but also your body. When stress-related hormones are released, your heart and breathing rates increase and your body's metabolism changes. Stress also makes you feel bad physically, causing muscle tension and altering sleep and eating habits. Moreover, long-term stress and severe anxiety can affect your babies. Studies with singleton pregnancies have shown that pregnant women with extremely high levels of anxiety and stress are more likely to experience complications such as early birth and low birth weight. There are also indications that severe maternal stress and anxiety can decrease blood flow through the uterus. Women who experience a serious life changing event, such as a death of a family member, may be at greater risk for pregnancy complications. There is also some evidence that women with multiple pregnancy are more likely to have depression during pregnancy and after birth. And if you have a history of an anxiety disorder or depression, you may be at even greater risk.

Take steps to recognize your worries. Seek help from your doctor or a counselor to sort out whether your concerns are manageable or out-of-control. Depression and anxiety disorders can be treated during a multiple pregnancy without risking your health or that of your babies.

BALANCING YOUR CONCERNS

Here are some suggestions on how you can balance having enough concern without allowing worry to overwhelm you as you go through your multiple pregnancy:

- Become informed. Ask questions and educate yourself about your multiple pregnancy, especially if you have complications
- View your pregnancy as special, not abnormal. Focus on having a positive attitude about your pregnancy and your babies, and don't be afraid to enjoy the good parts of this experience.
- Believe in your body's ability to provide for your developing babies, and envision yourself as a nurturing, safe haven. Communicate your love to your babies by talking, reading, and singing to them.
- Enjoy watching your body grow, and be proud of the incredible way your body is nurturing your babies.
- Be assured of your body's ability to give birth to your babies, whether through a vaginal or a cesarean delivery. No matter which way they arrive, your health and the well-being of your babies are most important.

- Have confidence in your health care providers. Take an active role in your pregnancy, and cooperate in your plan of care. If you don't understand the reasons for a treatment or plan, ask for explanations.
- Consult with a perinatologist (a high-risk pregnancy specialist) if you have complications or want more advice or a second opinion.
- Prepare for possible problems by learning about their warning signs and how they are treated. This can help you regain a feeling of control. Always focus on doing your best, and don't get discouraged thinking you or your body has somehow failed.
- If or when problems arise, be flexible. Carefully examine your options, and then move ahead with your decision. Don't dwell on what might have happened. Instead, be comfortable knowing that you are doing your best. Picture yourself as handling difficult situations well.
- Communicate as a couple or family about the pressures that you experience. If you like to write, keep a journal of your thoughts and feelings. Save it for your children!
- Talk about your concerns with others who have had similar experiences. It helps to know you aren't alone in your worries. You'll find great support from members of multiples clubs and other multiple birth support organizations.
- Eliminate unnecessary stress in your life. Decrease the noise level in your home or workplace by turning off the television or radio or keeping your door closed. Simplify your lifestyle, and cut out responsibilities and activities that drain your time and energy.
- Use relaxation techniques to help with stress. Nurture yourself with special treats such as a new outfit, a massage, or a dinner out with your husband.
- If you are experiencing severe stress, anxiety, or depression, tell your doctor. A counselor or psychologist can help you

manage your worries and fears and work out a plan to decrease stress.

- Rely on your faith. Use the power of prayer or meditation and the sense of security and calmness it can bring to help you handle your worries.

FINDING SUPPORT

One of the best ways to deal with your anxieties and emotions is to share them with others who have had those same feelings. When you are expecting multiples, you instantly become part of a wonderful community of multiple birth families. Multiple pregnancy creates an instant bond with others who also have multiples. You'll find support through informal friendships as well as organized clubs all across the nation and the world. Take advantage of this support during your pregnancy as well as after your babies are born.

Look through the list of national and international multiple birth support organizations in the Resources at the end of this book, and contact the groups that interest you. Locally, you may have to seek out opportunities to meet other parents of multiples. Hospitals, doctors' offices, and community health nurses can help you locate support groups. Wherever you find support, you'll discover that parents of multiples are happy to offer their time and share their experiences. It won't be long until you'll feel very much a part of this special family.

Singleton moms don't get it. For all the well-meaning friends I have that had only one baby at a time, they do not understand the difficulty of having two babies that want and need you at the same time. The physical and emotional stress of having multiples is only understood by one who has been there. I would not have survived the first year without the help of another twin mom. Together, we complained, rejoiced, whined, and cried over the difficulties of staying home with two babies—and those talks were the cornerstone of my sanity.

In the days ahead, be sure to enjoy the special things that you'll experience. When you face detours, or have to make an unexpected side trip, try to see a bright side. Look forward to the rest of your pregnancy and to the end, when you take your babies home. You'll look back in amazement at how fast the time went by. So plan ahead, take lots of pictures, and enjoy this special experience!

Chapter Four

Multiple Pregnancy Nutrition: Eating for Everyone

Although there are some things about your pregnancy that you cannot change, what you eat and how much weight you gain *are* within your control. Research has shown clearly that an expectant mother's nutrition and pregnancy weight gain are powerful contributors to her babies' birth weights. Birth weight is an important factor in babies' health and survival. In other words, by eating the right kinds of foods and gaining weight in pregnancy you can make a significant difference in your babies' health and well-being.

WHAT ARE YOU EATING NOW?

Healthy eating is easy once you know what to include and how much to eat. You can be sure that this is *not* the time to lose weight, but you don't need excessive weight gain either. You may be eating many of the right foods already. Take a few minutes to write down what you ate during the past twenty-four hours in the table on page 40. Don't forget to include all your beverages and that snack you had midmorning or before going to bed.

As you read the rest of this chapter, refer to your list to see where you are succeeding and where you need to improve. Be sure to talk with your doctor if you have a history of an eating disorder, because you need support in eating and gaining weight.

Beakfast	_____
Mid-morning Snack	_____
Lunch	_____
Mid-afternoon Snack	_____
Dinner	_____
Bedtime Snack	_____

NUTRITIONAL RECOMMENDATIONS FOR MULTIPLE PREGNANCY

Currently, there are no universally approved *recommended dietary allowances* (*RDA*) for multiple pregnancy. Because of this, various professionals and groups have proposed a variety of nutrition plans. Most of these nutritional guidelines are based on the RDA for singleton pregnancy, adding calories and nutrients in various amounts. Some health care professionals advocate multiple pregnancy diets with very high calorie intakes. Others emphasize adding supplemental nutrients, vitamins, and minerals. But more research is needed to clearly define the number of calories and specific amounts of nutrients needed for multiple pregnancies. The following nutritional guidelines are based on generally accepted recommendations. Talk with your doctor or dietitian about the specific nutritional needs for your multiple pregnancy.

Calories

Calorie is another word for fuel or energy. Foods contain calories that are used as fuel by the body. The two main fuel/energy sources of foods are carbohydrates and fat. The special demands of pregnancy require an extra 300 calories each day for one baby, and for a multiple pregnancy, you need more calories to meet the needs of additional babies. With a twin pregnancy, you would need at least 2,700 calories each day, with a triplet pregnancy, at least 3,000 calories, and so on. Underweight women often need more calories because of their already low body weight. If you are overweight, don't assume that you can skimp on eating and calories. You still need to eat enough to meet your babies' growth and development needs, but your calorie requirements may be different. Calories and nutrition also change depending on your activity level and any special needs such as gestational diabetes.

Most women are shocked at the idea of needing so many calories. In a culture as diet-conscious and obsessed with being thin as ours is, it's hard to imagine eating as much as a marathon runner! It isn't unusual for a busy nonpregnant woman to take in only about 1,200 calories each day, and now she is being asked to more than double that intake.

Although it is easy to get 3,000 calories from fast food, sweets, and soda, these aren't healthy calories. Your healthy eating plan should include a variety of foods including whole grains, fruits, vegetables, proteins, and fat. These foods provide the necessary energy, protein, vitamins, and minerals for the development and growth of your babies and for your own needs. For example, if you are tired all the time, it may be because you haven't been eating enough. You will probably feel better and have more energy once you are taking in enough calories and eating the right kinds of food.

The Food Pyramid

For most people, counting servings is easier than counting calories. The food pyramid, similar to that on food packaging labels, shows six food groups and the number of servings needed in each group. The servings shown in Figure 4.1 are for a twin pregnancy. If you are pregnant with higher-order multiples, add at least one serving or increase the serving size in each group.

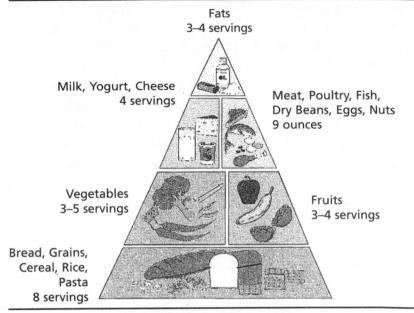

Figure 4.1   The Food Pyramid

Bread, Grains, Cereal, Rice, and Pasta   *8 servings*
One serving =

1	slice whole grain bread
½	hamburger bun
1	muffin or biscuit
½	bagel or English muffin
4–5	small or 2 large crackers
1	tortilla
½	cup cooked cereal
¾	cup ready-to-eat cereal
1	waffle or pancake
½	cup pasta or rice
3	cups popped popcorn
25	pretzel sticks

Grains are complex carbohydrates that are a major source of energy and provide vitamin B, minerals, and fiber. Taking in enough carbohydrates allows protein to be used for growth rather than for energy. You'll find it easy to get at least eight servings when you include a grain food with each meal and snack. Try to use whole grain products when possible for the fiber and extra nutrition. The Food and Drug Administration (FDA) requires manufacturers to fortify grain-based foods with folic acid, a B vitamin also known as folate or folacin. This vitamin is very important in the first trimester when the babies' spinal cords and brain tissues are developing. Many grain products are also fortified with minerals such as calcium and iron.

Fruits   *3–4 servings*
***One serving* =**
- ¾   cup juice
- 1   medium apple, banana or other fruit
- ½   cup fresh, cooked or canned fruit
- ¼   cup dried fruit
- 1   melon wedge

Fruits are another source of energy and a major source of vitamins. The carbohydrates in fruits are simple sugars that your body can use quickly. Fruits are rich in vitamin C, which is important in the growth of teeth and bones and helps maintain strong tissues and blood vessels. When you can, eat a piece of fruit rather than just a glass of juice so you'll get the extra fiber. Shop for citrus juices that have the bonus of added calcium, and choose juices that contain 100 percent juice rather than juice beverages that are mostly water and sugar.

Vegetables   *3–5 servings*
One serving =
- ½   cup cooked or chopped raw vegetables
- 1   cup leafy raw vegetables
- ¾   cup vegetable juice

Vegetables are excellent sources of vitamins A and C. Vitamin A is important for healthy nerves, skin, bones, and vision, and in placental function. Dark green leafy, yellow, or orange vegetables contain beta-carotene, which your body changes to vitamin A. These natural beta-carotene forms of vitamin A are recommended rather than preformed sources of the vitamin. Although studies have not determined the amounts, it is believed that consuming excessive amounts of preformed vitamin A in pregnancy is linked to birth defects. Because of this risk, never take supplements of vitamin A unless directed by your doctor. Accutane, a prescription acne medication, is high in vitamin A and should not be used in pregnancy.

Choose vegetables with a variety of colors and textures. Eat vegetables raw (after washing well), or steam them quickly to retain their vitamins and fiber. If fresh vegetables aren't available, choose frozen rather than canned vegetables, as canned products usually have added salt and many nutrients can be lost in processing. Some of the newer juice products include vegetable juices mixed with citrus to provide vitamins A and C.

Dairy products (see facing page) are wonderful sources of calcium and protein. An 8-ounce glass of whole, 2 percent, or skimmed milk contains about 285 milligrams of calcium and about 8 grams of protein. Calcium is important for your babies' developing bones and teeth and in the function of your heart, nerves, and muscles. The National Institutes of Health recommend 1,200 to 1,500 milligrams of calcium for a singleton pregnancy. With the extra demands of several developing babies, you'll need more cal-

Milk, Yogurt, and Cheese   *4 servings*
One serving =

1	cup milk
1	cup yogurt (not frozen)
1	cup pudding (made with milk)
1½	cups ice cream, ice milk, or frozen yogurt
1½	ounces natural cheese
2	ounces processed cheese
1½	cups cottage cheese
4	tablespoons Parmesan cheese

cium, at least 1,800 milligrams. If you do not take in enough calcium through your diet, your babies may use the calcium stored in your bones, and this can increase your risk for osteoporosis in later years. Some doctors recommend calcium supplements for women with multiple pregnancies, especially if they are unable to drink milk. Calcium citrate supplements are more easily absorbed than other forms.

With today's focus on fat, many women have questions about milkfat content. If you have been drinking skim or nonfat milk and are having trouble gaining weight, try using 2 percent or whole milk to add calories. Be sure to use only pasteurized dairy products because of the risk for bacterial contamination.

If you do not drink milk or eat any dairy products, you'll need some form of calcium supplementation. Ask your doctor to recommend the type of supplement you should use. You must also increase the amounts of other proteins and fluids in your diet to replace what you do not get from dairy products.

Many dairy products also contain vitamin D, which helps your body use calcium. Your body can make its own vitamin D when you are exposed to sunlight. Like vitamin A, vitamin D is stored in your body and excessive amounts can be dangerous, so never take supplements unless prescribed by your doctor.

**Meat, Poultry, Fish, Dry Beans,
Eggs, and Nuts** *9 ounces*
One ounce =
- 1   egg
- ½   cup cooked beans
- 2   tablespoons peanut butter or
      3 tablespoons peanuts
- 1   cup walnuts, almonds, or cashews
- 5   small shrimp or clams
- 1   ounce sardines with bones

Three ounces =
- 1   chicken breast half
- 1   hamburger patty
- 1   fish filet or 5 fish sticks
- 1   pork chop

Meat, poultry, fish, dried beans, eggs, and nuts contain proteins and vitamins that are essential for building tissues. Protein is important in the growth of your uterus, placentas, breasts, and blood. Animal foods also are good sources of iron, zinc, and B vitamins, as are beans, nuts, and seeds. Tofu (made from soybeans) and white beans also supply some of the calcium you need. Some nuts, like almonds, are good sources of vitamin E. All of the B vitamins are important in the health and development of nerves, skin, hair, eyes, and skin.

Nine ounces of protein-dense food provide about 60 grams of protein, the amount recommended for a singleton pregnancy. When you add to this the protein you get from other foods such as dairy products, you can easily take in 80 to 100 grams of protein each day. Portion sizes vary depending on the type of food. A 3-ounce portion of meat, pork, or fish is about the size of the palm of your hand or a deck of cards. An egg is equivalent to a 1-ounce serving.

Although fish is a good source of protein, you should avoid swordfish and shark as these fish often contain high levels of mercury, which is dangerous for developing babies. Fresh tuna may also contain mercury levels above the FDA limit for human consumption, so it would be wise to limit this as well.

Do not use protein powders or nutrient additives unless directed by your doctor or dietitian. These supplements are often promoted at health food retailers and body-building and sports facilities; however, the use of excessive protein supplementation has not been proven to help with fetal growth or substantially increase maternal weight gain. More importantly, one study found a slightly increased risk of neonatal death with the use of high-protein supplements.

Fats   *3–4 servings*
One serving =
- 1   teaspoon margarine, butter
- 2   teaspoons salad dressing
- 1   teaspoon oil
- 2   tablespoons sour cream
- 1   tablespoon cream cheese
- 1   teaspoon mayonnaise
- 1   slice bacon

Although many people today are cutting down on fat intake, fat is a necessary nutrient in pregnancy. Fats are a concentrated source of energy, carrying the vitamins A, D, E, and K, which are important in cell structure. If you include nuts, margarine, salad dressing, oils, and cheeses in your diet, you'll be getting enough fat to meet your needs.

Snacks

One of the best ways to take in enough calories and nutrients is to eat a nutritious snack between meals and before bedtime. As your pregnancy progresses, you might find it hard to eat three large meals because you don't have much appetite, or room for a lot of food at one time. It often helps to change your meals and snacks around so that you are eating several small meals a day. Some women find they do better by nibbling all day long, and when they get up in the night. Make each bite rich in nutrition and energy using proteins and carbohydrates. Even if you aren't hungry, do your best to eat what you can. Keep snacks handy in your purse and at your desk or workplace. Here are some nutritious snack suggestions:

- Cheese and crackers
- English muffin or bagel topped with cheese
- Half of a lean-meat sandwich on whole wheat bread
- Half of a chicken salad pita sandwich with lettuce and tomato
- Whole grain waffle, toast, or graham crackers with peanut butter
- Trail mix (nuts, dried fruit)
- Flour or corn tortillas with cheese, rolled and heated
- Popcorn
- Breadsticks, rice cakes, pretzels with cheese dip
- Bowl of cereal with milk
- Milkshake
- Banana with peanut butter
- Tomato with cottage cheese
- Cream soup and crackers
- Balanced nutritional supplement drink, such as Carnation Instant Breakfast, Ensure, or Boost

For variety, add one of the following:

- Fresh or canned fruit (orange, apple, grapes, strawberries, kiwi, banana, melon, or applesauce)

- Dried fruit (such as apricots or raisins)
- Frozen fruit juice bars
- Vegetable juice
- Vegetable soup
- Fresh vegetables with dip

Sample Menu

Here is an example of a menu for one day that includes approximately 2,700 calories and a variety of foods to provide the necessary protein, vitamins, and minerals. See Appendix B for additional menus that provide appropriate calories and nutrition for you and your babies.

Breakfast
1 cup bran cereal
1 cup strawberries
1 cup milk

Midmorning snack
¼ cup cottage cheese
1 cup sliced peaches
6 whole wheat crackers

Lunch
3 ounces roast beef on
2 slices whole wheat bread with
1 teaspoon mayonnaise
1 cup garden salad with 1 tablespoon dressing
1 cup milk
1½ cups ice milk or frozen yogurt

Midafternoon snack
2 tablespoons peanut butter
4 graham crackers
1 apple

Dinner

3 ounces chicken with Parmesan cheese

1 cup wild rice

½ cup green beans

½ cup squash

1 cup grapes

1 whole wheat roll

1 cup milk

Bedtime snack

1 ounce turkey on

1 slice wheat bread

1 teaspoon mayonnaise

6 ounces vegetable juice

SUPPLEMENTING YOUR DIET

Because food is the best source for nutrients, your focus should be on eating healthy foods rather than canned nutrition, pills, or supplements. However, there are times when pregnant women need supplements because they cannot take in enough vitamins and minerals from their diets.

Prenatal Vitamins

Think of prenatal vitamins as a form of nutritional insurance. They do not take the place of food, but they do ensure that you are getting the necessary nutrients each day. Never take an extra dose of your prenatal vitamins or take regular multivitamins. Some multivitamins contain excessive levels of vitamins that can be dangerous to you and your babies. Don't panic if you miss or occasionally are unable to take your prenatal vitamins. If they make you nauseous, try taking them at night, with food, or ask your doctor for an alternative brand. If you just can't handle them at all, ask your doctor about taking only folic acid supplements in the first trimester. You can add the prenatal vitamins when the nausea goes away.

Folic Acid

Prenatal vitamins also contain folic acid, and many doctors prescribe additional supplements of this important B vitamin. Folic acid is needed for red blood cell production and for the synthesis of deoxyribonucleic acid (DNA), the building blocks of your genetic code. Because low levels of folic acid are associated with neural tube defects such as spina bifida, many foods are now fortified with folic acid. Natural foods containing folic acid include lentils, beans, and spinach. Pregnant women need at least 400 micrograms of folic acid daily from fortified foods, vitamin supplements, or a combination. This is in addition to the naturally occurring folic acid they obtain from a varied diet.

Iron

Many doctors also recommend iron supplements for women with multiple pregnancies. A woman carrying twins is about two and one-half times more likely to have iron-deficiency anemia than a woman with a singleton pregnancy. About half of women with higher-order multiples have anemia. Anemia is associated with a higher risk of preterm birth and low birth weight babies, as well as causing fatigue. Iron-rich foods include red meat (the best source), whole grain breads and cereals, dark meat chicken, egg yolks, dark green leafy vegetables, and dried fruits. Take your iron supplements between meals with citrus juice to help your body absorb the iron more effectively. Avoid taking iron with tea, milk, or coffee as these decrease absorption.

Other Minerals

Some practitioners also recommend magnesium supplements for pregnant women. There have been several studies that found improved singleton pregnancy outcomes, including lower incidences of preterm birth, less maternal hospitalization, less maternal hemorrhage, and lower incidences of low birth weight and small for gestational age babies with magnesium supplementation. However, the method of these studies has been questioned, and further trials are needed, especially in multiple pregnancy. Additional clinical studies are needed to determine if zinc supplements can improve pregnancy outcomes.

Nutritional Supplements
There is evidence that balanced protein/energy nutritional supplements are helpful in maternal weight gain and fetal growth. Balanced supplements are those in which protein provides less than 25 percent of the energy (calorie) content. Examples of such balanced supplements include Boost, Ensure, Equate, Resource, and Carnation Instant Breakfast. Studies have found that use of such balanced supplements may help reduce the risk of stillbirth and neonatal death.

FLUIDS

Drinking plenty of fluids during your multiple pregnancy is important for several reasons. You need fluids to maintain the large amount of circulating blood. In addition, if you become dehydrated during your pregnancy, you are at increased risk for preterm contractions and urinary tract infections. Because you need fluids for digestion, you can become constipated if you drink too little fluid. Although you do get fluids from many foods and through other beverages, your body also needs water each day. One way to make sure you are drinking enough is to fill a thermos or water bottle with 48 to 64 ounces of water. Sip on it throughout the day with your goal to finish it by bedtime. Another tip is to drink a cup of water with each meal and snack. Avoid the empty calories in soft drinks. Instead, flavor your water with a squeeze of lemon or a splash of fruit juice, or drink carbonated water. Check with your doctor about how much fluid you need to take in. Too much water can be dangerous in some conditions and with certain medications.

VEGETARIANS

Multiple pregnancy is not the time to be a casual vegetarian. Serious vegetarians should pay close attention to their diets, especially their protein intake. Although proteins can be obtained by combining complex carbohydrates, animal foods are the best source. Vegetarians who eat dairy, eggs, and fish usually can obtain enough protein; however, vegans, who consume no animal products, should pay careful attention to protein intake and receive vitamin B$_{12}$ supplements. If you are a vegetarian to any degree, request a nutritional consult with a dietitian who can help you plan a diet with sufficient protein intake.

DIABETES

If you are a pregnant diabetic or develop diabetes during pregnancy, called *gestational diabetes,* you'll need specialized medical nutrition therapy. Diabetic management uses diet, or diet combined with insulin, to meet the calorie and nutrient needs of mother and babies without increasing blood glucose to unsafe levels. A registered dietitian can help you choose foods and plan your meals to keep your blood glucose within safe levels. Some women may need insulin in addition to their diabetic diet to keep blood glucose in control. See Chapter Eleven for more information on diabetes in pregnancy.

EATING DISORDERS

Women with a history of eating disorders such as anorexia or bu-limia must be especially careful in pregnancy. Because of the strong focus on food and weight gain in pregnancy, some women who have been anorexic or bulemic may find old feelings and urges re-turning. And the decreased calorie intake associated with a current eating disorder can result in poor weight gain and may lead to nu-trition-related birth defects, poor fetal growth, low birth weight, and preterm birth. However, pregnancy can give women with eat-ing disorders the motivation to eat well and change their eating habits for their babies, if not for themselves. Be sure to tell your doctor if you have a current or past eating disorder. Professional teams of counselors, dietitians, and doctors can work with you to manage your care.

FOOD ADDITIVES

Caffeine

Coffee, tea, many soft drinks, and chocolate all contain the stimu-lant caffeine. Caffeine is also present in many over-the-counter medications and in drugs advertised as stimulants. Although stud-ies are conflicting about the risks of caffeine use in pregnancy, some have shown that women with heavy caffeine intake are more likely to have increased pregnancy complications, especially low birth weight babies. Caffeine crosses the placenta and is transferred through breast milk. As a stimulant, caffeine can increase the heart rates of mother and babies. Caffeine decreases iron absorption, making anemia more likely, and it also works as a diuretic, making you lose some of the fluids you take in.

Because of these effects, you should limit the amount of caf-feine you consume. Decrease your caffeine intake slowly, over several days, to prevent withdrawal headaches. Substitute healthy fluids without caffeine, such as water, milk, and fruit juices.

Artificial Sweeteners

Because multiple pregnancy is a time to gain weight, not lose, artificial sweeteners and diet products aren't needed. However, if you are a diabetic, talk with your doctor about which sugar substitutes are best to use in pregnancy. Otherwise, it's best to avoid these and all artificial substances.

Aspartame is an artificial sweetener sold under the names Nutrasweet and Equal; and is an ingredient in many low-calorie foods and beverages. The FDA has approved aspartame as a safe food ingredient for the general population, including pregnant women. The American Academy of Pediatrics also advises that aspartame is safe for both the mother and developing baby. The only exception is for women with an inherited metabolism problem called phenylketonuria (PKU), who cannot properly metabolize phenylalanine, a major component of aspartame.

Saccharin, another artificial sweetener, is known to increase risks of cancer in children exposed in utero, and it should not be used in pregnancy.

The FDA approved a new sweetener called sucralose in 1998 for use in a wide variety of foods and drinks. Sucralose, sold under the trade name Splenda, is made from sugar and has been approved for use in pregnancy.

FOOD-BORNE ILLNESSES

Some foods can be unsafe in pregnancy if not carefully cleaned or cooked. Raw or undercooked foods, especially meats, often contain microorganisms such as *E. coli* that can cause serious illness. *Listeriosis* is a dangerous food-borne illness that can result in miscarriage, fetal death, preterm birth, or fatal neonatal infection. *Toxoplasmosis* is acquired by eating infected, uncooked meat, or by inhaling or ingesting cells of the organism excreted in cat feces. Babies can develop eye and brain problems from toxoplasmosis infection during pregnancy. Avoid all contact with cat litter and talk with your doctor about testing for toxoplasmosis if you are a cat owner.

Practice common sense in food choices and preparation. Keep cold foods cold and hot foods hot. All fruits and vegetables should be washed well to remove contamination from organic fertilizers and pesticides. Cook all animal products thoroughly to destroy bacteria, and avoid unpasteurized milk as well as raw meat, poultry, eggs, and seafood, including sushi. Also avoid Mexican-style soft cheeses such as queso blanco and asadero, and other soft cheeses such as feta (goat cheese), Brie, Camembert, and blue-veined cheeses like Roquefort, which can contain the *Listeria* bacteria.

HOW ARE YOU EATING?

Now go back to your list of the foods you ate in the past twenty-four hours. Can you identify the grains, fruits, vegetables, proteins, dairy, and fats? Which nutrients are you doing well with? Are there areas you need to add or change? How many extra servings do you need to add for each area? If you are having difficulty planning a diet or eating enough, ask your doctor for a nutrition referral. A consultation with a registered dietitian can help you choose foods and plan your meals within your food preferences and budget.

Sometimes a detailed nutritional evaluation is needed for women with complicated multiple pregnancies. Women with very high multiples or those on bed rest may need to change their caloric intake. Your doctor can calculate your energy needs by conducting a basal metabolic rate study, which accurately determines how many calories your body uses to breathe, circulate blood, and perform its basic functions. One woman pregnant with triplets had a daily basal metabolic rate of over 1,800 calories while on complete bed rest. This didn't count the 500 or more extra calories necessary for the growth of her babies!

WEIGHT GAIN

One way to know if you are eating enough is by your weight gain. There is a clear link between a mother's pregnancy weight gain and the birth weights of her babies. As a general rule, babies born to a mother who gains enough weight in pregnancy weigh more at birth than the babies of a mother who gains too little. This is an important principle for multiple pregnancy. Because multiple birth babies often are born prematurely, they tend to be small and have low birth weights. By gaining weight early in pregnancy, a mother can help her babies have higher birth weights despite being premature. In addition, early weight gain helps build up energy stores for the mother, which are used for her own increased needs in late pregnancy. Of course, there are situations that affect babies' birth weights despite good maternal weight gain. Sometimes the placentas do not function effectively to deliver enough nutrients to one or more babies. Also, certain conditions, such as twin-to-twin transfusion syndrome, can cause poor fetal growth. In spite of these problems, gaining enough weight in pregnancy can help your babies be as healthy as possible.

If your babies are growing appropriately in pregnancy, it usually means you are getting the right nutrition and gaining weight as well. At first, babies grow even if the mother has poor weight gain. The wonderful design of a woman's pregnant body makes this protective ability possible. The food and nutrients you take in are used for the babies' needs first, and then they are used to meet your body's needs. If you do not eat enough for your babies, your body supplies their needs from its own reserves. In the long term, your body can become depleted of important stores of iron, calcium, and protein. Babies ultimately can stop gaining and lose weight. By gaining weight, you maintain your body's supplies and establish stores that you might need for late pregnancy, birth, and later for breastfeeding.

How Much Weight to Gain

There are many opinions about the right amount of weight that women should gain with a multiple pregnancy. Some doctors don't address the issue unless they feel a woman is not gaining at all. Others suggest gaining extreme amounts of weight, but extremely high weight gain goals are unrealistic for many women. You are more likely to succeed in gaining weight if you have a moderate, achievable goal. And much of the research that has been done has found that optimal health and birth weights of babies occur with moderate weight gain amounts. Table 4.1 gives guidelines for multiple pregnancy weight gain that may help improve infant birth weights and infant outcomes.

These guidelines are for women with average height and weight. Women who are petite, underweight, or have a small frame should try to gain on the high side of the weight range. Women who are overweight also need to gain weight in pregnancy to support their babies' needs.

The pattern and timing of pregnancy weight gain is also important. With twins, you should try to gain 24 pounds by the first twenty-four weeks of your pregnancy, or about 1 pound every week. After twenty-four weeks, strive for a gain of about 1¼ to one

Table 4.1. Weight Gain Guidelines	
Twins	40–45 pounds
Triplets	45–55 pounds
Very high multiples	Triplet weight gain plus ten pounds for each additional baby.

and 1½ pounds each week. For triplets, the goal is to gain about 36 pounds by twenty-four weeks. Because higher-order multiples nearly always arrive several weeks preterm, gaining weight early is especially important.

Steady weight gain all through pregnancy is the goal for average-weight women. Especially for underweight women, studies have found that weight gain in the first half of twin pregnancy contributes most to increasing infant birth weight. Many women have nausea and poor appetite in early pregnancy and lose weight at first but catch up quickly after the nausea goes away. Don't panic if you haven't gained enough to meet these weight gain goals. It's never too late to make a positive change.

Where Does the Weight Go?

Most of the weight you gain is from the special structures of pregnancy, the extra circulating fluid, and the weight of the babies themselves. The remaining weight is stored for your energy needs in late pregnancy, birth, and afterward for breastfeeding. Table 4.2 gives you an idea of how your weight gain will be distributed.

Many women worry that they will never lose the weight they gain in pregnancy. However, most women find that large pregnancy weight gains are lost within two years after birth. For now, focus on the wonderful internal changes that are happening—the

---

Table 4.2 Average Weight Gain Distributions for Twin Pregnancy at Thirty-Eight Weeks

Babies	5½–6 pounds each
Uterus	2–3 pounds
Placenta(s)	1½ pounds each
Amniotic fluid	2 pounds for each baby
Breasts	2½–3 pounds
Fluid volume	6–8 pounds
Mother's body stores	8–9 pounds
Approximate total	40 pounds

development and growth of your babies and your body's ability to nurture them. Your hair, skin, and nails are often at their best because of your healthy diet and the hormones of pregnancy, so flaunt your best features and enjoy being big and beautifully pregnant.

> I tried really hard to follow the diet plan recommended by the dietitian. I gained 40 pounds by the time I was thirty-seven weeks, and fifteen of those weeks I was on bedrest. That weight just fell off in no time after the girls were born.

Chapter Five

Your Changing Body

Multiple pregnancy is physically very different from pregnancy with one baby. Women who have had both say there is no comparing how they feel with these pregnancies. Many of the normal physical changes of pregnancy are more intense in a multiple pregnancy—discomforts arrive sooner and often are more annoying. In just a short time, many women find everyday activities much harder to accomplish. How you respond to these changes can make a difference in how you feel and in the outcome of your pregnancy. Some women find it hard to slow down with a multiple pregnancy, but it is important that you do. This chapter discusses the physical changes that occur in multiple pregnancy. It also covers how your lifestyle and activities can affect the outcome of your pregnancy and the health of your babies.

> I loved my pregnancy until about month five, just after learning I was having twins. I concentrated on eating healthy, hydration, and rest, but I quickly learned the differences between singleton and multiple pregnancies. I would watch my pregnant neighbors out walking or playing tennis, and I could barely make it to the end of the driveway. I had to sit frequently, and very few people fully understood the physical difficulty. I had to discontinue favorite activities very early, even singing in our church choir, because I couldn't stand for long periods of time.

YOUR AMAZING UTERUS

As your uterus expands to accommodate two, three, or more babies, it can grow very dramatically. As early as the eighth week of twin pregnancy, a woman's uterus is nearly double the size it is with just one baby. After the twentieth week in a singleton pregnancy, the number of centimeters from the fundus (top) of the uterus to the pubic bone roughly equals the number of weeks. Thus, at twenty-seven weeks gestation, a woman with one baby should measure about twenty-seven centimeters. With a multiple pregnancy, the uterus grows more rapidly and is often four or more centimeters ahead of gestational dates. For example, a woman with twins at twenty-seven weeks can measure 31 centimeters, and women carrying higher-order multiples grow even faster! But all this expansion is important—it means your babies are growing too. You may find your uterus grows at a steady pace, or that it has growth spurts followed by plateaus. Whatever growth pattern your uterus takes, it's exciting to see your body make these amazing changes.

> I'm growing so fast I forget how big my belly is and I keep bumping into doors and countertops.

OUTFITTING YOUR
FAST-GROWING BODY

Finding comfortable clothing that fits can be a challenge with your rapidly growing body. You will probably need maternity garments much sooner than if you were carrying just one baby. Standard maternity clothes that fit at first may not be big enough in late pregnancy, especially if you are having higher-order multiples. If you need to dress for business, try shopping in the large-size women's department. If you are not working outside the home, look for casual, loose-fitting garments. Remember that your abdomen is not the only part that grows—your breasts and hips get bigger, too. Stay away from restricting waistbands and fussy clothes. If you have visions of looking like a circus tent, remember that comfort may soon be more important than appearance!

> When I was twenty-four weeks along, I went shopping for a pair of jeans. I am normally a size six or eight, and when I found that size eighteen maternity jeans wouldn't fit, I just gave up. I was content to live in a size XXXL drawstring sweat pants for the rest of my pregnancy.

A good bra is important during pregnancy to help support your heavy breasts. Bra support also helps reduce back strain and minimize any breast tissue stretching and sagging. Because your body is changing so fast, buy only one or two bras at a time. You might want to choose nursing bras so you can wear them later for breastfeeding. Avoid underwires, and look for breathable fabric, such as cotton.

Many women find their shoes quickly become tight, often as a result of swelling. Your shoe size might increase by a half size or more near the end of pregnancy. Avoid high heels that can throw off your balance and put a strain on your back and pelvic ligaments. Wear sensible shoes that slip on and off and don't require ties, as it may become virtually impossible to reach them later in pregnancy!

> I marveled at my enormity, and after gaining 52 pounds, I had no wardrobe. I could only fit into my husband's largest shirts and elastic shorts or tent-shaped dresses. Strangers were very bold to tell me, "You must be ready to go any day now," and they'd stand speechless when I'd tell them I had over three months left. I can't say I hated my body though. I lost the weight quickly, recovered from the terrible havoc on my stomach, and I see it all as an achievement that produced two perfectly healthy babies.

DIGESTION IN EARLY PREGNANCY

One of the first discomforts many women experience in multiple pregnancy is *morning sickness.* This nausea, queasiness, and vomiting may begin by the fourth to sixth week from your last period and can last through the first fourteen to sixteen weeks of pregnancy. For some women, the sickness isn't just in the morning but all day and all night—and for some it lasts throughout the pregnancy. Even if you don't have nausea, you may have very little appetite, and it is quite common to not gain weight during this time. Although morning sickness is normal, it's not a pleasant way to start your pregnancy.

It isn't clear why nausea is more common in women with multiple pregnancies, but it may be related to the increased levels of the hormone *hCG* (*human chorionic gonadotropin*). These levels can be as much as ten times higher than for a singleton pregnancy at the same gestational age. Progesterone, another hormone, increases in pregnancy and can affect the motility and the tone of your gastrointestinal tract. Food just doesn't move through as quickly or as smoothly.

> I was never sick. The only thing that ever bothered me was brushing my teeth. Having that foam fill up my mouth made me gag. Even now, years later, I still have some of that sensation.

Fortunately, not everyone feels awful. Some women have little or no morning sickness and sail through the first trimester, eating and gaining weight. If you aren't so lucky, do your best to eat nutritious foods when you can. Many women find it helpful to eat frequent, small meals, rich in carbohydrates and low in fat. Others use the time-tested trick of eating crackers before getting out of bed. Mixing liquids and solids sometimes makes meals less likely to stay down; so if this is a problem for you, try drinking your fluids between meals. Also, learn to avoid those foods that trigger nausea. You might find it helpful to have others prepare your meals when you are feeling queasy. Finally, a protein/carbohydrate bedtime snack such as cheese and crackers may help prevent morning nausea.

> I always interpreted that yucky feeling as needing to eat. So
> I ate constantly and never went anywhere without food in
> my purse.

A few medications can help relieve severe nausea, but you should take these only with your doctor's approval, as medication used in the first trimester of pregnancy can affect your developing babies. You may want to try drug-free therapies such as acupressure or seasickness bracelets. A new device called ReliefBand was recently approved by the FDA for pregnancy nausea. This is a wristband that uses low-level electrical signals to stimulate certain nerves in the wrist and is available by prescription. Also, ask your doctor about taking gingerroot or vitamin B_6 supplements, which are reportedly helpful with nausea.

> My dietitian recommended unfrosted cinnamon Pop-Tarts. I
> don't know why, but they really helped stop the nausea.

If you are completely unable to keep food or liquids down, or you are vomiting so much that you are dehydrated and urinating very little, you should call your doctor. A few women develop a severe form of morning sickness called *hyperemesis gravidarum*. This can be very serious and can result in fluid and electrolyte imbalances as well as kidney and liver problems. Hospitalization usually is needed to replace lost fluids and calories, and for severe cases, some doctors use intravenous therapy with *total parenteral nutrition* (*TPN*). Others recommend placing a tube through a woman's nose into her stomach to slowly pump in nutrients.

DIGESTION IN LATER PREGNANCY

Later in pregnancy, your growing uterus pushes your digestive tract into different positions. Your stomach and diaphragm are moved upward, and your intestines are pressed against the sides and the back of your abdomen. This, along with the effects of the hormone progesterone, contributes to slow movement of food through your digestive tract, possibly making you feel full all the time. Having heartburn and reflux of foods from your stomach into your esophagus can make you feel miserable as well. Constipation can also be a problem.

Most women find that frequent small meals are easier to digest than a few large meals. If you have heartburn or reflux, try sleeping with the head of your bed elevated, and avoid lying down right after eating. Check with your doctor before using antacids or other medications for heartburn. Severe reflux often can be treated with medication. If constipation is a problem, make sure you are drinking plenty of fluids and eating lots of fiber-filled vegetables and fruits. Do not take laxatives or use enemas because they can irritate your intestinal tract and possibly stimulate uterine contractions.

URINATION

In early pregnancy, your uterus tilts forward and presses on your bladder, making you feel as if you need to urinate constantly. In a singleton pregnancy, the uterus rises after the first trimester, relieving the pressure until late in pregnancy. With multiples, your uterus grows so quickly that you may not get this relief. The weight of the heavy uterus limits your bladder's ability to expand as it fills with urine. Many women say that their bladders always feel full, even after they urinate. In addition, the large uterus presses on the ureters, the tubes that connect your kidneys and bladder. These changes can result in a greater likelihood of urinary tract infections in multiple pregnancy, so it's important to watch for warning signs. Call your doctor if you have more frequent urination; burning or pain; dark, concentrated urine; or fever. Urinary tract infections can lead to serious kidney infections and preterm labor. To help keep your urinary system running smoothly and reduce the chances of infection, be sure to drink plenty of fluids each day and relax as you urinate, allowing your bladder to empty completely.

SHORTNESS OF BREATH

As your uterus enlarges, there is less and less space for your lungs to expand. In a singleton pregnancy, the diaphragm (the large muscle separating the lungs and the abdominal cavity) rises as much as 4 centimeters. It is thought that the diaphragm moves higher in a multiple pregnancy. Pregnancy requires extra oxygen, and your breathing rate increases to compensate, even when you are at rest. More rapid breathing and less room to expand can leave you huffing and puffing with normal tasks. If you find yourself winded with very little effort, slow down and allow yourself more time to get where you need to go. Break down large tasks into smaller jobs that don't require as much effort. If you have difficulty breathing, or chest pain, call your doctor; this may be a sign of a serious complication.

FATIGUE

Many women struggle through the first few weeks of pregnancy feeling absolutely exhausted. If you are working, you may fall asleep the minute you come home. This is perfectly normal! Your body is making enormous changes to adapt to the needs of your babies. This tiredness usually diminishes after the first trimester, when you begin to have more energy and stamina. Women carrying only one baby usually enjoy this energy boost until the last few weeks of pregnancy. Not so when you have a multiple pregnancy, as your developing babies place extra demands on your body. Bearing the extra weight of the amniotic fluid, placentas, and babies tires you as well. Many women with twins begin to feel fatigued again around the twenty-fifth week of pregnancy. This happens earlier if you are having higher-order multiples. You may find that as each week passes, it becomes more of an effort to climb stairs and do chores and your normal activities.

Don't let this discourage you. Instead, listen as your body tells you that you need to slow down. Taking several rest breaks throughout the day can help. This means stopping, putting up your feet, and closing your eyes for fifteen to thirty minutes. These catnaps can rejuvenate you and give you the energy you need to make it through your day. As you get further into your pregnancy, you'll find yourself looking forward to your rest breaks. Full-fledged naps are even better. Allow yourself to be a couch potato or a lady of leisure with a multiple pregnancy.

> I don't feel like I ever had the "blissful second trimester" that all my pregnancy books talked about. I went from the exhaustion and morning sickness of the first trimester, felt good from sixteen to nineteen weeks, and then I was so big that my experience was more like jumping right to the third trimester.

INSOMNIA

Despite being tired to the point of exhaustion, some women suffer from *insomnia*—being unable to sleep at night. Getting comfortable in bed is a challenge with active babies and a big abdomen. Once you begin feeling your babies move, at about twenty weeks, their constant movements may keep you awake. One expectant mom described her triplets as having a nightly pow-wow inside her. Turning over with a huge belly is a great effort, and you may wake up several times a night to go to the bathroom.

There are several ways to cope with not being able to sleep. Don't allow yourself to become overtired. Doing too much can backfire and result in muscle aches and overactive babies. Establish a bedtime routine such as taking a warm shower, eating a healthy snack, and emptying your bladder. Other helpful tips are using clean, well-fitting sheets, keeping your room dark and cool, using a sleep machine that creates noise—such as rain or ocean waves to drown out other sounds—and aromatherapy. Don't forget to place a night light on the way to the bathroom and remove throw rugs to prevent falls.

In bed, try placing pillows behind you, in front of you, and between your legs, as well as under your head. Many women find a large body pillow is helpful. Also, tucking a small pillow under your abdomen helps support its weight. You should try to sleep on your left side as much as possible. This is the most efficient position for circulation. Your right side is fine, too, but avoid lying directly on your back. The weight of your uterus can compress the large blood vessels in your abdomen, causing your blood pressure to drop when you stand up as the blood volume quickly changes. Also, prolonged compression of these blood vessels can reduce blood flow to the placentas and increase swelling. If you can't sleep in any other position than on your back, try elevating your upper body on pillows or sleeping in a recliner that is partially reclined. You can also place a pillow behind your back and roll slightly to one side.

In very late pregnancy, you may be unable to get comfortable in any position. An egg-crate mattress pad may be helpful. Some women have resorted to special circulating air mattresses or waterbeds. Dads often move out to the sofa, just to get a few uninterrupted hours of sleep.

Finally, don't panic if you can't get a full night's sleep. Resting and napping during the day can help you make up for lost sleep. And, as every new mother has learned, this is practice for when your babies come home.

ACHES AND PAINS

With the added weight of your growing babies, there are bound to be more than the usual aches and pains associated with pregnancy. Some discomforts are due to the physical changes associated with your enlarging uterus, while other aches and pains can result from doing too much. Since some discomforts can be related to pregnancy complications, be sure to talk with your doctor about any pain or change in sensation that you experience.

Round Ligament Pain
Several ligaments support your uterus within your pelvis, and as your uterus grows, these ligaments stretch and may spasm. This is often the cause of *round ligament* pain, often described as shooting pains down into your groin area. You might be awakened in the night with round ligament pain, just from turning over. To get up from lying down, roll to your side and push yourself up with your arms to a sitting position, and then bring your legs down over the side of the bed or sofa. Avoid making sudden movements or twisting your body which can pull a round ligament. At home, a bed rail with long supports under the mattress is helpful. If you are in the hospital, request that a bar be mounted over your bed. This gives you leverage to change positions more easily.

Backache
The *broad ligament* suspends the uterus within your pelvis. As your heavy uterus tilts forward, it pulls on these ligaments. In turn, the broad ligament can tilt your whole pelvis forward, making an

accentuated *S* curvature of your spine. Backache is a common result. Be careful about your posture, and avoid letting your back sway forward. When you walk or stand, tuck your hips under and allow your pelvis and legs to support the weight of your pregnancy, not your back. Warm showers, gentle back massage, and medication if advised by your doctor may also help relieve back pain.

Many women find that the pelvic rock exercise helps relieve back pain. To do this, get down on the floor on your hands and knees. Slowly and gently tuck in your abdominal muscles to flatten out the curve of your back. Relax, but don't allow your back to sag or fall back down sharply. Do this several times in a slow rhythm, rest, and repeat. You can also do a pelvic rock while standing.

You might want to invest in a maternity supporter, which you can find at most maternity stores. A maternity supporter is not a girdle but is specially designed to relieve some of the pressure from the weight of your uterus and help with backache. Look for a supporter that has wide firm bands that can be adjusted as you grow, rather than one with stretchable bands. Some have a moldable insert for extra back support.

Backache can be a normal discomfort of pregnancy, but it can also be a sign of preterm labor. You must be alert when your back begins to hurt in a different way than usual, or when the backache comes and goes, or when you are having other signs such as increased vaginal discharge. See Chapter Ten for more information on preterm labor. Call your doctor if you have a severe backache, if it feels different from backaches you've had before, or if it is not relieved by your usual methods.

Leg Cramps

There are various theories about the cause of these sharp charley-horse cramps in your legs. They are most likely due to pressure of your uterus on your leg nerves as well as circulatory changes. Whatever their cause, leg cramps can be a very annoying discomfort. For relief, try massage or stretching exercises.

Carpal Tunnel Syndrome

Carpal tunnel syndrome (*CTS*) sometimes occurs in multiple pregnancy. It is thought that increased weight gain and swelling in pregnancy causes compression of the median nerve in the hand and wrist. This results in pain, numbness, and tingling of your thumb, second, third and part of the fourth fingers. These symptoms can occur in one or both hands and usually go away after delivery. Carpal tunnel syndrome tends to occur more often in women over thirty who are having a first pregnancy and can occur postpartum, often associated with breastfeeding. Treatment usually involves splinting the wrist at night, while severe cases may require surgery to relieve the compression.

BLOOD VESSEL CHANGES

The pressure of your heavy uterus on blood vessels in your pelvic area can cause *hemorrhoids* to develop or worsen. These varicose veins of the rectum can be quite painful, and staying off your feet is usually the best treatment. You may also notice veins in your legs enlarging or an increase in broken blood vessels and spider veins. Avoid thigh-top and tight knee-high hose, which can aggravate these conditions. Your face may appear flushed and the palms of your hands often redden as a result of a large increase in blood flow in pregnancy. Some women also notice swelling of their gums, which can lead to pregnancy gingivitis. This inflammation can become infected, so good dental care is important in pregnancy.

DIASTASIS RECTI

The rapid and extreme growth of your uterus can cause *diastasis recti,* a harmless separation of the tissues between your abdominal muscles in the front of your abdomen, usually beginning in the second trimester. Some women have described feeling "unzipped" when they notice this. Although this feels strange it is not harmful.

ITCHING

Nearly every pregnant woman experiences itching, especially on the skin of her abdomen. But itching can also result from other conditions which may be more serious. Itching is a common result of the skin on your abdomen stretching. Most women find relief in oatmeal baths, using regular oats tied in mesh or a bag made from pantyhose and swished in the bath water. Keeping your skin soft and preventing dryness with lotion or creams may also help. But be sure to tell your doctor about any itching you have, because the two other sources of itching can require medical intervention.

One other possible cause of itching is a condition called *pruritic urticarial papules and plaques of pregnancy* (*PUPPP*), which can develop in late pregnancy. With PUPPP, a reddened rash with bumps and scaly patches develops on your abdomen and may spread to your buttocks, arms, and legs. PUPPP is thought to be related to increased abdominal size, which may explain why it is more common in women with higher-order multiples. The itching can make you miserable and is usually treated with doctor-prescribed antihistamines or steroids. Fortunately, PUPPP usually goes away within one to two weeks after delivery.

Another itching problem in pregnancy is caused by changes in your gall bladder function. The physical and hormonal changes of pregnancy can slow the movement of bile, resulting in a condition called *cholestasis*. Cholestasis causes a build-up of bile salts in your blood and skin, and itching results. There is no rash from this condition, only a generalized itching. Cholestasis is more common in multiple pregnancy and can be dangerous because jaundice (yellowing of skin) can develop, and the risk of preterm birth and fetal loss can increase. Medications may be needed to reduce the bile salts and can help with itching. Fetal monitoring with nonstress testing or other surveillance is often used, and in some cases, early delivery is advised.

CIRCULATION

Women having multiples have nearly twice the amount of circulating blood as women with singleton pregnancies. Your body handles this large amount of blood volume in several ways. For example, your heart rate increases slightly, and it has to work harder to pump the larger amount of blood.

Some of this extra fluid can settle in your tissues and appear as *edema* (swelling) in your ankles and feet at the end of the day. This is not unusual, especially in late pregnancy. The pressure of your heavy uterus on the blood vessels of your pelvis also contributes to swelling. Drink plenty of fluids, but do not restrict your salt intake. Limiting dietary salt has not been shown to be an effective treatment for edema. Overall or sudden swelling, especially in your face and hands, could be a sign of high blood pressure of pregnancy. Call your doctor if you have more swelling than usual or if you have a sudden weight gain of several pounds. See Chapter Eleven for more information on high blood pressure.

Another result of increased blood volume is *anemia* (iron deficiency). Iron is important in forming red blood cells that carry oxygen throughout your body and to your babies. Anemia also makes you feel tired and sluggish. Although your body makes more red blood cells in a multiple pregnancy, it usually is not enough. Your hemoglobin level (the concentration of oxygen-carrying cells) can often be low because the extra fluid dilutes the quantity of these cells. Although prenatal vitamins contain iron, additional iron supplements often are needed to treat anemia, and these can be constipating and can cause nausea. Slow-release forms of iron tend to be less troublesome.

SKIN CHANGES

One of the first things many women notice in pregnancy is the wonderful glow of their skin. Complexion problems often clear, and hair and nails grow and look fabulous. Many women notice darkening of their areolas (area around the nipples) and the appearance of a dark line called the *linea nigra* down their abdomen. Another common, more visible skin change is dark pigmentation on the face called *chloasma*. Although chloasma usually improves after pregnancy, sun exposure can worsen the pigmentation, so use sunscreen to help minimize the darkening.

The development of *stretch marks* can be distressing. These are thin pink or purple lines that appear on your abdomen, hips, breasts, and thighs. Rapid growth, stretching of the skin, and high levels of estrogen are thought to contribute to stretch marks. Although many women get stretch marks with multiple pregnancy, not everyone gets them, even with a huge abdomen. A number of creams and products claim they prevent stretch marks, but they only help keep your skin soft and moisturized. If you do develop stretch marks, try not to get upset. Although the lines do not go away, the dark coloring fades over time. Think of them as mementos of the wonderful job your body did in growing your babies.

The changes that come with pregnancy do bring discomforts, but they are usually manageable. It helps to remember that pregnancy doesn't last forever.

> I really did enjoy being pregnant with twins in spite of the extra discomforts. I'll always remember what it was like to feel and see them moving and try to figure out which baby was which.

Chapter Six

Adapting Your Lifestyle with a Multiple Pregnancy

Although many of the complications and risks of multiple pregnancy are beyond your control, you can make changes in your lifestyle. Your work, exercise, social activities, sexual relations, substance use—these are modifiable aspects of your life that affect, and are affected by, your pregnancy.

WORKING OUTSIDE THE HOME

Combining a multiple pregnancy and a job can be complex. Depending on your activities on the job and any additional pregnancy risk factors, you may or may not be able to continue working. Be realistic about the physical and emotional demands of your job and its activities. Women who have home-based businesses also need to be conscious of their self-imposed demands. Here are some questions to ask yourself:

- What do you physically do each day—standing, sitting, lifting, climbing stairs, bending frequently?
- Do you have a long, stressful commute?
- Is your employment hazardous—are you exposed to chemicals, x-rays, or other dangerous substances?

- Are you frequently required to travel by air or car?
- What kind of hours do you work, each day and each week? Do you work weekends?
- On the job, are you able to take frequent breaks for bathroom, snacks, water?

Some occupations, including nursing, teaching, food service, and hairdressing, can require long hours and excessive physical demands. Research has identified a number of activities and work environments that are linked to preterm labor and birth and poor pregnancy outcomes. These include standing for long periods of time, a long work week, heavy lifting (more than 20 pounds), and exposure to environmental stress such as cold, very loud noise, hazardous materials, or toxic substances. Military duty and assembly line work are also associated with poor pregnancy outcomes. Exposure to chemical agents, including pesticides, lead, mercury, and organic solvents that are common in cleaners, paints, and paint thinner, can be *teratogenic* (cause abnormal development) to unborn babies. Although concerns have been raised about the safety of video display terminals (VDTs) in pregnancy, a large study by the National Institute for Occupational Safety and Health found no association between VDT use and pregnancy loss. However, sitting for long periods of time in front of a computer terminal can restrict blood flow to the uterus and cause back strain.

Women expecting twins may be able to work through much of their pregnancy as long as there are no complications. However, most women are ready to stop work or cut back their hours around twenty-four to twenty-eight weeks of pregnancy. Women with higher-order multiple pregnancies generally need to stop working much earlier, around twenty weeks. If you have the luxury of not needing to work, quit your job now. You may not realize how much stress your job places on you until you stop working.

Don't be hesitant to tell your employer you have a high-risk pregnancy. You both can benefit by communicating up front that you need to make changes in your job. Your employer will be more willing to accommodate your needs if you already have some ideas and suggestions. Be candid about the risks of a multiple pregnancy and what your potential limitations might be. Don't try to minimize your needs now and have to ask to change again later. Look for ways to contribute as long as possible. Can you move to a different area of the company or take on other responsibilities? Can you do more phone work? Can another employee take over your travel responsibilities? Can you telecommute? Can you change your hours? Is going part-time or job-sharing possible? Going from ten-hour days to four-hour days can make a big difference in how you feel and possibly allow you to work longer.

> I had sailed through my twin pregnancy—both babies growing well and I was working full time. Then my blood pressure shot up and I had to quit.

Modify your work environment as much as possible for comfort. Use a stool instead of standing, or put a box under your desk to prop up your feet. Take frequent stretch breaks and, if possible, find a way to lie down for fifteen to thirty minutes at least twice a day. Make sure that you have snacks and plenty to drink at your desk or work area.

> At twenty-four weeks I am still working, but getting significantly more uncomfortable by the minute, so I'm not sure how long this will last.

Ask about maternity insurance and disability plans. Some disability plans cover high-risk pregnancy with a doctor's recommendation. If you're considering a change to part-time work, be sure to check into company policy regarding disability benefits because they might be different from what you have as a full-time employee. Your employer may offer other benefit plans, such as unpaid leave.

If you do not plan to return to work after your babies are born, let your employer know. By offering to train a new employee before you leave, everyone profits.

If you are concerned about job security because of your high-risk pregnancy, there are federal laws that provide protection for pregnant women against workplace discrimination. These laws apply in certain circumstances and have restrictions based on the number of employees. Some states also have enacted laws that apply to employers with smaller workforces. The federal Pregnancy Discrimination Act, which was added to Title VII of the Civil Rights Act, applies to employers with fifteen or more employees. Under this law, an employer must treat pregnancy, childbirth, and related medical conditions just as it would treat other temporary medical conditions or disabilities. If special accommodations are provided for an employee with a disability such as a broken arm or leg, comparable accommodations also must be provided for a pregnant employee with limitations or disabilities. The Family Medical Leave Act of 1993 applies to employers with fifty or more employees and guarantees certain employees up to twelve weeks of unpaid, job-protected leave for eligible reasons, which include pregnancy disability. Consult an attorney to learn about your individual employment rights.

Always keep in mind that your health and the well-being of your babies is your number one priority. You may find that working creates such a strain that any advantages are clearly outweighed. Finances may be an issue, but compromising your pregnancy is never worth the extra dollars.

HOMEMAKERS AND CARING FOR CHILDREN

Homemakers and mothers with other children also need to be aware of the demands of these full-time jobs. Many of the physical movements involved in cooking, cleaning, and caring for small children can be very taxing. For example, vacuuming is a stressful and physically demanding activity. Something as simple as doing laundry requires frequent bending and lifting. It is more difficult when your laundry facilities are not on the same floor or are in a different building. If you are a cleaning fanatic, start now to change your expectations. A spotless house is not very important in the big picture. If you can get the basics done, let the rest go. Ask others to do the hardest tasks, or teach older children to help with the chores that you can't do. If you can afford paid help, hire a service or a housekeeper to clean thoroughly every couple of weeks.

Limit meal preparation to the least time-consuming menus, and consider using a grocery delivery service. Fast food is not always healthy, but you can often find complete, nutritious meals at reasonable prices in the grocery deli. Limit your shopping trips by making a list and quickly getting only the things you need. Someone else can do heavy shopping. When friends visit, ask them to come with a meal for the freezer. Even if you don't need it now, it will come in handy once the babies come home!

Caring for small children is an endless task. Their needs and demands for attention don't stop just because you are pregnant. A twenty-five-pound toddler rarely understands why you can't bend down to pick him up any longer. Many children cannot comprehend why their schedules and activities must change. Even older preschoolers and school-age children who do understand react in different ways: some are eager to help while others become resentful and act out.

Children thrive on routine, and disruptions can upset them. Continue your children's routines as much as possible, and maintain a consistent schedule. If they are still taking naps, this is a good time to join them. They'll love the time you spend with them, and you'll benefit, too. If you are greatly restricted in your activity, try to meet your child's requests with a bit of creativity. Teach a toddler to use a stool to join you on the bed or sofa. Have a reading time or a special television time set aside each day. Encourage your older children to do their homework by your side. Arrange for carpools for your children's activities now and for the first few months after your babies are born. There will be plenty of time later to return the favors. If you plan to start children in a preschool or mother's day out program, it might be better to start them now rather than waiting. They could feel rejected if they are sent off to a new school when the babies come home.

If you have considered hiring someone to help when the babies come home, find out if they can start early. You'll probably enjoy the help with the chores and household responsibilities. Au pairs and nannies need to get to know your older children before they take on the task of the new babies.

Share your daily routine and activities with your doctor to help identify the areas that can increase your risks for problems. Work together with your family to make accommodations in your lifestyle so that your risks are minimized.

EXERCISE

Many women take part in active exercise programs and recreational fitness before they become pregnant, and it is true that exercise during pregnancy can help relieve some of the associated discomforts. Also, many studies have shown that, in a low-risk pregnancy, exercise does not harm the unborn baby. Although some research indicates that women who exercise have an easier time in labor, there is no proof that exercise improves pregnancy outcome.

Women with singleton pregnancies usually can continue regular exercise programs and their normal activities throughout pregnancy. But because of the increased risks with a multiple pregnancy, you'll need to modify many activities or stop some altogether. Most doctors recommend decreasing the length and intensity of exercise in the second trimester of a twin pregnancy. If you have complications, such as preterm labor or hypertension, your doctor will probably prohibit all exercise. Women with higher-order multiple pregnancies have much greater risks for complications. They usually have more restrictions on their activities than women expecting twins.

Here are some principles to keep in mind about exercise in pregnancy:

- Many of the physical changes of pregnancy affect your stamina and energy. These include an increased heart rate and decreased intake of oxygen.
- The weight of your uterus and breasts change your center of gravity and can affect your balance, making you more unsteady on your feet.
- Hormones of pregnancy can relax your ligaments, making them more susceptible to injury.
- Becoming overheated, especially in the first trimester, can be dangerous for your developing babies. Do not use hot tubs, saunas, or steam rooms, and drink plenty of fluids before and during exercise.
- Exercise uses calories, especially carbohydrates, which are an important energy source in pregnancy. You need to replace these burned calories for adequate weight gain.
- Activities that involve lying on your back or standing motionless for long periods of time can bring about a sudden drop in blood pressure.

Examine your motivations for wanting to exercise. Many women are concerned that if they stop exercising, they will gain too much weight and become fat. Indeed, the image of a thin, athletic woman is in stark contrast to the woman pregnant with twins who has gained 40 pounds.

I had a history of anorexia and I was terrified of gaining weight. I knew that I should stop exercising, but I was afraid of what I would look like if I did.

Remember that pregnancy weight gain has a great impact on the birth weights and health of your babies. Accepting the new, bigger you may mean readjusting your body image to incorporate the amazing changes and growth of your body. Try to refocus your mental picture from your nonpregnant body to one of blossoming mother and growing babies, and remember that this is a temporary change. After recovering from the birth of your babies, you can resume your exercise routines and get back into shape.

Talk honestly with your doctor about your current exercise regimen, including what you do, how often, and how long you exercise. Discuss your pregnancy specifically and ask for activity guidelines. You may be able to continue some activities as long as you have no risks other than your multiple pregnancy. Most women begin to reduce the amount and frequency of exercise on their own because they have less energy and stamina as pregnancy progresses.

If you have not exercised before, do not begin now. If you have exercised regularly, do not introduce new exercises or increase your activity level. You should eliminate all high-impact exercises and activities that require you to move quickly or twist abruptly or that have a risk of falling. These include rollerblading, water skiing, diving, downhill skiing, rock climbing and rappelling, competitive or mountain cycling, and horseback riding. The use of free weights can also be dangerous because pregnancy alters your center of gravity and balance. In addition, you should not lift more than 20 pounds unless advised otherwise by your doctor. Avoid any activities that pull or strain your abdominal or pelvic muscles, such as sit-ups or double leg lifts.

Low-impact walking and recreational swimming are generally safe activities for women with twin pregnancies who have no additional risks. Water provides a wonderful buoyancy and helps minimize the weight of the babies and relieve many pregnancy discomforts. You should avoid strenuous lap swimming.

Nonimpact conditioning exercises do not burn calories and are generally considered safe in multiple pregnancy. Some can be helpful for women on bed rest as well. These exercises help maintain muscle tone of specific areas of your body and can help relieve some pregnancy discomforts. The pelvic rock exercise described in Chapter Five is an example. Gentle arm and shoulder circles can help strengthen your upper back and arms. Stretching your arms above your head can help relax some of the muscles in your shoulders and rib cage and may help with indigestion. Smooth calf stretches and gentle foot circles can help relieve leg cramps. To help maintain the tone of your pelvic floor, do Kegel exercises by alternately tightening and relaxing the area around your urethra and vagina.

Another option for exercise is pregnancy yoga. This incorporates gentle stretching with mental relaxation. Check with your doctor first, and make sure that the yoga instructor is trained in the special needs of pregnancy.

Pregnancy massage is a wonderful therapy that has been used in other countries for years. Some of the benefits of pregnancy massage include increased circulation and muscle tone, which can reduce swelling and discomfort, and increased relaxation and relief of stress. Check with your doctor about massage and ask for recommendations of certified therapists. It is essential that the therapist have special training in pregnancy massage. There are certain deep pressure points in the feet and lower legs that can stimulate uterine contractions. A certified pregnancy therapist is aware of this as well as the special needs of pregnant women.

Finally, don't become discouraged about having to limit your exercise. While exercise may help you feel better about your body, no level of exercise during pregnancy has been conclusively demonstrated to improve perinatal outcome.

SOCIAL ACTIVITIES

Now is the time to streamline your social calendar. Once your babies are born, you won't have time to participate in clubs, organizations, or volunteer work, and you don't need the stress of these commitments during pregnancy. Begin to reduce your current responsibilities, and learn how to say no when asked about future activities. Most people are quite understanding about the demands of having several babies. Taking a leave now doesn't mean you are quitting, only that your participation is on hold. You may be surprised at how relieved you feel when you turn over your projects to someone else. Do participate in parents of multiples club meetings when possible; these can be a great support to you before and after your babies arrive.

Find ways to socialize with your friends and family without a lot of effort on your part. Limit your entertaining to home-centered activities where everyone helps provide the food. Rather than going out, have food brought in and watch a movie together.

INTIMACY AND SEXUAL RELATIONS

Sexual intimacy during pregnancy is a private subject most couples are reluctant to discuss with others, including their doctors. However, it is important to bring up this topic, even if your doctor does not. Pregnancy can bring about changes in sexual comfort and desire. Some women have increased sexual desires, while others are totally uninterested. Surprisingly, some men find women more desirable during pregnancy but may be afraid that lovemaking may harm the babies.

In general, sexual intercourse is safe in pregnancy, as long as you are not experiencing complications. However, you may need to limit sexual relations in multiple pregnancy because of the increased risks for preterm labor. It is known that uterine contractions often follow sexual activity. Here are some things to consider about sexual activity in a high-risk pregnancy:

- Female orgasm involves contractions of the muscles of the pelvis and the uterus.

- Nipple stimulation increases the production of the hormone *oxytocin*. Pitocin, a drug used to induce labor, is a synthetic form of oxytocin. When a woman undergoes a contraction stress test (CST) in late pregnancy to determine how her babies respond to contractions, nipple stimulation or Pitocin is used to produce contractions.
- Prostaglandin is a hormone contained in male ejaculate (semen). This is the same hormone used to soften a woman's cervix to induce labor.

Although it is unclear whether preterm labor is directly caused by sexual activities, the potential is present. You should not have sexual intercourse or other sexual activity if your amniotic sac is ruptured or leaking, if you have preterm contractions or bleeding, or if your cervix has softened, dilated, or shortened. Instead, look for other ways to express your love such as hugging and embracing that do not include sexual actions. As a couple, be open with each other and discuss your needs. Putting aside sexual activity for a few months may not be difficult when you consider the risks.

TRAVEL

Although traveling is usually safe in pregnancy, multiple pregnancy may limit how and when you can travel. Long commutes to and from work can be stressful, whether by car or public transportation. Because of the increased risks for preterm labor and other complications in multiple pregnancy, you should avoid long-distance travel. Instead, encourage friends and family to visit you.

In the car, always wear your seatbelt. Beginning in early pregnancy, place the lap portion of your seatbelt low, across your hips and upper thighs. Never place the belt over your abdomen. If the shoulder portion of the seatbelt cuts into your neck, adjust your seat. You might need to move your seat and adjust the steering wheel position as your abdomen gets bigger. Remember that you must wear a seatbelt even in a car with an air bag.

If long-distance travel is necessary, avoid sitting for long periods of time, as this can cause pooling of the blood in your legs and increase the risk of blood clots. Most doctors recommend getting up and walking around for several minutes at least every two hours. Be sure to eat and drink plenty of water, especially on airplanes where the air is dry. Particularly when you travel to a foreign country, you might want to ask your obstetrician to help you identify an obstetrician or perinatologist there. It would also be wise to take along a copy of your medical records.

LIFESTYLE HAZARDS

Most women are aware of the general adverse health effects of alcohol, cigarettes, and recreational drugs. But these substances are even more dangerous when used during an already high-risk pregnancy.

Alcohol

The use of alcohol in pregnancy is linked to fetal alcohol syndrome (FAS), which includes mental retardation, low birth weight, and abnormal facial development. Other malformations are also linked to alcohol consumption. The amount and timing of alcohol use required to produce these abnormalities are unknown, but it is known that alcohol in your bloodstream easily crosses the placentas to your babies in the same concentration. The only safe option is to totally avoid all forms of alcohol (including beer, wine, and liquor) before conception and throughout your pregnancy. Also avoid beverages that are promoted as nonalcoholic, as these still contain small amounts of alcohol. Even in celebration, resist the temptation of a social drink, and ignore any advice about its relaxing effects.

Smoking

Smoking is clearly linked to poor pregnancy outcomes. Women who smoke in pregnancy are more likely to have preterm birth and low birth weight babies. Smokers have twice the rate of miscarriage than nonsmokers. *Placental abruption* (separation of the placenta from the uterus), *placenta previa* (low placental location), premature rupture of membranes, and stillbirth are more common in pregnant smokers. Complications and poor outcomes increase with the number of cigarettes smoked. Secondhand smoke is thought to increase the risks of poor fetal growth and low birth weight. Smoking and secondhand smoke are also associated with sudden infant death syndrome (SIDS).

If you are a smoker, begin now to reduce how much you smoke. Your ultimate goal should be to quit completely and permanently. Ask your doctor about smoking cessation programs and support groups. Do not use any form of nicotine replacement such as gum, a patch, or nasal spray without your doctor's recommendation. These contain nicotine, one of the harmful substances in tobacco. Because secondhand exposure to smoke also increases your risks, do everything you can to reduce your exposure at home and in your workplace.

Illegal drugs

Marijuana, cocaine, crack, LSD, heroin, and other street drugs have significant dangers in pregnancy. Like alcohol, these cross the placenta and expose your babies to the effects of the drugs. However, it is difficult to show the effects of one particular drug since abusers often use several drugs along with alcohol and tobacco. Although marijuana use in pregnancy has not been shown to cause birth defects, it can lead to decreased birth weights. Cocaine use is linked to increased rates of miscarriage, preterm birth, low birth weight, and birth defects. Placental abruption can occur after inhaling or injecting cocaine. Moreover, babies can become addicted and often experience severe, painful withdrawal after birth. Drug abuse, especially intravenous drug use, is also associated with HIV infection. Using any such drugs can have devastating implications for you and your babies. If you are a casual drug user, stop immediately. If you are addicted, tell your doctor so that you can get the help you need to stop.

Over-the-Counter and Prescription Medications

Be sure to tell your doctor about all medications you take regularly or occasionally. Nearly all substances, including prescription drugs and over-the-counter medications, cross the placenta from your bloodstream to your babies. Although some medications can be used safely in later pregnancy, very few are safe in the first trimester when babies' organs are forming. Some drugs are known to cause birth defects and should never be used in pregnancy. These include isoretinoin (Accutane), an acne drug; tetracycline, an antibiotic; warfarin (Coumadin), an anticoagulant; and others. Some prescription medications for conditions such as asthma, epilepsy, psychological disturbances, and high blood pressure may need to be changed to a safer alternative.

Even some herbal preparations can be dangerous in pregnancy. Evening primrose oil and castor oil can stimulate uterine contractions, and cohosh can bring about cervical softening. Check with your doctor before using any herbal remedies, including herbal teas. Many have unknown effects in pregnancy.

WHAT IS REALLY IMPORTANT?

Think about all the demands and activities in your life right now and make a list. This list might include pregnancy discomforts, doctor's visits, your job, home, exercise, other children, spouse, pets, other family members, social activities, and religious services. You can use these to make some decisions about your lifestyle and to recognize where your pregnancy and your babies fit into your life and priorities.

Chapter Seven

Prenatal Care for You
and Your Babies

Prenatal care is a joint effort, with you and your health care providers working together to help you have the healthiest possible pregnancy. You'll probably see many different health care professionals during your pregnancy. Some, like your obstetrician, are part of every aspect of your pregnancy, while others have specific roles at various times. Your role is to actively participate by asking questions, learning all you can, and following the plan of care you develop together.

CHOOSING A CARE PROVIDER

Because of the increased risks of multiple pregnancy, early and regular prenatal care is vital. Your care providers must have specialized knowledge and skills to provide the care you need for your unique circumstances. The American College of Obstetricians and Gynecologists and the American Academy of Pediatrics recommend a board-certified obstetrician as the appropriate care provider for an uncomplicated twin pregnancy. Women with more complicated pregnancies may need to see a specialized obstetrician called a *perinatologist*. Certified nurse-midwives frequently care for women carrying twins in collaboration with a qualified obstetrician. While the main focus of nurse-midwifery is the care of uncomplicated pregnancies, nurse-midwives are often able to give expectant parents of multiples extra time and individualized teaching, as well as emotional support. Other care providers also contribute to pregnancy care, including nurses, technicians, and counselors. You'll need to choose a doctor or health care team as soon as you learn you are pregnant.

Ask all prospective care providers to share their philosophy of multiple birth care, their views on bed rest, how they decide on the route of delivery of multiples, and how many sets of multiples like yours have been under their care.

Obstetrician

Choosing an obstetrician is an important task. This is the health professional that directs your care throughout your pregnancy and most likely will be the one to deliver your babies. Talk with other women who have had multiples, ask for their recommendations, and consider interviewing several doctors. Look for a doctor who has experience caring for women with multiple pregnancies. You might even find a doctor who is a parent of multiples. Ideally, choose someone who uses a team approach in multiple pregnancy care, taking advantage of the skills and expertise of other health care professionals.

If you learn you are having multiples after you have already started prenatal care, talk with your doctor about his or her experience with multiple pregnancy and about any changes that should be made in your care.

> I discovered I was having twins fairly late—at nineteen weeks. Although my family practitioner told me of some of the risks of twin pregnancies, I think I was in a fair amount of denial about how difficult it can be to carry twins. I switched to a regular obstetrician who had delivered twins

before but was not well versed about several of my complications. I truly believe a high-risk obstetrician [perinatologist]
would have picked up on some my problems before they became as serious as they did.

Occasionally, you may find that you and your doctor are not
a match because of personality, differences of opinion, or other reasons. You'll be seeing your doctor frequently and you need to feel
comfortable with one another. You also need to feel confident in
your doctor's knowledge and ability to answer your questions. If
you do not feel that your doctor is right for you and your needs,
consider finding another care provider.

PERINATOLOGIST

Women with complications or a medical problem in addition to a
twin pregnancy, and any woman carrying higher-order multiples,
should also consult with a perinatologist. This is an obstetrician with
extra training who is board-certified in the specialty of maternal-fetal
medicine. Since many perinatologists are affiliated with regional or
high-risk perinatal centers, you may need to travel to another hospital or another city for consultation. The perinatologist works with
your obstetrician to perform specialized procedures and make recommendations for your care. Some perinatologists provide primary
obstetric care for certain multiple pregnancy cases, but most act as
consultants

> The doctor that we had chosen at our preferred hospital
> moved out of town, and when we learned we were having
> multiples, we decided that the reputation of a good perina-
> tologist and excellent NICU [neonatal intensive care unit]
> were far more important than our earlier preferences of the
> hospitals.

Certain health maintenance organizations (HMOs) and provider networks limit your choice of doctors and specialists. If a qualified provider is not available within your network, you should contact your health insurance company to discuss your options.

If you live in a small town or a great distance from a hospital that provides high-risk perinatal care, find out how your doctor would handle referral and transport if needed. Women with triplets or more may need to consider a temporary move closer to the high-risk facility. There may be situations when you must weigh the risks and benefits of location and the best care.

> Our doctor's office and hospital are almost an hour from our home (even longer during rush hours), which is not what I would have chosen if we weren't having multiples. Although we are tired of the long drive, and I am somewhat fearful of the long drive while in labor, it is all worth sacrificing in order to have the best situation for our babies.

Other Care Providers

It is common to rotate seeing other health care professionals as part of your prenatal care. This gives you different perspectives on your care and the chance to meet the other members of the practice in case one of them is on call when you deliver. However, a major disadvantage of seeing different providers is a loss in the continuity of your care, so most women prefer to see one consistent care provider.

Obstetric nurses are often your first line of communication with your doctor's office. It helps to learn the names of the nurses and begin to establish a relationship with them at your early visits. Some offices and clinics employ staff with different levels of training, including registered nurses, licensed practical nurses, patient care assistants, and physician's assistants. Perinatal nurse practitioners are registered nurses with additional training in high-risk pregnancy care. They can give you some direct care as well as coordinate your care among the providers.

Other professionals offer specialized care in consultation with your obstetric care providers. Ultrasound technicians perform routine ultrasounds in the obstetric office and in special ultrasound facilities. Perinatologists perform detailed ultrasound exams and prenatal diagnostic testing such as amniocentesis and chorionic villus sampling. Genetics counselors are specially trained to help you understand the risks and benefits of genetic and chromosome testing. Registered dietitians are available to help with nutrition counseling and meal planning. Perinatal educators offer classes and specialized education for multiple birth families. Social workers are available to advise you on financial concerns and coordinate government benefits and community services. Psychologists and counselors can help with stress and worries.

The perinatal case manager is another professional who is an important part of your care. This is usually a nurse who coordinates consultations and services and can be a wonderful advocate for you. Some case managers work for insurance companies, while others are employed by hospitals. Contact your health insurance company to find out if a high-risk pregnancy case manager is part of your benefits package. The role of a case manager is to assess your needs and work within your insurance contract to maximize your benefits. Examples of some of the support that case managers can provide include recommending specialists and nutritional consults; authorizing payment for custodial care, special medical equipment, and comfort measures, such as egg crate mattresses, shower chairs, wheelchairs, or a hospital bed; and reimbursement for special multiple birth classes.

YOUR FIRST PRENATAL APPOINTMENT

Schedule your first appointment as early in your pregnancy as possible. If your multiple pregnancy resulted from infertility treatments, your infertility doctor might monitor your pregnancy through the first trimester. But you can schedule your first appointment with your obstetrician before your final infertility visit. This helps smooth the transition between doctors and allows you to start your prenatal care as soon as possible. It also allows time to discuss any prenatal testing that you need in early pregnancy. Encourage your husband to attend this appointment with you, as well as future appointments.

At your first prenatal visit, expect to spend an hour or more relating your complete history and having a physical exam. You'll be asked about your medical and family history as well as past pregnancies. Be sure to discuss your diet, any discomforts, and your work, exercise, and activities. If you have a history of an eating disorder, be sure to mention this. It is also important to let your doctor know if you have a personal or family history of depression, especially postpartum depression, as this is more likely with multiple pregnancy. And, talk privately with your doctor or other health care provider if you have concerns about your personal safety. Domestic violence against women is a problem that knows no cultural or economic boundaries and may become worse during pregnancy.

Your complete physical exam includes a general medical assessment, height, weight, blood pressure, breast exam, pelvic exam, cultures for sexually transmitted diseases, and a Pap smear if needed. Your uterus is assessed for its size, and fetal heart tones are checked, often with an electronic device. Usually, an ultrasound examination is done to confirm the number of babies—and their chorionicity, heart rates, and positions—and to estimate gestational age. You'll be given a due date for your pregnancy. This date is sometimes referred to as the estimated date of confinement (EDC) and equals forty weeks or 280 days from your last menstrual period. Although many multiples are born before forty weeks, always use the forty-week EDC as your due date. If you use an earlier date, it might be confusing for other care providers.

At your first visit, you usually receive prescriptions for prenatal vitamins, folic acid, and iron supplements. You also undergo several laboratory tests, including hemoglobin or hematocrit (red blood cell count), Rh factor and blood type, antibody screen, rubella (German measles) titer, and urine testing for protein and glucose. You may also be offered testing for HIV, hepatitis B, and toxoplasmosis. Genetic screening for sickle-cell disease, Tay-Sachs, and other genetic problems is available if your history indicates a need.

This is a good time to talk with your doctor about an overall plan of care. You can discuss the various options for prenatal testing and arrange consultations with specialists and other professionals. It may be helpful to request a nutritional consultation with a registered dietitian. Find out how to contact support groups and whether prenatal classes for multiples are available. Many doctors provide an information packet with details about office policies and hospitals.

Make arrangements for prenatal education and parenting preparation classes as soon as possible. You should attend these classes in your early second trimester and complete them by your twenty-fifth week. If you wait, classes may be full or you'll be unable to attend if you have complications or are on bed rest. If you are having higher-order multiples, attend classes earlier.

PRENATAL CARE

There is no standardized schedule for the number and timing of prenatal visits for women with multiple pregnancy, but in most cases, you'll be seen more frequently than a woman with a singleton pregnancy. Visits usually occur about every four weeks at first. By twenty to twenty-four weeks, or the middle of your second trimester, they can increase to every two weeks. Weekly prenatal visits are typical beginning in your third trimester. These visits are reassuring; and if you feel the need to be seen more often, let your doctor know. Between visits, write down your questions and any concerns you want to discuss.

First Trimester—
Conception to Fourteen Weeks

The first three months of pregnancy pass very quickly. Most women are in their fifth or sixth week when they have a positive pregnancy test, leaving time for only one or two first trimester appointments. After your first visit, you'll be seen briefly for the following assessments during this time:

- Blood pressure
- Weight
- Urine dipstick for glucose, ketones, and protein
- Fetal heart tones

Many women have little appetite, nausea, and sometimes vomiting during these first weeks. Be sure to tell your doctor if you are having problems eating and describe what you are able to eat each day.

Prenatal tests that may be performed during your first trimester include a screening ultrasound. If needed, chorionic villus sampling or early amniocentesis can be done late in the first trimester. See Chapter Nine for more information about prenatal testing.

Early Second Trimester—
Fifteen to Twenty-One Weeks

The second trimester is a busy time. Your appointments are scheduled every two to three weeks, and you may be seeing several care providers. At your prenatal visits, expect the following routine assessments:

- Blood pressure
- Weight
- Urine dipstick for glucose, ketones, and protein

- Fundal height (measurement in centimeters from your pubic bone to the top of your uterus)
- Fetal positions and fetal heart rates

You might need additional blood work to test for anemia. If you have a family history of diabetes or other factors that increase your risk for diabetes, you'll probably have a glucose screening test around sixteen to eighteen weeks.

If you have a monochorionic placenta (a single placenta with one chorion shared by two or more fetuses), you'll have frequent ultrasounds, beginning around sixteen weeks, to watch for signs of fetal growth problems and twin-to-twin transfusion syndrome.

A cervical check done at eighteen to twenty weeks helps establish a baseline record of the size and condition of your cervix. This assessment is done during a vaginal examination or with an ultrasound probe. Your doctor can compare later cervical checks with this one to see if any changes have occurred.

You may want to schedule a consultation with a perinatologist during this time to discuss prenatal diagnostic testing. Maternal serum alpha-fetoprotein testing to help detect neural tube defects is done between fifteen and nineteen weeks. A detailed (Level II) ultrasound performed by twenty weeks helps determine the number and location of placentas and amniotic sacs and can screen for some birth defects. Amniocentesis is usually done in the early second trimester.

Let your doctor know when you begin feeling your babies move (called the *quickening*), usually sometime in the first part of your second trimester. Some women begin to feel faint flutters around the sixteenth week, while others first feel movement closer to the twentieth week. Mothers of higher-order multiples have reported feeling their babies move as early as eleven and twelve weeks. As your babies change positions during pregnancy, you feel their movements in many different places. You might feel kicking under your ribs and punching on your bladder, or simply overall squirming. Many mothers can tell which baby is which by the location of kicks, and often report feeling the lowest baby's movements more than the others.

Review your diet and weight gain with your doctor at each visit. If you are having trouble gaining weight, request a consultation with a dietitian. Be sure to bring up any discomforts or difficulties you are having. If you are especially tired, you could be anemic or simply pushing yourself too hard. Also, let your doctor know about your current level of exercise and activities at work and home. Many women begin to feel the effects of their pregnancies in their daily activities during this time. You may need to begin limiting your work hours or change your schedule and activities.

Now is the time to learn about preterm labor and begin watching for the warning signs and symptoms. Ask your care providers to help you learn how to feel for contractions and what to watch for. If you are unsure you are having contractions, it is always better to call and be checked than to ignore the symptoms. Chapter Ten has more information on preterm labor.

Begin your search for a doctor to provide health care for your babies once they are born. Find out if your hospital has a *neonatologist,* a pediatrician who specializes in the care of sick and premature newborns. A neonatologist is usually in charge of your babies' care if they are premature or have problems at birth. Look for a pediatrician for well-baby care who has experience caring for multiples and premature babies. Ask if the office has any special policies for multiples, such as discounts or joint appointments. Some pediatricians make house calls for higher-order multiples when they are very young. This relieves some of the burden of taking several babies to the doctor for their checkups and immunizations.

If you haven't already decided to breastfeed your babies, learn about the benefits of this perfect baby food. Talk with a lactation consultant, usually a nurse with special training in breastfeeding support, and take a breastfeeding class. If your babies are small or premature and can't breastfeed at first, you can pump your milk and gradually make the transition to breastfeeding. Do not use any methods for "toughening" your nipples to prepare them for breastfeeding. These techniques do not work, and nipple stimulation can bring about preterm uterine contractions. See Chapter Twenty-Two for details about breastfeeding multiples.

Late Second Trimester—
Twenty-One to Twenty-Eight Weeks

During this time, most women have prenatal appointments every other week and then weekly. The same routine assessments mentioned in the previous two sections are done at each visit. In addition, glucose screening is recommended for all women between twenty-four and twenty-eight weeks. You continue to be carefully assessed for signs of high blood pressure of pregnancy during this time. If your blood is Rh negative and antibody negative, you'll be given Rhogam at twenty-eight weeks to prevent Rh sensitization in case one or more of your babies is Rh positive.

Your doctor monitors your weight and the pattern of your weight gain. By twenty-four weeks with twins, most women should have gained about twenty-four pounds. Continue to keep your doctor aware of your activities and any discomforts you have.

Many doctors do a cervical check at each visit to watch for subtle changes that can increase your risk for preterm birth. Be sure to describe any contractions, vaginal discharge, or other sensations, as well as how often these occur and what you think is causing them. You may be tested for fetal fibronectin or the hormone estriol, which can help predict preterm labor. Some women begin home uterine activity monitoring for contractions, especially those with higher-order multiples.

You may have an ultrasound done each month to assess fetal growth, amniotic fluid levels, and placental function. Many doctors recommend nonstress testing in the late second trimester for women with complicated twin pregnancies and higher-order multiples.

Third Trimester— Twenty-Eight-Plus Weeks

Routine assessments continue at your visits, which are usually weekly. You are also checked for anemia and signs of high blood pressure problems, and you are likely to have cervical examinations at each visit. If you have risk factors for group B streptococcus infection (GBS), a culture is done in the middle of this trimester or if preterm labor begins. Weekly nonstress tests often begin by thirty-two weeks earlier if you have complications. Your doctor might also want a biophysical profile test to evaluate the well-being of your babies. See Chapter Nine for more information on prenatal testing.

Begin talking with your doctor about delivery. Discuss the time frame for when it is best for your babies to be born. Know where and when to go to the hospital. If you're a candidate for a vaginal birth, find out how your doctor, as well as other members of the practice, manage various birth situations. Find out where your babies will be delivered—in a labor and delivery or birthing room, or in a surgical operating area. Be sure to discuss your options for pain management in labor and the type of anesthesia that will be used if needed. Ask about hospital policies for visitors and who can be present at your delivery.

PRENATAL EDUCATION

Prenatal education classes help you prepare for pregnancy, birth, and the early care of your babies. Because you might develop complications that limit your activity, be sure to schedule all classes in the first part of your second trimester, before twenty-five weeks. Both expectant parents can benefit from prenatal education. Attending as a couple is a wonderful way to share in the excitement as you learn together.

Regular childbirth preparation or prenatal education classes designed for singleton pregnancies are helpful but usually do not cover all the information you need when you have a multiple pregnancy. Look for special classes for multiple pregnancies, such as the Marvelous Multiples Course. This program is available nationally and provides specialized education about multiple pregnancy, birth, and care of multiple newborns. If multiple birth classes are not available in your area, ask your nurse or the childbirth education department to help you find information or other classes that meet your needs. Find out if private classes are available if you are already on bed rest.

> I took a prenatal class offered by my hospital called Marvelous Multiples. It was so helpful. They talked about recognizing preterm labor and how to tell if your water is broken, and they prepared you for what to expect if you have to have a C-section. They brought in two sets of parents with twins for us to ask questions. The part I liked best was being in a class with ten other moms who were experiencing the same thing as me and were as big as I was. My hubby liked being with ten guys who were going through it, too.

Also, you might want to take other classes such as breastfeeding, baby care, infant CPR, and special father-to-be classes such as Boot Camp for New Dads. Lamaze classes are geared for women with low-risk pregnancies who want to prepare for a medication-free delivery; however, the relaxation and breathing techniques taught in these classes are helpful. Once you are in your last weeks of pregnancy and you are planning an unmedicated vaginal birth, you might want to find a class that offers just these labor-coping skills.

Be sure to arrange a hospital tour that includes a visit to the a hospital tour that includes a visit to the *neonatal intensive care unit*

(*NICU*). About half of twins and most higher-order multiples are in the NICU for some part of their care. An advance tour can help prepare you for some of the sights and sounds of this sometimes overwhelming place. It is also reassuring to know that specialized care is available if needed for the care of your babies.

Do your best to keep every appointment with all your health care providers. Attend classes to help you learn about your pregnancy and prepare for the birth of your babies. Your participation in your care and learning about your pregnancy and birth can help your babies have the best chances for a healthy outcome.

Chapter Eight

Fetal Growth
and Development

From the moment your babies begin life with the union of sperm and egg, they are truly a miracle. Occurring within you is an incredible process as tiny cells join, multiply, and become unique human beings. The twinning process itself is another of life's wondrous processes. It is an extraordinary experience to have several babies forming and growing at the same time within you. Throughout pregnancy, your babies continue developing into the individuals they will ultimately become. This chapter covers some of the important changes and stages in fetal development and growth and how these occur with multiples.

THE BEGINNING OF PREGNANCY

The start of the pregnancy calendar begins with the first day of your last menstrual period. Approximately two weeks later, ovulation occurs, followed by conception. If you took ovulation medications or used assisted reproductive technologies to conceive your babies, ovulation may not have happened on the 14th day of your menstrual cycle. These medications and procedures can change the timing of the entire cycle. So count back about 14 days from the actual day your ovulation occurred, or the day you took medication to release the mature eggs, or the day your egg retrieval was performed. Use this date as the first day of your last period, count back three months, and then add 7 days. For example, if your menstrual period started on May 12, subtracting three months gives you February 12, and adding 7 days makes February 19. This date should be close to forty completed weeks, or 280 days, the average length of a full-term pregnancy. If you like, you can mark a calendar to show each week. Although most multiple pregnancies do not go to the full forty weeks, always use the forty-week date as your "official" due date.

Your due date can change if early pregnancy ultrasound shows that the babies are more developed or not as far along as your dates show. This is quite common, especially if your periods were irregular or you used infertility medications to get pregnant. Fertility procedures and medications can alter the timing of conception as well as implantation and embryo development.

SINGLE FETAL DEVELOPMENT

Here is a look at normal fetal development throughout pregnancy. Remember that each baby is unique and the timing and phases of development are approximate. Development begins with conception at the end of the second pregnancy calendar week, approximately day fourteen.

At conception, the egg and sperm cells unite to form an embryo. Almost immediately, the embryonic cells begin to multiply into four, then eight, then sixteen cells, and so forth. This continues until there are the billions of cells that make up the human body.

About five days after conception, the embryo's trophoblast cells begin forming the early pregnancy structures. The yolk sac nourishes the embryo until its own circulatory system is functioning many weeks later. The outer trophoblast cells attach to the inner wall of the uterus by about the tenth day after conception. These cells form layers that eventually develop into the placenta with the chorionic and amniotic membranes.

By the fourth week, or two weeks after conception, the embryo is only 1 to 2 millimeters long. Three specialized layers of embryonic cells have emerged. These develop into the unique organs and tissues of the body. At about five weeks' gestation, or three weeks after conception, a well-defined gestational sac surrounds the embryo. By the sixth week, the embryo has a tiny heartbeat that can be seen on ultrasound as brief flickers of light. As early as seven to eight weeks gestation, movements of the embryo can be seen.

Organ development occurs very quickly in the embryo. By the eighth week, the head, spinal column, and arms and legs are apparent. The heart has four distinct chambers. The brain develops rapidly, and by the ninth week it has detectable brain waves. The internal ovaries or testes are formed by the tenth week. By this time, all the vital organs and body structures are formed, but they still continue to develop and grow. The embryo is now called a fetus.

By the eleventh week, the fetus has a larynx and vocal cords and can make sounds. Fingernails are forming. In the twelfth week, ultrasound can detect the stomach, bladder, and liver. The lungs begin to inhale and exhale amniotic fluid, and the baby is about 1½ to 2 inches long. In the fourteenth week, swallowing and sucking movements occur. By now the baby is about 3 to 4 inches long and weighs about 2 ounces. Fingerprints are present by the sixteenth week. Many women begin feeling fetal movements around this time. Lanugo, a fine, silky body hair forms by week eighteen. By week twenty, the structures for hearing are developed.

Dramatic growth occurs over the next few weeks. By the end of the second trimester, at about twenty-seven weeks, the baby is about 10 to 11 inches long and weighs approximately 2 pounds. Lungs produce surfactant and are mature by the thirty-seventh week. Fat begins to be deposited, and the baby puts on weight rapidly, reaching approximately 7 pounds by forty weeks.

MULTIPLE FETAL DEVELOPMENT

Overall, fetal development of multiples occurs just as with a single-ton baby, but there are some differences at the very beginning. Division of the first forming cells can result in identical twins. When the division occurs in the first three days, each baby may have its own separate placenta and amniotic sac, just as fraternal multiples do. When division occurs on the fourth through the seventh days after conception, the babies share one placenta but have separate amniotic sacs. This is the most common combination, occurring in about two-thirds of identical twins. Division after eight days results in babies that share the same placenta and amniotic sac. This rare event only occurs in about 1 percent of identical twins. Later divi-sion is very rare and can result in conjoined or Siamese twins.

During pregnancy, multiples grow in a slightly different pat-tern from singletons. Normal growth of singletons speeds up after thirty weeks gestation. Typically, the growth of twins is similar to singletons up until about the thirty-second week, when it begins to slow. Higher-order multiples begin this slow-down earlier—around twenty-eight to thirty weeks for triplets and around twenty-six to twenty-eight weeks for quadruplets. It isn't clear why this happens, but it may be due to competition for nutrition, decreases in pla-cental blood flow, or crowding in the uterus.

Other factors can contribute to slowing of growth and lower birth weights in multiples. The race of the babies is one factor. In African American twins, the growth slow-down after thirty-two weeks is slightly less than in white twins. The sex of multiples affects birth weights as well. Female twins tend to weigh less than female singletons and less than male twins. The type of placental struc-ture also affects growth. Multiples that share a placenta tend to weigh less than those with individual placentas. Some multiples have slower than expected weight gain in pregnancy. This is called *intrauterine growth restriction* (*IUGR*). It can occur in one or all babies and is more common with problems such as *twin-to-twin transfusion syndrome* (*TTTS*). See Chapter Eleven for more information on IUGR and TTTS.

The highest average birth weights occur at about thirty-nine weeks for twins and thirty-seven weeks for triplets, compared with forty-one weeks for singletons. A twin often weighs about a half pound less than a singleton at thirty-two weeks. Compared with a singleton, a triplet typically weighs 1 pound less at thirty-two weeks and more than 2 pounds less at thirty-eight weeks.

Although small babies can have problems, multiples can actually have better health at slightly lower birth weights. Retrospective studies of complications and perinatal deaths in multiples have found the ideal birth weight to be approximately 2,500 to 2,800 grams (5½ pounds to 6 pounds 2 ounces) for twins; 1,900 to 2,000 grams (4 pounds 3 ounces to 4 pounds 6 ounces) for triplets; and 1,400 to 1,500 grams (3 pounds to 4¼ pounds) for quadruplets.

INTRAUTERINE BEHAVIOR

Ultrasound provides fantastic views of the behavior of multiples before birth. Touching, kicking, embracing, sucking on each other, and kissing between twins have been documented. Babies can respond to touch as early as the end of the seventh week. The first intrauterine contact between multiples occurs as early as the tenth week. Between the twelfth and sixteenth weeks, mothers and ultrasound technicians have noted an increase in interplay and interaction of twins and higher-order multiples. Around the sixteenth gestational week, mothers report seeing their babies "help" each other, by offering a thumb to suck or touching a cheek during a stressful time. Around thirty-two weeks, many mothers report more "calm" time, but when the babies are awake, their activity is more apparent and uncomfortable.

Singleton babies can touch their own faces and bodies with their hands before birth. But multiples can touch each other and feel touch inside the womb giving them the ability to comfort each other and regulate their environment together. Multiples often exhibit a synchrony in sleep and awake states before birth, with similar movements and heart rate accelerations because of their shared environment and contact. It is thought that multiples have more frequent periods of fetal activity than singletons. And those that share a placenta tend to have earlier and more frequent interactions than those with separate placentas. This makes sense because they are physically close together and have more opportunities for contact. Some babies in the set may be more active than the others. The movement of one baby can wake and stimulate the others. Mothers often report feeling movement of one baby more often than others, especially the lowest or presenting baby.

Although they have a common intrauterine experience, infant twins do show differences in activity, irritability, resistance to soothing, and sleeping behavior. These similarities and differences are partially based on whether the babies are identical or fraternal. Identical twins seem to share more common behavioral traits after birth than do fraternal twins. Behavioral differences among babies may also be due to physical factors. For example, intrauterine growth restriction in one twin can result in differences in infant behavior. Babies who are hospitalized for different lengths of time also have different behaviors.

Sharing a womb is a unique experience and creates special emotional needs for the babies. Many professionals believe that because multiples are used to the continuous presence and touch of the other baby or babies, they should continue this contact after birth. The practice of *co-bedding* of multiples uses the principles of intertwin stimulation—a reciprocal relationship of interactions throughout pregnancy. Co-bedding is also based on the knowledge of multiples' synchrony in sleep and awake states caused by their intrauterine contact and physiologic interdependence. In other words, babies who are conceived together, develop together, and are born together need to stay together. Co-bedding is also an integral part of developmental care of premature babies because it helps babies feel more secure and decreases stress. Simply put, co-bedding multiples makes sense because the babies still need each other! For more information on co-bedding in the NICU, see Chapter Twenty.

Chapter Nine

Prenatal Diagnosis and Testing in Multiple Pregnancy

Today's technology provides many ways to monitor your pregnancy and assess the health of your unborn babies. Although no test is completely accurate, prenatal diagnosis and testing offer you and your care providers valuable information about the health of your babies. These tests and procedures can help in planning your care and in anticipating your pregnancy outcome.

It is likely that you'll be offered several different tests and procedures at various times throughout your pregnancy. Genetic testing is often recommended for multiple pregnancy, especially if you are at increased risk for chromosome or genetic problems because of a family history or maternal age. Birth defects occur in about 3 to 4 percent of the general population. The causes of most birth defects are unknown. About 7 to 8 percent of birth defects in the general population are genetic or inherited, such as Duchenne muscular dystrophy or Tay-Sachs disease. Chromosome abnormalities, such as Down syndrome, account for about 6 percent of all birth defects. About 20 percent of birth defects are due to a combination of factors. A small number of birth defects are due to exposure to teratogens such as alcohol. Based on national statistics, birth defects are about 18 percent more likely in multiples than singletons. The increased rate depends on many factors—including zygosity, race, and sex—and may be as much as 2 to 3 times higher for certain populations. Generally, birth defects are more common in monozygotic twins, males, and whites.

The most common birth defects in multiple pregnancy include heart defects, gastrointestinal tract abnormalities, and neural tube defects. With fraternal multiples, each baby has an independent risk for a particular problem, and usually only one baby is affected. Identical multiples have a higher risk for structural birth defects than fraternal multiples and one or more may be affected depending on the cause.

Generally, multiples have a higher risk for birth defects because of the additional babies and the fact that many mothers of multiples are over age 30 when the risk for birth defects naturally increases. Some researchers have calculated that a woman over age 30 carrying twins has a similar risk of a chromosome abnormality as a woman 2 years older with a singleton pregnancy. Because of these increased risks, many women carrying multiples are offered prenatal diagnostic testing.

Some prenatal diagnostic tests can be done in the doctor's office, whereas others need specialized equipment and skills found in the hospital. You may need to travel to a high-risk perinatal center for very specialized procedures. Certain tests and procedures do have risks; however, many are risk free. When a test carries risks, explore with your doctor whether the benefit of the information that can be gained outweighs these risks. Many tests give you advance notice of problems that can be prevented or treated. Sometimes the information learned from test results is simply a particular piece of data. And sometimes tests do not provide enough information to make a clear diagnosis, so other tests are needed.

ULTRASOUND

Ultrasound is an amazing technology that uses sound waves to create a picture. It can reveal much about the world inside your uterus. These fascinating pictures have detected multiples cuddling each other inside the uterus as well as sucking their thumbs, smiling, and even waving. Currently, most ultrasound scans are in black and white, but color imaging is now available that permits more detailed interpretation and diagnosis. Most ultrasound machines use two-dimensional scanning that shows a real-time photograph of the structures being examined. However, ultrasound technology is advancing rapidly, and three-dimensional scanning is being used in some centers. This type of imaging is especially helpful in diagnosing birth defects and detailing features that may be associated with chromosome abnormalities.

A basic ultrasound examination is a screening tool for your doctor to roughly estimate fetal growth, amount of amniotic fluid, and to see the fetal positions, movements, and heartbeats. A very detailed examination, sometimes called a Level II ultrasound or targeted imaging for fetal anomalies (TIFFA) study, is often recommended for multiple pregnancies. An obstetrician trained in maternal-fetal medicine (perinatologist) usually performs this type of ultrasound exam. Detailed measurements and assessments are made of each baby and your placentas, amniotic sacs, uterus, and cervix. An abdominal probe and often a vaginal probe are used for the exam, which can take up to two hours.

The Level II ultrasound includes nearly every internal organ and structure of each baby. The brain, spinal column, structures of the heart and lungs, diaphragm, stomach, bowels, kidneys, and urinary system are carefully visualized. Measurements include the length of limbs and circumference of each baby's head and abdomen. Facial features and the positioning of hands and feet are also noted. The placentas are examined and measured, and where each umbilical cord inserts into the placenta is determined. Pockets of amniotic fluid are measured to estimate amniotic fluid volume. Finally, the uterus is examined, along with the cervix to detect any signs of cervical change.

Early pregnancy ultrasounds can help identify the number of placentas, chorions, and amnions. In later pregnancy it is harder to visualize the thin membranes because the babies are larger and there is less amniotic fluid. Throughout the remaining months, you'll have additional ultrasound exams to check for fetal growth and to monitor any problems with the babies, placentas, or amniotic sacs.

In the first eighteen weeks of pregnancy, ultrasound is very accurate in determining gestational age. The crown-rump (head to buttocks) length and the biparietal (side-to-side) diameter of the baby's head are measurements that can estimate gestational age within a few days. Fetal growth and weight are also estimated by measuring the long bones of the babies' legs and the head circumference. Measurements are more difficult as the babies get bigger, making weight estimates less accurate.

Many physical abnormalities can be detected with ultrasound from eighteen to twenty weeks gestation although some are visible earlier in pregnancy. Ultrasound is able to detect almost three-fourths of major abnormalities, such as those of the central nervous system, musculoskeletal system, and urinary system. Less than half of heart abnormalities and minor malformations in other systems can be identified with ultrasound. Characteristics of chromosome abnormalities such as Down syndrome also may be noted. The presence on ultrasound of extra fingers, heart defects, or a thickening of the neck folds can suggest an abnormality, but chorionic villus sampling or amniocentesis is needed to accurately diagnose genetic or chromosome abnormalities.

Fetal growth can be tracked with ultrasound to identify weight that is lagging in one or more babies. The effects of twin-to-twin transfusion syndrome (TTTS), in which babies share blood vessel connections in the placenta, can also be monitored. Ultrasound is also used for cervical measurements and to detect signs of preterm labor, including funneling inside the cervix and cervical thinning and dilatation.

There are no documented risks of diagnostic ultrasound, but it isn't a perfect tool, and incorrect diagnoses can happen. Some problems cannot be seen on ultrasound, or what appears as an abnormality sometimes turns out to be nothing. Today's ultrasound technology allows us to see much more than we are currently able to understand about unborn babies. With time, the knowledge of how internal structures look and change throughout pregnancy will catch up with the technology. Until then, think of ultrasound as a wonderful tool in pregnancy care that can provide an enormous amount of information.

ALPHA-FETOPROTEIN

Alpha-fetoprotein (AFP) is a protein produced in the fetal liver. When a baby has an open break in the covering of the brain and spinal cord, called a *neural tube defect* (*NTD*), large amounts of this protein are released into the amniotic fluid and into the maternal circulation. High levels of AFP in your blood can mean a baby has an NTD, such as spina bifida.

Screening for AFP is usually done between sixteen and eighteen weeks of pregnancy and requires a blood sample from you. A test can also be performed on a sample of the amniotic fluid during an amniocentesis. Although increased levels of AFP can mean that an NTD is present, these tests frequently have false positive results. Sometimes the laboratory test is inaccurate, and if a woman is farther along or earlier in her pregnancy than was thought, AFP results can be incorrect for her dates. Some women learn they are having multiples when their AFP levels are high, because two or more babies are making the protein.

It is more difficult to use AFP testing as a screening tool with multiple pregnancy. The normal AFP level for twins is about two times the normal singleton level. For triplets, the average AFP level is approximately three times the average singleton level, and even higher for quadruplets. There has not been enough testing to determine specific normal AFP levels for very high multiples. AFP levels can remain elevated for many weeks following a multifetal reduction procedure, making the test inaccurate. The AFP test is sometimes part of a multiple marker blood screening. Other markers include hCG (human chorionic gonadotropin) and un-conjugated estriol. In singleton pregnancies, these markers may help predict chromosome abnormalities such as Down syndrome; however, this association has not been fully researched in multiple pregnancies.

Ultrasound is recommended with any abnormal AFP result. If ultrasound cannot explain why the AFP level is abnormal, amnio-centesis is usually offered. There is some evidence that women with unexplained abnormal AFP levels are more likely to have pregnancy complications such as placental abruption, high blood pressure, preterm labor, and low birth weight. Research has found that 50 to 70 percent of NTDs can be prevented when women receive enough folic acid (a B vitamin) before and during pregnancy. A minimum of 400 micrograms of folic acid daily is recommended.

Although AFP testing is not flawless, it can provide some re-assurance. And if problems are identified, having this knowledge can help you make decisions and allow you to receive early, spe-cialized care.

CHORIONIC VILLUS SAMPLING

Chorionic villus sampling (*CVS*) tests for the presence of certain chromosome abnormalities and genetic defects (excluding NTDs like spina bifida) and is performed at the end of the first trimester of pregnancy, at about ten to twelve weeks gestation. Chorionic vil-lus sampling requires the removal of small pieces of the chorionic villi, which are part of the early placenta and have the same chro-mosome makeup as the baby.

There are two methods of CVS. The transcervical method uses ultrasound to guide a thin tube through a woman's vagina and into her cervix where the villi are gently removed with suction. For a transabdominal CVS, a needle is inserted through a woman's ab-domen into the uterus, much like an amniocentesis. Most women feel only a small twinge or cramping during the procedure, and some cramping and bleeding are common for a few days following CVS. Results of CVS are usually available within two weeks.

Using CVS with multiple pregnancy is complex. It may be necessary to use both the transcervical and transabdominal techniques to test all the placentas. It is sometimes difficult to distinguish placentas that are fused or have thin separating membranes, making the sampling less accurate. Amniocentesis often is recommended when results are inconclusive. With multiples, the rate of miscarriage after CVS is about 3 percent compared to about 1 percent with a singleton pregnancy.

AMNIOCENTESIS

Amniocentesis is another prenatal test for genetic and chromosome abnormalities. Women over the age of thirty-three and those with a previous genetic abnormality or a family history of genetic problems often choose to have an amniocentesis. The risk for chromosome abnormalities increases with a mother's age and because there are more babies in the pregnancy. Amniocentesis can be performed as early as twelve to fourteen weeks gestation but usually is done at about fifteen to eighteen weeks. The procedure involves removing a small amount of fluid, about an ounce, from each baby's amniotic sac. Using ultrasound to view the needle and the positions of the babies, the doctor inserts the needle through the mother's abdomen into her uterus and to a pocket of amniotic fluid. Most women say they feel a sharp cramp when the needle is inserted.

> The sensation of the needle going through the skin, then the muscle, then the uterus was weird! I nearly jumped off the table for the first stick, but I was much more prepared for the second.

With multiples, each sac must be entered and some fluid removed. Often a harmless blue dye is injected into the first sac to prevent confusion when fluid is drawn from a second sac. Fetal cells in the amniotic fluid are grown in the laboratory and tested. The chromosomes within the cells can be studied under a microscope, and tests for specific genetic diseases and the presence of AFP can be performed. Results take about two weeks.

After amniocentesis, you may have cramping as the uterus and tissues heal. Some women also leak amniotic fluid, and there is a risk of infection. The risk for miscarriage after amniocentesis with twins is about double that for a singleton. With higher-order multiples, the risk is greater. In most cases, the risk of pregnancy loss with amniocentesis is slightly higher than the normal risk of miscarriage at the time when amniocentesis is done.

In late pregnancy, amniocentesis may be recommended to test the maturity of your babies' lungs. When the proportion of two substances, lecithin and sphingomyelin, in the amniotic fluid is 2:1 or higher, the babies' lungs are considered mature. In most cases, multiples have the same degree of lung maturity, so only one amniotic sac needs to be entered for this test.

NONSTRESS TEST

The *nonstress test* (*NST*) uses a fetal heart rate monitor to observe the heart rates of your babies. The NST is considered reactive (normal) when the babies' heart rates increase fifteen beats per minute, two times during twenty minutes. A nonreactive (abnormal) NST is noted if there are decreases in the babies' heart rates or no increases with their movements. This can mean your babies are not receiving enough oxygen because of cord compression, low amniotic fluid levels, or poor placental function. However, lack of activity can mean that one or more babies are in a normal sleep cycle. Some doctors use fetal acoustic stimulation (FAS) to "awaken" sleepy babies so that they are more responsive. With FAS, an artificial larynx or other sound device is placed on a mother's abdomen and activated for a few seconds. Sometimes the movement of one baby is enough to stimulate the others. Studies have found no hearing loss in children exposed to FAS during pregnancy. It is thought that the amniotic fluid and the fluid inside the middle ear help muffle the sound.

Nonstress testing is often used to monitor babies who have poor growth, *twin-to-twin transfusion syndrome* (*TTTS*), or placental problems, or when the mother has gestational diabetes. In late pregnancy, NSTs might be done frequently to watch for signs that the placentas are aging or not functioning effectively. A nonreactive NST may require the preterm delivery of your babies.

Another related test is the *contraction stress test* (*CST*). This test uses medication such as Pitocin or stimulation of the mother's nipples to cause contractions. The babies' responses to the contractions are monitored for signs of distress. Because of the risk of preterm labor with multiples, the CST is not commonly used. Often, a spontaneous CST can occur when a mother has a contraction on her own during an NST, and the babies' responses can be documented.

BIOPHYSICAL PROFILE

The *biophysical profile* (*BPP*) is an ultrasound test that combines several assessments. These assessments include amniotic fluid volume, fetal breathing movements, fetal body motion, and fetal tone. Sometimes the results of an NST are also used with the BPP. Each assessment area scores two points for full function, so a normal BPP score, including the NST, is ten. To accurately assess each multiple, a complete BPP can take an hour or more. A BPP is used when an NST result is questionable or additional information is needed and is often used with higher-order multiples because of the difficulty in separately monitoring each baby with an NST. If one or more of your babies scores low on the BPP, it can mean your babies' health is at risk, and preterm delivery might be necessary.

DOPPLER FLOW ULTRASOUND

Doppler flow ultrasound uses sound waves to measure blood flow. The sound of moving blood produces waveforms on the ultrasound screen that reflect the speed and amount of blood moving through a blood vessel. This is a helpful tool in monitoring blood flow through your babies' umbilical arteries, aortas, and brains as well as your uterine arteries. Color-coded imaging gives clearer pictures of the blood flow pattern, and a new technique of Doppler angiography allows improved imaging of smaller vessels. Doppler flow studies are helpful in detecting fetal heart problems. These studies are also used when there is poor fetal growth due to conditions such as maternal high blood pressure or TTTS.

FETAL MOVEMENT

Another method of monitoring your babies' well-being is by keeping track of their movements or kicks. Kick counting is simple to do, has no risks, and can be done anywhere, anytime. Fetal movement is a good indicator that the babies are doing well. When there is poor placental function, not enough blood is transported across the placenta and a baby does not have the energy to move.

You might want to set aside some time each day to count your babies' movements. A good time is after an evening meal, as babies are often more active after you eat. Rest on your left side on a sofa or bed, and have a pen and paper nearby. Each time you feel a movement, a kick, or just a small roll, mark it down. Try to do this at the same time each day. For most babies, five or more movements per baby per hour are considered a good response. Sometimes it's hard to tell which baby is moving, so a total of ten movements for twins and slightly more for triplets are expected. Some mothers report that their babies' movements change to a calmer, less frenetic action after about thirty-two weeks. Don't panic if you don't feel movement all the time. Babies do have periods of sleep when they may be inactive. However, if you notice a change in your babies' movement patterns or don't feel as many kicks as you have before, call your doctor. Fetal monitoring or ultrasound can help detect any problems.

DECISION MAKING

You have the right to decide whether to use any of these tests. It is important to remember that test results are not 100 percent accurate, nor do tests tell about every possible problem you or your babies might have. Your doctor, along with a perinatologist and a genetics specialist, can provide information about your personal risks and which prenatal tests may be helpful. Some couples are reluctant to pursue invasive tests such as amniocentesis or CVS. They feel strongly that they would not terminate their pregnancy if a test reveals a birth defect and do not want to incur the risks of the procedure. Even if pregnancy termination is not something you would choose, testing can give you and your doctor valuable information. Remember that many tests are not invasive and have minimal risks, or are without risk. Sometimes early diagnosis of a problem can allow interventions during pregnancy to correct or reduce the risks for your babies. Also, knowing in advance gives you time to prepare yourself emotionally. Finally, remember that the vast majority of pregnancies are normal, and finding out that your babies are fine is very reassuring.

• • •

PART II

The Joys and Challenges of Being High Risk

This section explores the most common problems that can occur with multiple pregnancy and how those problems are managed. You may be tempted to skip over this section because it's scary to think that something might go wrong with your pregnancy. Although no one wants to imagine such a possibility, ignoring it won't make it go away. There is no doubt that some women sail through a multiple pregnancy without problems, but there are many others who have complications.

The truth is, multiple pregnancy is high risk. A woman's body is made to carry only one baby at a time, and having multiples often pushes the bounds of the natural design. This makes complications and unexpected situations more likely than with a singleton pregnancy. However, it's not the end of the world! Having a high-risk pregnancy doesn't guarantee a negative experience, nor is it a sign that you or your body has failed. Instead, you can use this situation to your advantage. Knowing problems are more likely encourages you to be more cautious and alert to the warning signs. It also gives you opportunities to reduce the likelihood and the severity of some complications. You can improve the chances of having a healthy pregnancy and babies by making positive changes in your lifestyle and getting the best possible care.

THE FACTS

Nearly every pregnancy complication that can occur with a single
baby is more likely with twins and higher-order multiples. Here are
some of the risks.

Twin Pregnancy Risks

- Average gestational age at birth is thirty-five to thirty-six
  weeks.
- Two and one-half times more likely to have preterm labor
  than singleton pregnancy.
- Seven times more likely to have preterm birth from
  twenty-eight to thirty-one weeks; about 6 percent of
  twins.
- Nearly six times more likely to have preterm birth from
  thirty-two to thirty-six weeks; about 45 percent of twins.
- Two and one-half times more likely to have high blood
  pressure of pregnancy; about 20 percent of twins.
- Three times more likely to have placental abruption (early
  detachment of the placenta).
- Mothers are 2.4 times more likely to be anemic; about 10
  to 25 percent of twins.
- Babies are seven times more likely to be admitted to the
  neonatal intensive care unit; about 50 percent of twins.
- Eight to nine percent have birth defects.
- Eight to ten times more likely to have low birth weight
  (less than 2,500 grams or 5½ pounds) or very low birth
  weight (less than 1,500 grams or 3¼ pounds).
- Average birth weight is 2,500 grams (5½ pounds).

Triplet Pregnancy Risks

- Two times more likely to have preterm labor than twin
  pregnancy, or five times more likely than singleton pregnancy.

- Average gestational age at birth is thirty-three weeks.
- Ninety to ninety-five percent are born before thirty-seven weeks.
- Twenty-five percent are born before thirty-two weeks.
- About 8 percent are born before twenty-eight weeks.
- One-third of mothers have high blood pressure of pregnancy.
- One-third to one-half of mothers are anemic.
- Four times more likely to have premature rupture of membranes than singleton pregnancy.
- Seven percent have birth defects.
- Ninety-two percent of triplets have low birth weight (less than 2,500 grams or 5½ pounds) and 35 percent have very low birth weight (less than 1,500 grams or 3¼ pounds).
- Average birth weight is 1,800 grams (about 4 pounds).

Quadruplet Pregnancy Risks

- Average gestational age at birth is twenty-nine and one-half weeks.
- One-half are born before thirty weeks.
- One-fifth are born before twenty-eight weeks.
- Average birth weight is 1,400 grams (about 3 pounds).

FACING THE FACTS

It is startling to read such statistics, but it is also comforting to know that most multiple pregnancies have good outcomes despite the problems. Go back and reread these statistics with a positive spin. For example, half of twins are born after thirty-six weeks and two-thirds of mothers expecting triplets *don't* get high blood pressure. Or, *only* 6 percent of twins are born before twenty-eight weeks and 91 percent *do not* have birth defects. In fact, some of these problems can be prevented or lessened. Even when a complication is unavoidable, it helps to understand what it is and why it happens. If you take the time to learn about problems and difficulties, you will feel that you have more control. Knowing about potential complications also helps you recognize warning signs and be more prepared for treatment, allowing you to be more involved in your care and giving you the confidence to ask questions. You can communicate more effectively with your care providers; and they, in turn, can take better care of you and your babies.

> I was fully involved in all the decisions about my care. I felt that I was part of the team and it made a difference in my outlook.

Some women with multiple pregnancies may be on bed rest or in the hospital, and many require medical interventions and cesarean births. These don't have to be terrible experiences, and they don't happen because somehow you have failed as a woman or mother. Rather, these interventions often are needed to ensure the health of you and your babies.

If you have complications, try to focus on the things that *are* going right. It is important to have a positive outlook on what may be very trying experiences. Sometimes you have to look hard to find some good or benefit, especially if problems are longterm, but you can celebrate the success of the day's treatments or simply the joy of feeling your babies move. Many medications and procedures can make you feel awful. So when there are unpleasant times, do what you can to minimize their effects. Don't be afraid to ask questions and tell your care providers how you feel. Sometimes it helps just to understand the medical reasons for your misery. By doing this, you'll be better prepared and find it easier to cope with difficult situations.

Certainly, don't let others influence you with horror stories or negative thoughts. Such things can keep you from looking forward to your pregnancy and your babies. A positive attitude can help you feel better and may even influence a bad situation. Talk to your unborn babies as they grow, and let them know how excited you are about having them. Tell your friends and family that you are on a mission to have healthy babies, and they can be a part only if they will help you accomplish this goal.

Chapter Ten

Preterm Labor and Birth

Of all the possible complications of multiple pregnancy, health care providers and expectant parents are most concerned about babies being born too soon. Preterm labor and birth (before thirty-seven completed weeks of pregnancy) are the most common complications in multiple pregnancy as well as in singleton pregnancy! About half of all twins and most higher-order multiples are born before thirty-seven weeks. The average set of twins arrives at thirty-six weeks, and triplets at about thirty-three weeks. Each additional baby in a multiple pregnancy can subtract another three weeks. Fortunately, many of these babies have healthy outcomes because of the tremendous advances in medical care. Compared with just twenty years ago, premature babies have much better survival rates. Babies at greatest risk are those born before thirty weeks gestation. These extremely preterm babies are much more likely to have serious and lifelong complications.

WHAT IS PRETERM FOR MULTIPLES?

Even though most multiples are born before thirty-seven weeks gestation, having your babies a few weeks early is not necessarily a prescription for disaster. For singleton babies, the best outcomes are when they are born between thirty-seven and forty-one weeks gestation. Many professionals feel that the window of time for the healthiest multiple birth babies is earlier than for singletons. For twins, this window is between thirty-five and thirty-eight weeks; for triplets, it is approximately thirty-five to thirty-six weeks; and for quadruplets, it is about thirty-four weeks. Studies have shown that perinatal death rates are lowest during this time.

Several physiologic mechanisms play a role in protecting preterm multiples. First, there are indications that lung maturity may occur earlier in multiples. This means that premature multiple birth babies may have fewer or less severe breathing problems compared with premature singletons. Second, late birth can have risks for multiples. There is evidence that stillbirth is more likely when multiples are carried very late in the pregnancy. Multiple birth placentas begin to age and become less efficient at circulating nutrients and oxygen to the babies as the pregnancy lengthens. Poor placental function can limit the nourishment of the babies. In turn, the babies often stop gaining weight, can lose weight, and are at risk of dying. By the thirty-eighth week, twin pregnancies need monitoring for signs of decreasing placental function. Monitoring should begin earlier for higher-order multiples. A woman with a triplet pregnancy rarely is allowed to deliver past the thirty-seventh week because of these risks.

Although there appear to be some advantages in multiples arriving a little early, this doesn't mean that premature multiples don't have problems. They can still have many difficulties related to prematurity. Talk with your doctors about the timing of your babies' birth, and discuss how to monitor the well-being of your babies throughout pregnancy.

WHY IS PRETERM BIRTH A CONCERN?

Premature babies are born before their bodies have finished maturing and developing, and nearly every organ system can be affected. The most common complication of preterm birth is *hyaline membrane disease* (HMD), or *respiratory distress syndrome* (RDS).

RDS develops because premature babies do not have enough *sur-factant,* a substance that allows their lungs to expand and contract easily. Without surfactant, their tiny airways stick together, making them work harder and harder with each breath. Eventually, they can no longer breathe on their own and need the help of a mechanical ventilator and extra oxygen. Usually, RDS improves over several days with treatment. Severe RDS can lead to chronic respiratory problems such as bronchopulmonary dysplasia, and even death.

Premature babies are at increased risk for other problems as well. Bleeding inside the brain, called *intraventricular hemorrhage* (IVH), can occur. Severe IVH can lead to developmental delays and mental handicaps. Cerebral palsy (CP) is more common in multiple birth babies. Although more research is needed to learn why CP occurs, most experts feel it is because so many multiples are premature. Premature babies are also at risk for *necrotizing enterocolitis,* a serious intestinal problem that can damage the baby's intestinal system and often requires surgery to remove diseased intestines.

Babies born preterm miss out on a mother's protective immunities that are transferred in the last part of pregnancy. This makes babies more susceptible to infection and disease. Breast milk contains similar immunities to those transferred in pregnancy, so breastfeeding or providing pumped breast milk can give your babies a wonderful advantage if they are premature.

Multiple birth babies are more likely to be smaller than singleton babies born at the same gestational age (the number of weeks of your pregnancy from your last menstrual period). This is significant because small babies are weaker and have less stamina. Twins are eight to ten times more likely than single babies to have low birth weight (less than 2,500 grams, or 5½ pounds) or very low birth weight (less than 1,500 grams, or 3¼ pounds). Low birth weight occurs in 92 percent of triplets, and 35 percent have very low birth weight.

Although technology has dramatically improved the care of premature babies, the best place for your growing babies is inside you. It has been estimated that for every day a baby remains in its mother's uterus before thirty-three weeks gestation, that baby may spend two days less in the neonatal intensive care unit.

CAUSES OF PRETERM LABOR

Compared to a woman with a singleton pregnancy, having twins makes you about two and one-half times more likely to have preterm labor and five to seven times more likely to have preterm birth. With triplets, your risks are twice that for twins. Monozygotic twins who share a placenta are more likely to be premature than are dizygotic twins.

No one totally understands why preterm labor occurs, but there are many suspected contributors. In multiple pregnancy, it has long been thought that a woman's large, overdistended uterus can trigger labor. Some think that the weight of the babies on the cervix stimulates labor. Urinary tract infections and dehydration can bring on contractions and lead to preterm labor. If untreated, certain vaginal infections can lead to preterm labor and birth. Rupture of an amniotic sac can stimulate preterm labor and lead to infection.

Other risk factors for preterm birth include medical problems such as diabetes and heart disease, a previous preterm birth, an abnormally shaped uterus, previous surgery on your cervix, exposure to diethylstilbestrol (DES), age younger than eighteen or older than thirty-five, and placental problems. Although these are factors you can't change, knowing they exist helps you be prepared.

Some preterm birth risk factors *are* within your control. Certain activities and lifestyles are associated with preterm labor and birth. Smoking, use of alcohol or other drugs, poor nutrition, and lack of prenatal care are associated with preterm birth and small babies. Studies have shown that standing for long periods of time, repetitious or monotonous work, and long work hours, as well as high levels of stress are associated with preterm birth. Sexual contact or stimulation can bring about preterm contractions in women at risk. Chapter Six has information about work, exercise, and activity—including sexual activity—and how to have a healthy, multiple pregnancy lifestyle.

SIGNS OF PRETERM LABOR

Fortunately, you can reduce some of your risks for preterm labor and birth by knowing what to watch for. The good news about preterm labor is that if it is identified early, it can often be stopped. Here are some warning signs:

- Recurring (often painless) contractions
- Menstrual-like cramps
- Pelvic pressure
- Backache
- Diarrhea or intestinal upset
- Vaginal discharge, bleeding, leaking or gushing of amniotic fluid
- A sense that "something isn't right"

Contractions

What is a contraction and how do you know if you're having one? A contraction is the tensing of the muscles of the uterus. If this is your first pregnancy, you probably have no idea what a contraction feels like. Even women who have experienced labor say that preterm contractions are different (often more subtle) from what they felt before.

Contractions can begin by the middle of your second trimester, as early as twenty to twenty-one weeks, and there have been reports of preterm labor at sixteen to eighteen weeks. Some contractions are frequent tensings of small areas or just one side of your uterus. These are called *uterine irritability contractions* and usually last less than forty seconds each. They often occur when you get up from a chair or when you need to urinate, and even when the babies move. Women with higher-order multiples are especially likely to have uterine irritability. These contractions can lead to organized preterm labor contractions. *Organized contractions* are an overall hardening and rounding of your uterus. Women often describe these as feeling the babies "balling up."

Many times, contractions are not painful; or, they may feel like menstrual cramps. You may not always feel them in the front of your abdomen—contractions can masquerade as a mild backache that is constant or that comes and goes. Pressure in your pelvis and thighs may also be a sign of preterm labor. Intestinal upset or diarrhea can be a sign of—and can aggravate—preterm labor, because as your intestines cramp and contract, your uterus can become irritable as well. Diarrhea can also lead to dehydration, which can increase contractions.

Contractions during pregnancy are sometimes called *Braxton-Hicks contractions.* In singleton pregnancies, these are common as the uterus "practices" for labor. However, in multiple pregnancy, these practice contractions can lead to preterm labor. Never ignore any contraction, no matter what it is called, or how it feels.

Even after reading these descriptions, you might be unable to tell when you are having contractions. The following plan can help you get to know your body and help you detect contractions. Set aside one hour twice a day, in the morning and evening. Lie down on your left side and find something quiet and relaxing to do, such as reading or listening to music. Place your hands on the top and sides of your uterus. To learn what a contraction feels like, find a spot on your uterus where there are no baby parts (bottoms, heads, elbows, etc.) and press gently. A noncontracted uterus feels like the soft part of your cheek when you press on it. A contracted uterus feels more like the hardness of your forehead. During this hour, keep your hands on your uterus and note if you feel any changes. You'll probably notice your babies moving, and you can sometimes feel your uterus tightening at the same time. Write down the times of any contractions or any other sensations. If you keep this record for several days, you might discover a pattern.

Maybe you'll notice more contractions in the evening and night than in the morning. Share your findings with your doctor.

It is reassuring to know that it is normal to have occasional contractions. Research has shown that women with multiple pregnancies often have more contractions than those with singleton pregnancies. However, an increase in the number of contractions is the most important sign of preterm labor. Remember that uterine irritability contractions can lead to organized contractions and preterm labor, and these should never be ignored.

Having more than four contractions in an hour is a warning sign, regardless of how strong the contractions are or how long they last. If this should happen, or any other symptoms of preterm labor occur, contact your doctor immediately and describe what is happening and how you feel. When you are dehydrated, your uterus often responds by contracting. So you will usually be instructed to drink a large glass of water and to monitor your contractions for another hour. If you still have contractions, insist on meeting your doctor in the office or in the labor and delivery area of the hospital. The doctor can check your cervix and observe your contractions on an electronic monitor. Don't wait until morning!

Vaginal Discharge

Any time you have a change or increase in the discharge from your vagina, you should notify your doctor. It is normal to have a small amount of clear or whitish discharge in pregnancy. This is a result of the increased blood supply and hormonal changes. A change in the color or amount of discharge (especially if it has a bad odor or causes itching) may mean an infection. Some infections, such as yeast, are quite irritating but not harmful to you or your babies. Other types of infections, such as bacterial vaginosis, may be linked to preterm birth if untreated.

A discharge that is thick or has a congealed texture may mean you have passed your mucus plug. This thick piece of mucus inside your cervix (the opening to your uterus) is a barrier to bacteria. Some women pass only small pieces of the mucus plug at a time; but once the plug is gone, there is less protection against infection. Passing this plug also may mean your cervix has started to soften or dilate.

If you see blood or streaks of blood in your discharge, you should notify your doctor immediately. If your cervix begins to soften and change, tiny blood vessels can break and allow small amounts of blood to mix with your vaginal discharge. This is sometimes called "bloody show" and can be a sign of labor. Bleeding may occur when an area of a placenta begins to weaken and detach from the uterus, called *placental abruption*. Sometimes bleeding occurs with *placenta previa*, when a placenta is attached low in the uterus over the cervical opening. Bleeding can be dangerous for both you and your babies, and it is important to seek care immediately.

Leaking or gushing of water from your vagina is a serious warning sign. When one (or more) of the amniotic sacs breaks, called *rupture of membranes*, amniotic fluid leaks out. This opens a route for bacteria and infection that can lead to preterm birth. See the section titled "Premature Rupture of Membranes" for more information. If you have questions or concerns about any vaginal discharge, always contact your doctor.

"Something Doesn't Feel Right"

Of all the warnings of preterm labor, your own intuition that something just isn't right is one of the most powerful. Your sense of feeling different today compared with yesterday can mean just as much as actually feeling contractions. Don't be afraid to trust your instincts about your body, and don't hesitate to call your doctor. Many women fear that they may look silly if they call and have nothing specific to report, but you may need to be assertive and insist on being seen.

> I couldn't put my finger on how I felt, I just knew that when
> I woke up that morning, I felt bad. I felt different than I had

other mornings. When I called the doctor's office, the nurse told me to rest and take Tylenol. After a couple of hours, I called back and insisted on coming to the office. At twenty-four weeks, my cervix had started to dilate.

PREMATURE RUPTURE
OF MEMBRANES

When an amniotic sac breaks open before thirty-seven weeks gestation, it is called *premature rupture of membranes (PROM)* or more specifically, *preterm premature rupture of membranes (PPROM)*. PROM occurs in about 5 to 15 percent of twin pregnancies and is more likely with triplets and other multiples. Rupture occurs most often in the presenting (lowest) amniotic sac, although it can occur in the other sacs. Normally, the amniotic membrane is very strong, but it may be weakened by factors such as smoking, early labor, premature cervical dilatation or shortening, bleeding, vaginal infections, and polyhydramnios (an excess of amniotic fluid) discussed later in this chapter. PROM can happen at any time in pregnancy, and it often leads to the preterm birth of one or more of the babies.

Be alert to the signs of membrane rupture. You might notice a slow leak or a sudden gush of watery fluid. Or you might feel a constant wetness in your panties. Amniotic fluid normally is clear and has a distinct, sometimes fruity odor. When your uterus is very large and heavy, you may have a hard time deciding if you have accidentally passed some urine or if it is amniotic fluid. If you are unsure, go to the bathroom and empty your bladder. Lie down for fifteen to twenty minutes, and then stand up again. If more fluid leaks out, it is probably amniotic fluid. Your doctor can examine a drop of the fluid under a microscope or test its pH to determine if your amniotic sac has broken. Never hesitate to call your doctor if you think your membranes have ruptured, even if it is a small leak.

Treatment of PROM depends on when it occurs and whether or not there is preterm labor or infection. In some cases, the sac may seal over, allowing the amniotic fluid volume to build back up. However, the ruptured area stays weakened and can break open again. You and your babies will be monitored carefully, and you will most likely be on bed rest in the hospital.

Once an amniotic sac breaks, there is an open route for bacteria and a risk of infection for you and your babies. Infection is dangerous and it can bring on preterm labor and birth. With PROM, there is about a 40 percent chance for infection of the membranes, called *chorioamnionitis*. Signs of chorioamnionitis include fever, uterine tenderness, and increased white blood cell count. Antibiotics are usually prescribed, but they may not be completely effective in treating the infection. Because chorioamnionitis is a serious infection, preterm delivery may be required.

Because PROM usually occurs before the babies' lungs are mature, corticosteroids can be given to the mother to help mature fetal lungs. However, there are risks in using corticosteroids with PROM because these drugs can hide signs of infection. Corticosteroids might not be given when PROM occurs past thirty-two weeks gestation. By this time, there is a lower risk for respiratory problems in the babies.

> My water broke at twenty-five weeks. We were totally unprepared. They gave me steroids, but we only had eighteen hours until the babies had to be delivered by C-section. Everything happened so fast, we hadn't even picked out names yet. We kept going over and over in our minds what we could have done differently. You feel so out of control.

If PROM occurs early in pregnancy, every day that passes without delivery is crucial to your babies' survival. In some cases, a week or more may go by before delivery is inevitable. And one week can make a huge difference in the outcome. However there are risks in waiting, including chorioamnionitis and placental abruption (separation of the placenta from the uterine wall). Because low amniotic fluid levels increase the chance for compression of the umbilical cord, the babies' heart rates may be monitored closely. When babies are born after PROM, they are more likely to have respiratory problems and infection.

A new surgical technique for PROM called amniotic repair has been successful in a few cases. However, this procedure is highly experimental.

PREDICTING PRETERM LABOR

When preterm labor is identified early, treatment can be started, and the birth of your babies can usually be delayed. All the signs and symptoms discussed so far are things you can identify, but only your care providers can detect some signs of preterm labor.

> My main concerns at first had to do with pain of labor and delivery, fear that I wouldn't get an epidural in time, and just hoping that the delivery would go well for both babies. However, when my doctor diagnosed me with premature cervical effacement, my main concern changed to the fear that I may be contracting and not feeling it, that I may go into labor extremely early, and concerns for the health of my babies if this happens.

Cervical Change
Cervical change is a serious warning sign of preterm labor. A normal cervix is about 3 to 4 centimeters long, is closed, and has thick walls. Continual contractions and pressure of the presenting (lowest) baby can cause your cervix to change. Over time, your cervix can soften, thin, and shorten (efface), and begin to open (dilate).

Studies show that when a woman's cervix is less than 2½ centimeters long, she has an increased risk for preterm birth. Generally, the shorter the cervix, the greater the risk for preterm birth. Another cervical change, called *funneling,* is a funnel-shaped widening of the end of the cervix nearest the uterus.

It is often hard to sort out the normal sensations of pregnancy from the warning signals. You won't usually feel changes happening in your cervix. Although some women report tingling or needle-like sensations, many are surprised to find out that their cervix has dilated or effaced. This is why it is important to have cervical examinations. Usually, a cervical examination is done at about eighteen to twenty weeks gestation as a baseline measurement and repeated regularly at future visits. Cervical examinations can be done two ways. One is an examination of your cervix using the doctor's gloved fingers to gently feel the length, softness, and any dilatation. The other is an ultrasound using a probe inserted into your vagina to measure the length of the cervix. Funneling can only be detected using ultrasound because it occurs inside the cervix.

> I began to notice an awkward feeling in my vagina, a fullness, sort of like a tampon was out of place. It was really bothersome and I called my doctor. It turned out to be just the pressure of the weight of my babies. The feeling stayed throughout my pregnancy, but they checked my cervix regularly to make sure I wasn't dilating.

Regular cervical examinations have been shown to be helpful in detecting cervical changes. These are done at every visit or as often as needed to keep track of cervical change. Cervical exams do not appear to increase the risk of infection or stimulate contractions, and they can be helpful in guiding your activity levels. Depending on how early in pregnancy cervical changes occur, you might need to limit your daily activities, which can mean just "getting off your feet" or as much as complete bed rest.

Tests to Predict Preterm Labor

Biochemical testing is now available to help predict your risk for preterm labor and birth. The *fetal fibronectin (fFN)* test can be used as early as twenty-two weeks. If you have signs of preterm labor, your doctor may recommend using this test. The test samples might have to be sent to a laboratory in a different city, and it could take forty-eight hours for results. In some locations, results are available in about an hour. Currently, these tests cost about $100 each, and some insurance plans cover the cost. The results can predict your risk for preterm labor and birth for about two weeks.

The fFN test detects fetal fibronectin, a protein found within the tissues of the plancental membranes that functions as a sort of "glue" to bind cells together. Fetal fibronectin normally is present in a woman's cervical and vaginal secretions until about 22 weeks gestation, when it disappears. Fetal fibronectin reappears in these secretions shortly before labor begins at term. When fFN reappears early, it means that there has been a disruption in the placental tissues. This can be due to inflammation, infection, or some other stress in the physical structure of the pregnancy. You'll need a vaginal exam to have this test so that secretions from your cervix and vagina can be collected. Fetal fibronectin testing has been shown to be accurate in twin pregnancies, and studies are being done to determine if higher-order multiple pregnancies might also benefit.

If the test is positive, a second test is nearly always performed. If a second test is also positive, it means that your risks are increased for preterm labor and birth during the next one to two weeks. This information can help guide your doctor in recommending treatments and medications to guard against preterm labor. The good news is that fFN testing is most accurate as a negative predictor. In other words, there is very little chance of spontaneous preterm birth within the next two weeks when the test results are negative. With negative results, you may not need medications or interventions. Regardless of the results, your doctor will watch you closely for any signs of preterm labor and may recommend testing again.

Another biochemical test for preterm labor prediction measures the level of estriol in saliva samples. Estriol is a hormone that plays a key role in labor. Although the test has been approved by the Food and Drug Administration (FDA), the American College of Obstetricians and Gynecologists (ACOG) does not recommend the test as a screening tool for preterm labor. ACOG cites problems, including a high percentage of false positive results and potential for significant additional costs and unnecessary interventions in prenatal care. The initial research on salivary estriol testing did not include known high-risk conditions such as placental abruption, premature rupture of membranes, incompetent cervix, intrauterine fetal growth restriction, and multiple pregnancy. However, clinical studies are currently underway with twin pregnancies, and the test may become a useful tool in the future.

Home Uterine Activity Monitoring

Some women just cannot tell when they are having a contraction. A large and stretched-to-capacity uterus can feel tight all the time. Or babies may move so much that it is hard to tell movement from contractions. This is especially true for women with higher-order multiple pregnancies. A system for monitoring contractions called *home uterine activity monitoring* (*HUAM*) uses an electronic transducer to record uterine contractions from your home. Twice a day, you strap the transducer around your abdomen, over your uterus. After an hour of monitoring, you send the contraction record over a telephone connection to a central monitoring station staffed by trained nurses. If there are too many contractions, the nurses consult with your doctor and call you with instructions.

HUAM is a useful tool and is often used with higher-order multiple pregnancies because of the very high risk of preterm labor. It is also used to follow women who are being treated for preterm labor at home, especially if they are taking medication to control contractions. While HUAM can identify contractions,

studies have not proven that HUAM alone prevents preterm births. HUAM is a diagnostic tool, and using the system can show an increase in contractions and help identify when intervention is needed. But it is not clear whether it is the actual monitoring or the nursing contact that identifies preterm labor. Talk to your doctor and health insurance company if you think you would benefit from HUAM.

TREATING PRETERM LABOR WITH MEDICATIONS

Fortunately, there are medications available to counter preterm labor and help delay the early birth of your babies. The medications used to stop the contractions of preterm labor are called *tocolytics*. They are not without risks, and their use must be individualized. Because women can respond differently, you may not receive the same medications as another expectant mother.

Betamimetics—Terbutaline and Ritodrine

Two of the most common tocolytics are terbutaline sulfate (Brethine) and ritodrine. These drugs work by interrupting the chemical and enzyme reactions that cause the uterine muscles to contract. Known as betamimetics, they are similar to asthma drugs. Ritodrine is not used as often as terbutaline, but it is the only medication the Food and Drug Administration (FDA) has approved for the treatment of preterm labor. As an asthma drug, terbutaline has not been given this approval but is frequently used "off-label" as a tocolytic.

Ritodrine is given as an injection or intravenously. Terbutaline can be given as a pill, as an under-the-skin injection, or through a pump that delivers small continuous amounts under the skin. The terbutaline pump (T-pump) allows control of contractions with a lower dosage of medication. Women with heart disease or severe high blood pressure should not use betamimetic tocolytics. These

drugs also affect glucose (sugar) metabolism and are not usually recommended for women with diabetes. Side effects result from the relaxant action of these medications on other smooth muscles in your body. These side effects include rapid breathing and a rapid heart rate, nausea, and feeling jittery and anxious. Effects on the babies include increased fetal heart rates and lowered blood sugar at birth.

Although betamimetic medications can treat preterm labor, taking them just as prevention is not effective. Betamimetics have risks, and it is very important to communicate regularly with your doctor about how you feel when taking these medications. Although rare, a dangerous complication is *pulmonary edema,* a build-up of fluid in your lungs. Women with multiple pregnancy have large amounts of circulating blood that makes them more susceptible to developing pulmonary edema. This is even more likely with higher-order multiples. Another problem with the use of betamimetics is that they become less effective when used continuously.

Betamimetics also increase blood glucose levels, especially if used with corticosteroids. Unstable maternal blood glucose levels can cause problems for pregnant diabetics or women with gestational diabetes and can affect newborns, as well. Because of these risks, betamimetics are not recommended for pregnant diabetic women.

Long-term use of betamimetics is controversial, and benefits for babies have not been clearly shown. In 1997, the FDA issued a statement on the use of terbutaline that concluded, "No benefit from prolonged treatment has been documented. In addition, the safety of long-term subcutaneous administration of terbutaline sulfate, especially on an outpatient basis, has not been adequately addressed." Most studies show betamimetics are effective on a short-term basis, long enough for corticosteroids to be given and take effect to mature babies' lungs. However, many doctors and patients feel there are benefits to longer use in certain cases and that the drugs can be used safely with close monitoring. As with all

medications, be sure to discuss with your doctors the risks and benefits of betamimetics and how they may be used in your individual situation.

Here are some potentially serious side effects of betamimetic medications. Notify your doctor immediately if you experience any of these symptoms:

- Dizziness or blackout
- Heart rate over 140 beats per minute
- Heart palpitations
- Frequent skipping of a heartbeat
- Irregular heart rate
- Chest pain
- Shortness of breath
- Extreme anxiety or restlessness

Magnesium Sulfate

Magnesium sulfate has been used for many years to treat preeclampsia, a high blood pressure condition in pregnancy. Magnesium sulfate is also a very effective medication for preterm labor. It works by competing with calcium in the muscle cells of the uterus. Without calcium, the uterine muscles can't contract. Although many doctors feel magnesium sulfate is the most effective treatment for preterm labor, they are often reluctant to give the amounts of the drug needed to stop labor because of the troubling side effects. Magnesium sulfate must be given intravenously, and hospitalization is necessary. Side effects include feeling flushed, nausea, vomiting, headache, and overall weakness. Very high doses can dangerously suppress your respiration, and your blood levels of magnesium must be monitored. Most women find that the side effects of magnesium sulfate usually go away in three to four days and agree that enduring few days of misery are better than the dangers of preterm birth.

Magnesium sulfate also is used when a woman no longer responds to betamimetic medications. A "mag sulfate vacation" allows your body time to clear the terbutaline and be more sensitive to its effects when restarted. Magnesium sulfate has valuable benefits for your babies. Studies have shown that a mother's use of magnesium sulfate before birth is associated with lower rates of intraventricular hemorrhage (IVH) and cerebral palsy in her babies.

Indomethacin

Indomethacin is a nonsteroidal anti-inflammatory drug (NSAID), a group of drugs that counter the prostaglandin (a hormone) action that causes contractions. Indomethacin is used to treat preterm labor for short periods of time before the thirty-second week of pregnancy. It should not be used if unborn babies have growth problems or low levels of amniotic fluid. Long-term use of indomethacin can affect babies' urine production and decrease the amount of amniotic fluid. Use of indomethacin after thirty-two weeks gestation can increase babies' risks for constriction of the major blood vessels around their lungs, called *pulmonary hypertension*. Indomethacin is given rectally or in a pill form taken by mouth. Side effects include gastrointestinal irritation and bleeding.

Nifedipine

Nifedipine is the generic name of a cardiac drug commonly known as Procardia. As a calcium channel blocker drug, it works to stop contractions by blocking calcium from entering muscle cells. Nifedipine is given by mouth as a swallowed pill or dissolved under the tongue. It is sometimes used along with betamimetic tocolytics. Side effects include headache, palpitations, and low blood pressure.

Corticosteroids

Over twenty-five years ago, it was discovered that giving a mother a corticosteroid medication before delivery helped her unborn baby's lungs produce more surfactant and have fewer severe breathing problems when born preterm. Since then, studies have shown other benefits of this medication, including decreased intraventricular hemorrhage (IVH), less necrotizing enterocolitis (NEC), and lower death rates of premature babies.

If you are at risk for preterm birth between twenty-four and thirty-four weeks gestation, you may be given corticosteroids. Women with higher-order multiples who are less than thirty-two weeks with a shortened cervix, preterm labor, or other signs of impending early birth are often given corticosteroids. Dexamethazone and betamethazone (Celestone) are most frequently used. Both are given by injection in several doses over forty-eight hours. The protective effects of corticosteroids reach their maximum forty-eight hours after the first dose and last about one week. Some studies have shown that multiple rounds of corticosteriods may be dangerous for mother and babies. This means the timing of the dosage must be carefully planned so the babies receive the greatest benefit at the optimum time. Many women with higher-order multiples have an increase in contractions after receiving corticosteroids. Some go into preterm labor and deliver their babies early. Because of this risk, careful assessments of the number of contractions must be made.

Because corticosteriods can affect glucose metabolism, gestational diabetics need careful assessment. Also, if one of your babies' amniotic sacs ruptures, corticosteroids can disguise signs of infection.

OTHER WAYS TO MANAGE
PRETERM LABOR

Medications are just one part of preterm labor care. You may also need other treatments and care in the hospital or at home. Some women are candidates for therapies such as cervical cerclage or a vaginal pessary. In some cases, a delayed interval delivery occurs when one baby is born but the others are not. Relaxation therapy is an effective strategy for handling stress and possibly preventing preterm labor and birth.

Hospitalization

Most women with preterm labor are admitted to the hospital, often in the labor and delivery area. This can be a scary as well as a reassuring time. Sometimes, events happen so quickly that you don't know what is happening. You'll have an IV and monitors to check your contractions and the babies' heart rates. Your doctor may examine your cervix to find out whether there has been any change and whether an amniotic sac has ruptured. Depending on the doctor's findings and the number of contractions, you may receive a tocolytic medication. Sometimes just getting one dose is enough to stop the cycle of contractions. At other times you may need more. Usually, you'll be restricted to your bed. Once contractions are under control, you are either sent home or moved to a different area of the hospital. Many large hospitals have special care areas for women with high-risk pregnancies. If you are moved to one of these high-risk antepartum units, you'll likely join other women with multiple pregnancies. Depending on your condition, you may need to stay in the hospital until your babies are born.

If your hospital is a small community hospital, without a neonatal intensive care unit (NICU), you may need to be transferred elsewhere. Most large tertiary hospitals (designated as high-risk centers) are equipped and staffed for managing high-risk mothers and babies. This can be frightening, especially if the hospital is many miles from home and family. However, when mothers are transferred before delivery, their babies can receive immediate specialized care, and the outcomes for babies delivered at tertiary hospitals are better than those delivered at smaller hospitals and then transported.

If you are able to go home, you still may need contraction monitoring and regular visits by home health nurses. Often you must continue on bed rest and medication, especially if your cervix shows signs of change.

Cervical Cerclage

Stopping your contractions and keeping the pressure of the babies off your cervix can slow changes in your cervix. However, a woman's cervix can begin to open even without contractions. An *incompetent cervix* is not strong enough to support the pressure of the babies and amniotic fluid. A surgical procedure called cerclage may be used to close up the cervix with a stitch, like a drawstring purse.

Although it seems logical that cerclage would be helpful for all women pregnant with multiples, studies have not shown that it prevents preterm birth. It is recommended only for true incompetent cervix. A rescue cerclage is sometimes used if a woman's cervix has begun to dilate very early in pregnancy. This is more likely with higher-order multiples because of the greater pressure on the cervix.

If you need a cerclage, you may be given tocolytic medications before, during, and after the procedure to guard against contractions. Antibiotics are also prescribed to help prevent infection. For the procedure, your bladder may be filled with a sterile fluid through a catheter. This helps push back the amniotic membranes from the cervical opening. Placing you in *Trendelenburg position*, with your head lower than your feet, also helps clear the opening. The doctor pulls down on your cervix using a clamp and stitches a synthetic band through the cervix near the internal opening. Either general or epidural anesthesia is used for cerclage.

Cerclage can be very effective if needed, but it has risks. During the procedure, the amniotic sac of the presenting baby can be nicked, causing leaking of amniotic fluid and opening a route for infection. The procedure can also bring about contractions. After a cerclage, your activity may be restricted and you should avoid all sexual activity. When time for delivery nears, the band is removed.

A vaginal birth is possible, although some women do need cesarean delivery. Scar tissue can slow the normal process of cervical change in labor, or the tissue can tear.

Vaginal Pessary

A vaginal pessary is a device placed in a woman's vagina to help support the weight of her pelvic organs. These devices have been used for years in older women with uterine prolapse and other pelvic weakness. A vaginal pessary is also used for a pregnant woman with an incompetent cervix or a retroverted uterus (tipped to the back), as well as to help relieve pressure on the cervix and the lower part of the uterus. There are reports that pessary use can delay delivery in multiple pregnancies with advanced cervical dilatation and low station of the presenting baby.

Delayed Interval Birth

Sometimes preterm labor or an incompetent cervix can lead to the birth of one or more babies, but not all of them. This is called *delayed interval birth*. Although it is possible to delay delivery of the remaining babies for days, weeks, and even months, there are many risks. Success depends on the cause of the first birth and whether there is infection, bleeding, or ruptured membranes. After the first baby or babies are delivered, the umbilical cord(s) are cut, clamped, and moved back into the uterus. A rescue cerclage is usually performed, and antibiotic and tocolytic medications are started. Bed rest in the hospital or at home is needed for the remainder of the pregnancy. There are risks to delayed interval birth, but it can allow the remaining babies more time to mature and have a chance for a better outcome.

Relaxation Therapy

Stress appears to play a role in preterm labor as well as other pregnancy complications. The exact process of how stress can lead to preterm labor and birth is unclear, but several theories exist. Stress results in the release of hormones that prepare the body for "fight or flight." Under stress, blood flow is decreased to the body's nonvital organs, including the uterus; and the heart rate, blood pressure, and breathing rates all increase. Relaxation therapy helps counter the effects of stress by increasing blood flow; lowering the heart and breathing rates, blood pressure, and the amount of oxygen used; and decreasing muscle tension. One study compared two groups of women at risk for preterm labor. One group practiced daily relaxation exercises while the control group did not use the exercises. The results showed that the relaxation group had longer pregnancies and babies with higher birth weights compared to the control group.

Whether stress is physical (such as discomforts of pregnancy or handling the effects of medications) or emotional (such as worry over your babies' health or concerns about finances), it has a negative effect on your body. There are many effective relaxation methods, including meditation, yoga, hypnosis, biofeedback, deep breathing, and progressive relaxation techniques. All help you minimize the physiologic effects of stress, reduce your anxiety level, and improve your perspective of stressful events.

Progressive Muscle Relaxation

Progressive muscle relaxation is a simple and effective technique that nearly everyone can use. It is done by isolating a muscle group, creating tension for several seconds, and then letting the muscle relax and the tension escape. This process is based on a principle of muscle physiology: When you create and then release tension in a muscle, the muscle must relax; and if allowed to rest, the muscle becomes even more relaxed. When you use progressive relaxation with all your muscle groups, you experience other positive effects throughout your entire body. With practice, you can relax more effectively in a shorter period of time. You can also work with a partner to help you relax various muscles in response to touch.

The technique is simple and is outlined in Table 10.1.

Table 10.1.   Progressive Muscle Relaxation

- Find a quiet place where you will not be disturbed. Dim the lights.

- Rest on your left side, supported by pillows.

- Take a deep breath through your nose or mouth. Hold it for a few seconds. Exhale slowly and fully through your mouth.

- Close your eyes. Let your body breathe comfortably and naturally.

- Raise your eyebrows up as far as you can and hold the tension. Now relax.

- Squeeze your eyelids tightly together. Now relax and open your eyes.

- Bite down and clamp your teeth together. Feel the tension along your jaw. Now relax.

- Bend your head forward as if trying to touch your chin to your chest. Feel the tension along the back of your neck. Now relax.

- Raise your shoulders as high as you can and notice the tension. Now let them drop all at once and relax.

- Take a deep breath, hold it briefly, and exhale slowly.

- Bend your right hand back at the wrist and briefly hold the tension. Now relax.

- Do the same thing with the left hand. Hold the tension and then relax.

- Tighten both hands into fists and hold the tension. Feel the tension spread up your arms toward the elbows. Now relax.

- Bend both arms at the elbows and raise your hands up to your shoulders. Tighten up the muscles in the biceps and hold. Now relax.

- Point your toes down. Now relax.

- Raise your right leg up in front of you and feel the tension build. Now relax.

- Do the same thing with your left leg and relax.

- Bend your toes up, pointing toward the ceiling, and feel the tension around your feet and ankles. Hold and then relax.

- Take a deep breath, hold it briefly, and exhale slowly.

- Once you are relaxed, picture yourself in one of your favorite, peaceful places. This might be the beach, the mountains, a vacation spot, or your front porch. Imagine the sounds, sights, feel, and smells of this relaxing place. As you think of your peaceful place, continue to relax.

REDUCING THE CHANCES
OF PRETERM LABOR—
WHAT CAN YOU DO?

You may feel quite helpless after learning about all the problems of preterm labor. Although some things are beyond your control, you do have many opportunities to make a difference for your babies. Now that you know the warning signs and how preterm labor is managed, you have a real advantage. Here are some other ways you can make a difference:

- Believe in yourself, that you are going to manage this pregnancy. Set your goals on achieving the optimum outcome, and don't settle for less.
- Eat well and gain enough weight in pregnancy to help increase your babies' birth weights and overall health. Read Chapter Four for more information on nutrition and weight gain.
- Make positive changes in your lifestyle that can reduce some risks. Avoid activities known to be dangerous, such as smoking and heavy work. Pick up on subtle changes by staying in tune with how you feel from day to day. Be aware of your body, and use good sense about your activity. Never push yourself to complete a task or do an activity when your body is telling you to stop.
- Stay in close touch with your care providers. Be assertive, and never be afraid to call them if you are uncertain about what is happening. Let your care providers know what you are doing and how you feel. Frequent communication and education can help identify preterm labor.
- Once in a while, release pent-up emotions with a good cry it can do wonders. There may be times when you feel completely overwhelmed and that your world is falling

apart. Talk with a member of one of the support organizations listed at the end of the book. They've been there and know how you feel.

- Learn and practice relaxation techniques. They'll be helpful now, for labor, and for life.
- Remember that complications can occur without warning, and in spite of everything you do. If you think you might be in preterm labor, try to stay calm because fear can increase contractions, and act as quickly as possible to get the care you and your babies need.

Chapter Eleven

Other Complications in Multiple Pregnancy

Although preterm labor and birth are the most common complications in multiple pregnancy, you may also encounter other problems. These include high blood pressure; gestational diabetes; problems with the amniotic fluid, placentas, and umbilical cords; twin-to-twin transfusion syndrome; and loss of one or more babies during pregnancy. Some of these complications can be quite serious, and if untreated, they can be dangerous for you and your babies. In most cases, there is nothing you can do to prevent them from occurring. Fortunately, however, there are treatments for many of these problems that can lessen their severity. And, when you know the warning signs and symptoms, you are more likely to get early treatment and improve your babies' chances for a better outcome.

HIGH BLOOD PRESSURE

High blood pressure (hypertension) can be a serious complication of pregnancy. The most common type is *pregnancy-induced hypertension* (*PIH*), sometimes called preeclampsia or toxemia. Approximately 15 percent of women with twins, about 19 percent of women with triplets, and 38 percent of those with quadruplets develop some form of PIH or related complication. If you have never had a baby before, your risk of developing PIH is even higher. PIH usually occurs earlier and is more severe in multiple pregnancies. It can also develop during labor and postpartum.

What Happens?

Although the exact cause of PIH is unknown, certain factors can increase your risks. These include multiple pregnancy, diabetes, hypertension when you are not pregnant, kidney disease, poor nutrition, PIH with a previous pregnancy, or a sister or mother who had PIH.

The process of PIH is complex and can affect many parts of your body. The beginning action of PIH is spasm or constriction of blood vessels, resulting in damage to their linings. When your body releases platelets and other blood cells to help repair the damage, these extra cells fill the vessels and limit blood flow. This leads to less blood circulating to vital organs including your brain, kidneys, liver, and uterus.

The three most common signs of PIH—high blood pressure, swelling, and protein in the urine—are related to the effects of blood vessel spasm. High blood pressure results when blood tries to pass through narrowed vessels. Edema (swelling) occurs when the damaged blood vessels begin to leak and fluid moves out into the tissues. Swelling also occurs when the kidneys are damaged by blood vessel spasm and can't filter waste products properly. This also causes protein to spill into the urine.

Other problems can develop as PIH worsens. When uterine blood vessels spasm, the blood supply to the babies is reduced. Over time, limited blood flow and reduced oxygen and nutrients to the babies can slow their growth. Placental abruption (separation of the placenta from the uterus) and fetal distress can also occur.

PIH can progress to a dangerous condition called eclampsia. With eclampsia, a woman can have seizures, bleeding in the brain, and coma caused by brain edema and restricted blood flow through the cerebral blood vessels. Severe PIH can also lead to liver damage due to blood vessel spasm and a condition called *HELLP* (hemolysis, elevated liver enzymes and low platelets) *syndrome.* Women with HELLP syndrome can have serious complications, including uncontrolled bleeding, placental abruption, kidney failure, pulmonary edema, and even death.

Signs and Symptoms

In multiple pregnancy, it isn't unusual to have a small amount of swelling in your feet and hands and even some small increases in blood pressure because of the large amount of blood volume in your body. But if swelling or blood pressure increases too much, it can mean that PIH is developing. Other warning signs of PIH are sudden swelling of your face and hands, headaches, blurry vision or seeing spots, sudden weight gain, nausea or vomiting, and pain under your breastbone or right side. Be sure to tell your doctor if you have any of these.

> Overnight my pregnancy changed. I started to swell like crazy and my feet grew two sizes. I was gaining one or two pounds per day. My blood pressure was up, too. I had preeclampsia.

Women with higher-order multiple pregnancies tend to have subtle or unpredictable forms of PIH. Rather than the usual signs of swelling or urine protein, there may be increases in liver enzymes and lowered blood platelet levels—changes that can only be checked by laboratory tests. Women with higher-order multiples are also at greater risk for HELLP syndrome. Because of these risks, your doctor will keep close watch on your blood pressure and swelling, and may do blood tests for platelet counts and liver enzymes.

> I gained 11 pounds in thirty-six hours and I felt bad. I knew something was very wrong. At the hospital I was diagnosed with HELLP syndrome and had an emergency cesarean delivery.

Prevention

There has been much research looking for ways to reduce or prevent hypertension in pregnancy. Studies have tried to find whether supplementing a woman's diet with substances such as calcium, magnesium, zinc, and fish oil have an effect on preventing PIH. However, much of this research has been with singleton pregnancies, and the data may not be applicable to multiple pregnancies. Other studies have concluded that low-dose aspirin does not reduce the risk of PIH in multiple pregnancies. Talk with your doctor about whether you are a candidate for preventive therapies, for while some of these therapies can improve outcomes, there may be adverse effects.

Treatment

How PIH is treated depends on when it develops, its severity, and how well your body responds to treatment. The earlier PIH develops in pregnancy, the more serious it can be for you and your babies. PIH can worsen quickly and may not respond to medications or other treatments, placing you and your babies in danger. Sometimes the only choice is to deliver your babies, even though they may be very small and premature.

Activity Restriction and Bed Rest

With multiple pregnancy, hospitalized bed rest is usually the initial treatment. In some cases, mild PIH can be treated at home with activity restriction or bed rest. Home health nurses may need to monitor your blood pressure and assess your swelling. Some women can do blood pressure measurement at home using a special machine that reads the level and transmits it to a nursing center. You will probably test your urine for protein and weigh yourself daily, as well as keep track of your babies' movements. When you rest, lie on your left side as much as possible, as this takes the pressure off the major blood vessels and helps increase blood flow and oxygen to your kidneys and placentas. See Chapter 12 for more information on bed rest.

If your condition worsens, you may need to be hospitalized because severe PIH often requires intensive treatment and monitoring. You may need to be transported to a hospital equipped to care for high-risk mothers and babies. In the hospital, your blood pressure, pulse, respirations, deep tendon reflexes, and fetal heart rates will be checked frequently. In many hospitals, an electronic blood pressure machine is used to frequently measure and record your blood pressure. You will have an IV and a urinary catheter in place to monitor your fluid intake and urine output and to check your urine for protein.

Alternatively, your urine is collected for a twenty-four-hour period to help determine how well your kidneys are working, how much medication is excreted, and how you are responding to treatment. Blood may be drawn to monitor liver enzymes and blood cell counts. Fetal heart rate monitors and nonstress testing might be used to assess your babies. It is often necessary to keep your room dimly lit and to restrict visitors and telephone calls to minimize stress and help you rest.

Medications

The most common medication used to treat PIH is magnesium sulfate, usually given in a continuous dosage through an IV. This is a very effective but potent drug, and the amount that builds up in your body must be monitored. Magnesium sulfate slows nerve-muscle reactions and dulls the central nervous system. It has many side effects that include feeling warm or flushed, nausea, vomiting, headache, and overall weakness. You will probably have blood drawn frequently to monitor your magnesium levels, because if too much of the drug accumulates in the cells, magnesium toxicity can develop, causing loss of reflexes, slurred speech, inability to move muscles, and difficulty breathing.

> They gave me magnesium sulfate for my high blood pressure. It's pretty awful stuff—I felt like I had a huge hangover, but it worked.

Other medications sometimes used to lower blood pressure include hydralazine, labetolol, and nifedipine. These drugs may be used as alternatives or along with magnesium sulfate to treat severe hypertension.

Because your babies may need to be delivered preterm, you may also be given a corticosteroid such as betamethasone to help mature your babies' lungs. For the maximum benefit, corticosteroids must be started at least forty-eight hours prior to delivery. Corticosteroids may also help with some of the effects of PIH, including low platelet counts.

Delivery with High Blood Pressure

How your babies are delivered depends on the severity of your PIH. Although a vaginal delivery is sometimes possible, cesarean birth may be needed because of potential complications, including placental abruption, prematurity, low birth weights, and fetal distress. The type of anesthesia for delivery also depends on many factors. Sometimes an epidural is possible, but epidural and spinal anesthesias are not generally used with HELLP syndrome because of the risk of bleeding, so general anesthesia is used.

> My PIH got worse by the hour and I had to have an emergency C-section at thirty weeks. Even though I had known for months before that a C-section was very likely, it was still alarming to have it happen so suddenly.

Your condition will be carefully monitored, and medication is often continued because PIH can occur even after delivery.

INTRAUTERINE GROWTH RESTRICTION

Although small multiples can be healthy, problems can occur if their intrauterine growth slows too much. Smaller than normal babies have a diagnosis of fetal growth restriction or intrauterine growth restriction (IUGR). At birth, the babies are classified as small for gestational age (SGA). This term is a comparison of the size and weight of babies to a standardized amount for a particular gestational age.

Several maternal factors can increase the chances for babies developing IUGR and being SGA. These include high blood pressure, diabetes, poor nutrition and low pregnancy weight gain, substance abuse, placental problems, maternal anemia, and maternal heart and lung diseases. Sharing a placenta and twin-to-twin transfusion syndrome also make IUGR more likely. In all these situations, the restricted growth occurs because there is too little nourishment reaching the baby.

Growth-restricted babies are at much greater risk for stillbirth and neonatal death. They are malnourished, have little body fat, and are weak because of poor muscle and body development. Decreased circulation can result in chronically low oxygen levels, and this can affect the function of all organs. The chance for problems is higher the earlier in pregnancy IUGR occurs. Babies who have had IUGR and are born prematurely are at greater risk for complications than with either condition alone.

What Is It?

IUGR is said to be present when the estimated weight of a multiple is less than the tenth percentile for a singleton fetus at the same gestational age—in other words, when more than 90 percent of all babies of the same gestational age weigh more than that baby. More than one-third of twins and triplets fit this description compared with less than 10 percent of singletons.

Usually, twins differ in their birth weights by about 10 percent or less. An example would be twins with birth weights of 5 pounds 7 ounces and 5 pounds 3 ounces. Multiples can have concordant IUGR, when all babies are small for their gestational age. Twins at thirty-seven weeks that weigh 3½ pounds and 4 pounds have concordant growth restriction because they are both smaller than the normal weight for that gestation. Sometimes one multiple is significantly smaller than the others. When the difference between the babies' weights is more than 25 percent, it is called discordancy. An example would be when one baby weighs 5 pounds 7 ounces and the other weighs 4 pounds. This difference is more significant the earlier it occurs. When the babies are very small, it takes much less actual weight difference needed to make 25 percent. For example, when one baby weighs 2 pounds and the other weighs 1½ pounds, the actual weight difference is only half a pound, but the percentage difference is very high.

About 5 percent of twins have discordant birth weights of 25 percent or more. The average weight difference among triplets is about 20 percent. Of triplets with discordance, about 30 percent have more than 25 percent weight difference, and 7 percent have more than 40 percent difference. Discordant weights are more likely with higher-order multiples, twin-to-twin transfusion syndrome, birth defects, and placental problems.

Detection and Treatment

Ultrasound is a valuable tool that allows measuring and estimating the weights of the babies. Ultrasound exams are done more frequently in multiple pregnancies to monitor for IUGR. Along with small size of the babies, one of the early signs of IUGR is low amniotic fluid volume, called *oligohydramnios,* which is calculated using measurements of pockets of amniotic fluid. (See the section titled "Oligohydramnios" to learn more about this condition.) If IUGR is suspected, fetal growth and amniotic fluid volume are tracked with regular ultrasounds. This is important to detect any worsening of IUGR. Ultrasound is also used to perform a biophysical profile that can help identify each baby's risk. See Chapter Nine for more details on this test.

Treatment of IUGR often depends on the cause. Babies with IUGR due to twin-to-twin transfusion syndrome may improve following amniocentesis of the other twin's amniotic sac. When IUGR occurs without a specific cause, treatment is more difficult.

Bed rest is often prescribed to increase uterine and placental blood flow and promote weight gain for the babies. In addition, increasing the mother's calories and adding nutritional supplements may help increase fetal weight.

There are some tough challenges in caring for multiples with severely discordant IUGR. Delivery may be the only option to save a small baby who is very sick; but this means all of the babies must be delivered, often preterm, putting them all at risk.

Early identification of IUGR and the improvements in technology have helped decrease some of the risks for these babies. Although preterm birth can add complications, many babies with IUGR do well. Most children who had IUGR as babies usually catch up in growth over time. As adults, they may be slightly smaller in height and weight if IUGR occurred very early or was severe.

GESTATIONAL DIABETES

Gestational diabetes mellitus (GDM), or diabetes of pregnancy, is a disorder of glucose (sugar) metabolism. While some studies have shown that GDM is more likely with twin pregnancy, other studies have found no difference. GDM occurs in about 2 to 7 percent of pregnancies with twins, 9 percent with triplets, and about 11 percent with quadruplets. Women with family histories of diabetes are more likely to develop GDM.

Your pancreas normally makes the hormone insulin, which regulates glucose levels. During pregnancy, the placenta also produces certain hormones—estrogen, human placental lactogen, and cortisol—that can cause your body to resist insulin. When your pancreas cannot produce enough insulin to keep up, blood glucose levels rise and are passed to the babies across the placentas. Babies are affected because your insulin cannot cross the placentas, and they are unable to produce enough of their own insulin to manage the high amounts of glucose.

Detection of GDM is simple. For most women, a blood glucose screening test is performed between twenty-four and twenty-eight weeks of pregnancy. If this test is positive, a three-hour glucose tolerance test is needed. For this, you must fast the night before the test. The next morning you have a fasting blood glucose test and are given a special drink, such as Glucola, that contains 100 grams of glucose. Then you'll have blood drawn once an hour for the next three hours. If the results show your blood glucose levels are high, it means your body cannot handle glucose properly. If you are diagnosed with GDM, you are placed on a special diabetic diet with strictly controlled calories and carbohydrates. Request a consultation with a registered dietitian for help with planning your meals and snacks. Most women need to do home blood glucose testing using a finger-stick device. Some may need to take insulin if diet control is not enough to keep blood glucose levels normal.

Diabetes also affects your babies. High glucose levels can cause babies to put on large amounts of weight during pregnancy. Babies of diabetic mothers are more likely to have hypoglycemia (low blood sugar) and respiratory distress syndrome at birth. Mothers who do not control their diabetes increase their babies' risks for birth defects and stillbirth. Therefore, be diligent about your diabetic diet and carefully monitor your blood sugar levels.

GDM usually goes away after delivery, but your babies may need close monitoring after birth to watch for hypoglycemia and respiratory problems. Finally, if you have GDM, you are at greater risk for developing adult-onset diabetes later in life.

AMNIOTIC FLUID PROBLEMS

Surrounding each baby is an amniotic sac (membrane) containing amniotic fluid. This unique fluid plays an important role in the development and health of your babies. Amniotic fluid begins forming in the first trimester inside the gestational sacs. By the second trimester, the babies maintain the amniotic fluid volume in a cycle of swallowing the fluid and returning it through urination and lung secretions. Amniotic fluid is also returned to the circulatory systems of mother and babies by diffusing across the chorionic and amniotic membranes. About a liter of this fluid circulates through this system every few hours.

Normally, there is approximately 500 milliliters of fluid in each baby's amniotic sac. This amount varies depending on the gestational age, from about 200 milliliters to as much as 1,000 milliliters. Amniotic fluid helps cushion each baby and allows the umbilical cord to float free from pressure. Because of the vital role of amniotic fluid, the volume around each baby is monitored routinely with ultrasound. This is often referred to as the *amniotic fluid index* (*AFI*). The AFI is calculated based on ultrasound measurements of pockets of fluid. Too much and too little fluid can signal a problem with a baby's swallowing and excreting cycle or a problem with the circulation through the placenta.

Polyhydramnios

Polyhydramnios and *hydramnios* are terms used to describe excess amounts of amniotic fluid. This condition occurs in about 10 to 12 percent of all multiple pregnancies and is more likely in a multiple pregnancy when there is a single placenta with twin-to-twin transfusion syndrome (TTTS). Rh sensitization is also a cause of polyhydramnios. About 25 percent of babies with polyhydramnios have a birth defect.

Polyhydramnios can be worrisome because excessive amounts of amniotic fluid can overstretch the uterus, leading to premature rupture of membranes as well as preterm labor. Treatment of polyhydramnios depends on the amount of fluid and the reason for its overproduction or lack of reabsorption. Amniocentesis is often used to remove excess fluid and may be needed several times before delivery as fluid continues to build up.

Oligohydramnios

With *oligohydramnios,* too little amniotic fluid is in the amniotic sac. This condition develops for several reasons. Like polyhydramnios, it is more common when there is a single placenta with TTTS. Birth defects, especially in the kidneys and urinary system, can prevent a baby from producing and excreting urine, leading to low amniotic fluid levels. Poor placental blood flow can also result in decreased amniotic fluid production.

> At my first appointment with the high-risk clinic at about twenty weeks, the ultrasound tech found that baby A had significantly less fluid than his brother. There was also a big enough difference in the babies' weights that they suspected I had TTTS. From then on, I had weekly appointments and ultrasounds.

Babies with constantly low amniotic fluid levels may also have IUGR. Also, babies' lungs may not fully develop (a condition called pulmonary hypoplasia), and they may have other forms of abnormal development when there is not enough amniotic fluid. The most severe form of oligohydramnios is called the "stuck twin." When there is only a tiny amount of fluid in the amniotic sac, it shrinks down around the baby like a cocoon. This makes the baby appear to be stuck against the uterine wall.

How oligohydramnios is treated depends on the cause. It is not possible to add fluid to an amniotic sac. However, if TTTS is the cause, removing fluid from the sac with too much fluid by amniocentesis can stimulate the sac with oligohydramnios to produce more fluid. There are increased risks during labor with oligohydramnios. Without the cushion of fluid, the umbilical cord can become compressed, causing the fetal heart rate to slow. A technique called *amnioinfusion* can be performed during labor if the amniotic sac is ruptured. In this procedure, sterile fluid is infused into the uterus through a special catheter. The fluid cushions the umbilical cord, helping prevent its compression during contractions.

PLACENTAL PROBLEMS

Placentas play a vital role in the well-being of the babies, so it is important to understand how placentas function. The chorion, or outermost membrane of the placenta has villi—fingerlike structures that implant into the inner wall of the uterus. These chorionic villi are bathed in maternal blood supplied by the uterine arteries. Nutrients and oxygen from the mother's blood pass across these chorionic villi to the fetal membranes. The nutrients then pass to the baby through the blood vessels in the umbilical cord. In reverse, waste products from the baby's circulation go back across the chorionic villi to the mother's circulation to be excreted. When there is a problem with the membranes or in the placental circulation, these cycles are interrupted. The babies do not get the nutrients and oxygen they need and are unable to rid the wastes from their systems. When each baby has its own placenta, only the baby with the placental problem is affected. When babies share a placenta, each can be individually affected by placental problems.

Bleeding In Pregnancy

Bleeding occurs in approximately 2 to 6 percent of twin pregnancies and most bleeding is due to either placenta previa or placental abruption.

Placenta Previa

A placenta covering part or all of the internal cervical opening is called *placenta previa*. The condition is more common in multiple pregnancy, in women over the age of thirty-five, in women with a prior cesarean delivery, and in African American women. Diagnosis of placenta previa is often made early in pregnancy using ultrasound. Later examinations may show that the placenta has moved or migrated away from the cervical opening, but this is less likely when several placentas are crowding the uterine space. There simply isn't enough room for the placenta to migrate.

Cervical changes or preterm labor can disturb a placenta previa, causing painless bleeding. This is the most common sign of the condition and usually occurs in the second or third trimester. If this happens, you may be placed on bed rest at home or in the hospital to decrease pressure on the placenta. If you have lost a large amount of blood, you may need a blood transfusion. In some women, cervical cerclage can help prevent further blood loss. Bleeding often reoccurs when labor begins. In most cases, cesarean delivery is needed with placenta previa. Be sure to tell your doctor about any bleeding you have, even if it is painless.

Placental Abruption

The placentas normally detach from their implanted places in the uterus right after the birth of the babies. When part or all of a placenta separates from the uterus before this time, it is called *placental abruption*. Women carrying twins are about three times more likely to have placental abruption than those with singletons. Some risk factors for abruption, such as smoking and poor nutrition, can be changed. Other factors may not be preventable, including high blood pressure, polyhydramnios, and trauma to the mother's abdomen from incidents such as an auto accident, a fall, or physical abuse.

With placental separation, a large amount of blood builds up and pushes the placenta away from the uterus even more. Sometimes the separation occurs on the edge of the placenta, and blood leaks into the uterus and out the vagina. Because each baby is dependent on the placenta for its nourishment and oxygen supply, placental abruption can be a serious complication. At least half the placenta must remain attached for a baby to survive. *Chronic abruption* occurs when there are several small areas that separate over time. This may lead to IUGR and low birth weight. Partial abruption occurs when only part of the placenta separates. Partial abruption can be alarming, especially if two babies are dependent on that placenta. A complete abruption, when the entire placenta detaches, is life threatening for mother and babies.

There is usually pain with abruption, and sometimes it's severe and involves contractions. Be sure to call your doctor immediately if you are having any bleeding, especially if you have pain. Treatment of placental abruption depends on the severity of the separation, the amount of bleeding, and if the babies are in distress. The babies must be closely monitored, and they may need to be delivered preterm if abruption is life threatening. A cesarean delivery is usually needed for placental abruption.

Twin-to-Twin Transfusion Syndrome

Twin-to-twin transfusion syndrome (TTTS) is a complication of the placenta that happens when blood vessels in a shared placenta become joined. Occuring in about 15 percent of identical twins that share a placenta, TTTS can develop when there is a connection between the two circulations of the babies. Through this connection, one baby becomes a blood donor and the other a blood recipient. As the blood flows in one direction, the donor twin loses blood volume and can develop anemia, IUGR, and oligohydramnios. The recipient twin receives too much blood, grows larger in size, and can develop congestive heart failure, organ failure, and polyhydramnios. TTTS is not a birth defect and is not hereditary. It is not caused by anything the parents did or did not do and is not something that the babies are doing to each other.

TTTS only occurs in monochorionic placentas. The severity of TTTS is influenced by how the placenta is shared between the babies and the number and direction of connecting blood vessels in their placenta. This information can only be confirmed through placental analysis after the babies are born. The earlier in pregnancy TTTS begins, the greater the risks for the babies. The babies have a longer time to be affected by this disproportionate flow of blood, and it is too early to deliver them. Without treatment, the risk of death is as high as 80 to 100 percent for severe TTTS. If one baby dies during pregnancy, the surviving twin is at great risk for bleeding, causing brain damage or death. But fortunately, TTTS is not hopeless.

Detection

In the past, TTTS was not discovered until delivery, and many babies died. Today, there are effective ways to manage TTTS. Because of their risk of developing TTTS, all multiples with a monochorionic placenta should be carefully monitored with ultrasound throughout pregnancy by a perinatologist. If the babies begin to have growth problems, changes in the amounts of amniotic fluid, or their bladders are not visible on ultrasound, TTTS is often suspected. Frequent follow-up ultrasound exams are needed to watch for further changes. Other methods of monitoring include nonstress testing, biophysical profiles, and Doppler flow studies. The TTTS Foundation recommends that a woman diagnosed with a monochorionic placenta have weekly ultrasounds beginning with the eighteenth gestational week until the delivery of the babies to watch for the warning signs of TTTS. During labor and delivery, babies' heart rates should be closely monitored because the acute form of TTTS (when no warning signs have been present) can be triggered. If the babies show signs of distress, a cesarean delivery should be done immediately.

Treatment

The most common treatment for TTTS uses amniocentesis to remove some of the extra amniotic fluid from the larger, recipient baby. This reduces pressure on the uterus from the excess amniotic fluid and makes the mother much more comfortable. Amniocentesis can help prolong the pregnancy because overdistention from excess amniotic fluid often stimulates preterm labor. For unknown reasons, this procedure can help even out the fluid levels in the babies' amniotic sacs. However, amniocentesis only treats the symptoms of TTTS. The placental blood vessels are still connected, and the problem continues. Amniocentesis may need to be repeated several times during pregnancy as the fluid levels build up and lessen in the sacs. Removing large amounts of amniotic fluid must be done carefully because rapid decompression of the uterus can cause placental abruption. Amniocentesis can also bring about contractions, so this must be monitored closely. If the signs of TTTS seem to resolve with the use of amniocentesis, they may reappear in future weeks and cause serious problems again.

Another treatment for TTTS is laser surgery during pregnancy, a procedure first performed in 1990. An opening is cut in the uterus so that a laser can be inserted and directed at the placenta. The connecting blood vessels between the babies' umbilical cords are identified and cauterized, or sealed shut, by the laser light. Laser surgery goes directly to the source of the problem and is a one-time procedure, unlike amniocentesis treatment. If one baby dies due to TTTS, previous laser treatment helps protect the surviving baby from hemorrhage back through the connecting blood vessels. Laser surgery is only an option for the most severe cases of TTTS, when the warning signs are present at eighteen to twenty-six weeks. This procedure has significant risks and is still considered experimental by many. In addition to the risks of bleeding and preterm labor associated with surgery on the uterus, the laser may not be able to completely sever all the blood vessel connections in the placenta. Another risk is that healthy and normally functioning blood vessels can be sealed off. A European report of experience with over three hundred cases gives a survival rate of 55 percent to 60 percent, with at least one survivor in 75 to 80 percent of pregnancies. The risk of neurologic damage in surviving infants at one year of age is around 5 percent. Currently, only a few doctors are performing laser surgery. The TTTS Foundation can help parents with travel costs in certain cases.

If treatments to control TTTS are not successful, preterm delivery of both babies may be the only option for their survival. Both babies in a TTTS pregnancy are completely normal and healthy. They only become affected by what is happening in their shared placenta. There is tremendous hope for these babies, and they are worth fighting for. Having a condition like TTTS is very stressful because you have no control over what is happening inside you. You can find support and learn more from the Twin to Twin Transfusion Syndrome Foundation, an organization devoted to educating parents and health care professionals about TTTS (See "Resources" at the end of the book).

> Everything I read about twin-to-twin transfusion syndrome after I was diagnosed was depressing and basically gave me no hope. I want people to know that it's not an automatic death sentence for their babies. I was not a candidate for laser surgery so my perinatologist aggressively treated me with nine therapeutic amniocenteses. My babies were born at thirty-six weeks and are now healthy seventeen-month-olds.

UMBILICAL CORD PROBLEMS

Certain problems with the babies' umbilical cords are more likely with multiples. Conditions such as *velamentous cord insertion* and *marginal cord insertion* are more common, especially with a shared placenta. These occur when the umbilical cord develops on or near the edge of the placenta instead of at the center. When the cord does not insert correctly into the placenta, it can limit the transfer of blood and nutrients to the baby. Bleeding from the cord insertion site, called *vasa previa,* is also more likely. Ultrasound can sometimes show the location of the cord insertion.

When babies share a single amniotic sac, they are at risk for cord entanglement—the twisting and tangling of their umbilical cords. This occurs in as many as 70 percent of monoamniotic pregnancies. The movement of the babies in the sac during early pregnancy allows the cords to wrap around the babies and to become tangled or even knotted. This is a life-threatening complication, and nothing can be done to prevent it from happening. As many as 50 percent of babies with cord entanglement die in pregnancy. Because of these risks, close monitoring of multiple pregnancies with a single amniotic sac is very important. Ultrasound can help detect the locations and any shortening or tightening of the babies' cords. Early delivery may be needed if the babies' cords are becoming compressed from the entanglement.

FETAL LOSS—WHEN MULTIPLES DIE DURING PREGNANCY

It is something no one wants to think about or read about. Losing one or more of your babies is probably the worst imaginable experience. Yet it happens, and it is important to know what to expect if it happens to you.

Early Pregnancy Loss

The vast majority of pregnancy losses with multiples occur in the first trimester, sometimes before a woman even knows she is pregnant. She may dismiss bleeding as a heavy period and not realize she is still pregnant. She may carry on with a healthy singleton pregnancy, never knowing there were twins at the start. As early as the 1940s, it was suspected that more women were conceiving twins than were actually giving birth to twins. Early pregnancy ultrasound has shown that the theory of a "vanishing twin" actually does occur. This first-trimester loss happens in about one in five twin pregnancies and more frequently in higher-order multiples, often very early, before pregnancy is known. For no known reason, one or more of the gestational sacs stop growing and disappear. The loss can only be detected by ultrasound when there is no longer a heartbeat, or one of the gestational sacs is empty.

While there is no way to know whether this may happen to you, it is thought that multiples with a small gestational sac, small fetal size, and a slow heart rate are more likely to "vanish." Many women experience bleeding with an early pregnancy loss, but this can happen without any outward sign. In most cases, there are no complications for the mother or the other babies. However, because of possible blood vessel connections, there can be risks for a surviving baby that shares a placenta with the one that died. The twin that vanished is absorbed, and there is no visible evidence at delivery.

Because first-trimester pregnancy loss is the most common, most women and their doctors feel a big weight lifting once this time has passed. Some women wait until the end of the first trimester to tell people outside their immediate families that they are having multiples, as this can prevent having to deal with nosy or insensitive comments.

Later Pregnancy Loss

When loss of one or more babies occurs in later pregnancy, it is called an *intrauterine fetal demise* (*IUFD*). Sometimes the reason for the loss is known, such as a birth defect, chromosome abnormality, or congenital infection. Babies with monochorionic placentas have a three times higher risk of IUFD than those with individual placentas. Twin-to-twin transfusion syndrome and intrauterine growth restriction can also cause fetal death in monochorionic pregnancies. Although monoamniotic (one amniotic sac) twins are very rare, the risk of fetal death for these babies is very high due to cord entanglement.

Medical management of IUFD depends on many factors. The physical condition of the mother, the number of placentas, the length of gestation, and the condition of the surviving baby or babies must all be considered. If each baby has its own placenta, there is less danger to the surviving babies than if the placenta is shared. However, IUFD can increase the risks for neurologic damage in the surviving babies. When babies share a placenta and one baby dies, the surviving baby can bleed into the circulation of the dead baby through connecting placental blood vessels. This reduces the amount of blood circulating in the live baby. Oxygen delivery to the brain and kidneys of the surviving twin is affected in about 10 percent. The surviving twin is also at risk for cerebral palsy.

Because of the risks to the surviving babies, ultrasound, non-stress tests, and biophysical profiles are used to monitor them after an IUFD. Mothers may also need blood testing for coagulation abnormalities. If pregnancy continues for several weeks after the IUFD, there is an increased chance of a blood clotting complication called *disseminated intravascular coagulation* (*DIC*). Heparin can help stop the clotting, but in some cases, delivery is necessary to protect the mother and her surviving babies. Mothers may be given corticosteroids to help with fetal lung maturation if delivery is preterm. How the babies are delivered—vaginal or cesarean—depends on the condition of the mother and babies.

Grieving Your Loss

After seeing three sacs on ultrasound at six weeks, I had some spotting. My doctor thought this might mean one of the fetuses was "resorbing." Another ultrasound a week later confirmed those suspicions. At that time, I did not feel a sense of sorrow, but rather resolved the loss in my mind by promising to "come back for number three" using the frozen embryos we had stored. Later, though, when I learned we were having two boys, I felt a very strong wave of emotion and I sensed I had lost a little girl. It took about three or four days before I was able to work through this grief and be able to talk about the pregnancy again.

No matter when or why pregnancy loss happens, it is traumatic for everyone—parents, family, and friends, as well as the health care team. It wreaks emotional havoc on all your plans and dreams. When you find out one week you are having multiples and then, at the next ultrasound, learn you have lost one or more, it is like being on an emotional see saw. It's natural to fear losing your other babies or to blame yourself for causing this to happen or for not doing something to prevent it.

When loss occurs in later pregnancy, parents often feel a much deeper sense of loss and grief. After seeing their babies on ultrasound, learning they are boys or girls, naming them, and feeling their kicks and movements, mothers especially have a deep and binding attachment. Having multiples makes the grieving process even more complicated. When a twin or triplet dies, parents have not only lost a baby, they have also lost the completeness of the set of multiples. They grieve not only for the individual baby that died but also for the loss of the twinship or the specialness of multiples. When there is a surviving baby or babies, parents are completely torn apart emotionally. They feel deep sadness and ache for the baby that died. But at the same time they are relieved and joyful for the baby or babies they still have. Nothing can change the fact that they once had more babies—parents never forget about babies that die.

Delivery can be especially traumatic after a pregnancy loss. If the loss occurred early, emotions that you put aside can come flooding back. If the loss occurred later in pregnancy, you might have great anxiety about what will happen at delivery, what you may feel and see. Others who have experienced such loss have found several ways to manage these fears. Even though you think you could never bear to see the baby that died, doing so helps establish the reality of the death. Nearly all parents find that what they imagine is much worse than the real thing. Seeing the baby cancels out any doubts about whether this really did happen and helps you come to terms with your loss. Many hospitals have specially trained grief counselors or bereavement teams to help you during this time. They can offer recommendations that have helped other parents in the same situation, including the following:

- Name your babies.
- Have photographs taken of the baby(ies) that died, both individually and together with the surviving babies.
- Hold your babies and say goodbye.

- Plan a funeral or memorial service for family and close friends.
- Request that the Twin A or B sign on the surviving baby's crib not be changed.
- Let others know about your loss in an announcement that not only shares the births of all your babies but also tells of the loss.
- Contact a support group. Parents of multiples clubs may have members who can share in your loss. Also, contact the Center for Loss in Multiple Births (CLIMB), which provides telephone and written support for grieving parents of multiples, regardless of when the loss occurred (see "Resources" at the end of this book).

With all of the problems that can potentially happen in multiple pregnancy, it can seem hopeless. Try to remember that although these can happen, the majority of multiples are born healthy.

Chapter Twelve

Bed Rest

Bed rest has been used for many years to treat pregnancy conditions such as preterm labor, high blood pressure, incompetent cervix, ruptured membranes, bleeding, and fetal growth problems. About 20 percent of all pregnant women are put on bed rest for some portion of their pregnancy, and it is used even more frequently with multiple pregnancies. Using bed rest seems logical for many situations related to preterm birth because gravity increases pressure on the cervix when a woman is in an upright position. In some studies, women on bed rest were less likely to develop high blood pressure and had improved fetal growth. This is probably because high blood pressure reduces blood flow to the uterus and limits the amount of nutrients and oxygen to developing babies. Without sufficient nutrition, babies do not grow appropriately and often have low birth weight. Rest, especially in the left side-lying position, helps improve blood flow to the uterus and can help improve fetal growth.

Although bed rest is recommended for women with certain pregnancy complications, research has not been able to support the routine use of bed rest for multiple pregnancy, either at home or in the hospital. A common practice in past years was to routinely prescribe bed rest beginning at twenty-eight weeks. It was thought that because few infants survived before that time, bed rest would help prevent preterm birth after twenty-eight weeks. Although babies today are surviving at earlier gestational ages, using bed rest at any time just because a woman is carrying twins has not been found to prevent preterm labor or birth or improve perinatal outcome. Routine hospital bed rest for women pregnant with twins is not only ineffective and disruptive to family life, but it is very expensive for the family and the health care system. Despite the lack of supporting evidence, many care providers use arbitrary routine bed rest for all twin pregnancies.

The conclusions are not as clear for higher-order multiple pregnancies. Some research has shown positive effects of using bed rest for women with triplets and very high multiples. These multiple pregnancies have greatly increased risks for pregnancy complications, especially preterm birth. Because of their higher risks, most women carrying triplets have very restricted activity or bed rest. Those with very high multiples usually spend a significant part of pregnancy in bed at home and in the hospital. A common practice with higher-order multiples is to greatly reduce activity beginning at twenty weeks, and then begin bed rest at twenty-five weeks. Hospital bed rest may be needed at any time, especially if there are preterm contractions or cervical changes.

PROBLEMS OF BED REST

Why is bed rest such a controversial issue? In addition to the conflicting research, problems can arise with its long-term use, including physical stresses such as weight loss, muscle wasting, bone loss, deep vein thrombosis (blood clots), and cardiovascular deconditioning. You may experience weakness after just a few days of bed rest. Many women have compared it to the weakness after having the flu. Muscle spasms in the lower legs is a common complaint. Bed rest can become a vicious cycle. Lack of activity can make you feel sluggish and dull your senses. It can take away your motivation or energy to do the few activities that are allowed. Women often complain about their brains as well as their muscles going to mush. They have a hard time concentrating and completing tasks. Bed rest can also bring anxiety, hostility, and depression. Complete recovery from long-term bed rest can take many weeks after the birth of your babies.

> Having to recline for hours a day was isolating and depressing, but I took my job seriously: to keep those babies inside me for as long I could.

Be sure to discuss the use of bed rest with your doctor early in your pregnancy. Ask for your doctor's experience and recommendations for pregnancies like yours. Many doctors take a wait-and-see attitude, reserving bed rest for when there are clear indications, such as cervical change or preterm contractions.

If bed rest is recommended, ask for a clear definition of your restrictions. Bed rest can mean different things to different people. You may have thoughts of sleeping late and puttering around the house when your doctor means you must stay in bed twenty-four hours a day. Limited bed rest can mean rest periods in bed with the ability to get up to eat, take a quick shower, and, occasionally, take a trip in the car to the doctor's office. Strict bed rest can include only bathroom privileges. Be sure to clarify how you should be resting: on your left side, reclining, or sitting. Does bed rest have to be in the bed, or is the sofa or recliner also acceptable? Ask about taking a shower, using stairs, and getting up for meals.

Be honest with yourself and your doctor. If you are the type of person who just cannot slow down, you may need stronger restrictions. Without compromising your babies' health, work together to come up with a reasonable plan.

> My doctor figured out I was not going behave and that I always did more than I was supposed to do. Finally, he ordered complete bed rest, hoping that I would at least slow down. It was like a prison sentence for me, but it made me

realize how much I had been pushing myself. Eventually we
were able to come to an agreement on how much I could
do. I was happier, and he knew that I was resting enough.

HOW TO COPE WITH BED REST

At first, the idea of bed rest might sound inviting. After all, how
many chances do you get to spend your days lounging in bed,
catching up on reading, watching TV, and talking on the telephone? All too soon, though, reality sets in, and bed rest becomes
a test of endurance. There are many hours to dwell on your situation and to worry. It's natural to experience some denial, as well as
anger and guilt, about what is happening to you. Looking at the
same four walls twenty-four hours a day is not how most women
envision pregnancy.

Losing the ability to be in control is hard. Your job, household chores, and all your former responsibilities must be taken over
by others. It can be frustrating to watch these things being done,
often not the way you would do them. Try to accept that how
they are done is not really that important in the big picture. You
may also feel tempted to do things you should not. No matter how
legitimate or important these reasons may seem, always remember
your end goal of having healthy babies.

Bed rest affects more than you alone. It affects your mar-
riage, your relationship with your children, and your friends and
other family members. Everyone in your life is called on to make
sacrifices and changes in their routines and lifestyles when you are
on bed rest. It is helpful to have a family meeting to work out a plan
and contingencies. Sometimes it is easier for another person to take
charge of getting helpers and volunteers. That way you can enjoy
others' help without feeling obligated to return the favor.

Boredom is another major difficulty with bed rest. Try to establish a routine for each day. Wake up at the same time, eat your

meals at the same time, and plan activities for certain parts of the day. This can help time pass more quickly and reduce anxiety.

Bed Rest at Home

Here are some suggestions on coping with bed rest at home:

- Set up a bed rest survival station. Everything you need should be placed within reach or be accessible by remote control: telephone, television, VCR, stereo, computer. Keep a supply of videos on hand. Be cautious about the type of videos and television shows you watch. Extremely violent and emotionally draining programs can be stressful. A variety of books and magazines, crossword puzzles, needlework, or art supplies are also helpful. One mom began crocheting an afghan with a goal of completing a section each day in a different color. By the end of her bed rest, she had completed a beautiful blanket.
- Place a cooler with nutritious snacks and drinks beside your bed. If you can get up occasionally, use a small microwave placed across the room to heat leftovers.
- Keep a calendar and mark off each day. Celebrate each week or significant milestone with a special meal or allowed activity.
- Keep your internal clock on a schedule to avoid "bed lag." Make a plan that you follow each day—get up, shower, eat meals, and go to sleep at the same times. Open curtains and blinds in the morning to let in sunlight, and close them at night. Nap only when you really need to.
- Start a journal. Writing down your feelings and frustrations can be a release.
- Arrange your stacks of photos in albums or create memory books.
- Read books you've always planned to read, as well as parenting and baby books and magazines.

- Put on your makeup and real (but comfortable) clothes—
  it often helps you feel better about yourself. However, you
  may find that others are not as likely to see the need to help
  if you look less "sick."
- Encourage your friends to visit. When they come, have a
  small chore or task that they can do, such as a trip to the
  grocery store, returning videos or books, or running a load
  of laundry.
- In nice weather, have a sofa or lounge chair moved outside
  in the shade. Stay out of the sun because you can quickly
  become overheated and dehydrated. If you can ride a short
  distance in a car, go to a friend's house and use their bed or
  sofa. A change of scenery works wonders.
- Connect with organizations such as Sidelines and local
  parents of multiples clubs. Sidelines is a wonderful support
  organization for women on pregnancy bed rest. They support you by phone or e-mail with trained bed rest sur-
  vivors. Find out if your hospital has a support group.
- Use a laptop computer to surf the Internet. There are a
  number of informative Web sites and e-mail discussion
  groups for multiple pregnancy.
- Staying in touch with your boss and coworkers can help
  you feel you are still contributing. Unless it is too stressful,
  you may be allowed to do some work from home. One
  woman participated in teleconferences from her bed. At
  the office, she had a picture of herself placed at her seat in
  the conference room to remind everyone of who she was.
- Pamper yourself with a few luxuries. Hairdressers often
  make house calls, and getting your hair cut and styled can
  do wonders for your spirits. Have a friend or a professional
  manicurist give you a manicure and pedicure. Check with
  your doctor about having a regular massage with a professional therapist trained in the special techniques for pregnancy. These are relaxing ways to help you feel better about
  yourself.

- If you are on long-term bed rest at home, talk with your doctor about having a physical therapist come teach you exercises that you can do in bed. This service is covered by some insurance plans.
- Plan and supervise the preparation of your babies' nursery. You can pick out paint colors and wallpaper from your bed as well as choose the style of baby furniture.
- Focus on your babies. You'll have lots of time to communicate and bond with them. Talk and sing to your babies; they may respond to the sound of your voice, and it may be relaxing for you as well. Visualize them in their different positions and how comfortable they must feel inside you.
- Use relaxation techniques and music to soothe yourself and your babies.
- Write journals to each baby. It's good therapy for you and they may appreciate your thoughts some day.

I'm making a scrapbook for the babies. It starts with their ultrasound pictures when they looked like little lima beans, and I'm writing little stories beside each picture telling what it was like when we found out they were twins.

Bed Rest in the Hospital

Your activities are even more restricted if you are on bed rest in the hospital. You can use many of the suggestions given in the previous section in the hospital as well. If you'll be in the hospital for a long time, look for ways to make your room more comfortable and homey. Here are some suggestions:

- Bring pictures or artwork from home, a favorite lamp, a special blanket or comforter, or even a colorful rug that can be taped securely to the floor. A fan helps move stale air and can mask unwanted outside noise.
- Wear your own nightgowns as opposed to hospital gowns.

- When hospital food becomes unbearable, have friends bring in food or have food delivered from a favorite restaurant (unless you are on a special diet).
- Borrow or purchase a sound effects machine to drown out noises. Hospitals are not known for their tranquil and quiet nights. These machines often have sounds that are soothing to babies as well.
- Work with your nurses to plan minimal interruptions in your days and nights.
- If possible, take a bath and request clean sheets daily. Ask for or bring a foam egg crate mattress or sheepskin pad. Some hospitals provide air flotation mattresses, or you can rent one from a hospital supply store. Bring your own pillows and some colorful pillow cases.
- Request sessions with a physical therapist to help with muscle weakness. Although weight-bearing activities such as walking are the only true way to minimize weakness in muscle and bones, isometric and range-of-motion exercises help prevent stiffness and soreness.
- If your condition is stable, ask for a wheelchair to go outside to a courtyard or hospital roof garden with family. Stay in the shade where you won't get overheated or dehydrated.
- Plan an occasional "event," such as a popcorn or pizza party with a movie in your room.
- Ask to meet other women who are on pregnancy bed rest. Some hospitals coordinate a social hour for bed resting women, and others have support groups guided by a social worker or counselor.
- Some hospitals provide full or queen-size beds or a pull-out sleeper chair so your husband or other family member can spend the night with you.
- Plan something simple that you can do with a visiting child, such as storytelling, working on a project together, creating artwork that goes up on the walls, or making a book.

- If cabin fever gets too bad, or if you have a disruptive roommate, request a room change.
- If there is something that can be done or changed to help you feel better, don't be afraid to ask. Nurses are great advocates for their patients' needs and often can find creative ways to work around or through the system. Most hospitals make accommodations in their rules if you ask.
- Remember that nurses and doctors are human and respond to your kindness. You might have a friend or family member bring a treat for the staff to show you appreciate their care.

Chapter Thirteen
Multifetal Pregnancy Reduction

Some parents expecting multiples, especially triplets or more, find themselves faced with a difficult decision early in pregnancy. A procedure called *multifetal pregnancy reduction* has been used in recent years because of concern about the effects of preterm birth and other complications with higher-order multiple pregnancies. Multifetal pregnancy reduction is the planned termination of one or more fetuses in a multiple pregnancy. The rationale is that reducing the number through the sacrifice of one or more fetuses can help save the lives of the others. Reduction is controversial and emotionally stressful for families and for health care providers.

Fetal reduction was first recorded over twenty years ago when it was performed for a twin pregnancy in which one baby had a fatal genetic condition. Today, multifetal pregnancy reduction frequently is offered to women carrying three or more babies. Because very high multiples are nearly always born early, they are at greater risk for long-term problems of prematurity. These problems include respiratory difficulties, serious neurologic and learning disabilities, and developmental delays. When there are fewer babies, the pregnancy often lasts longer and the risk of these problems is reduced. However, this is not a simple issue, and there are many factors that make the decision very difficult.

It is important to understand the terminology. The term *selective reduction* often is used but may not be an accurate description of the procedure. With selective reduction, specific fetuses are designated for reduction rather than randomly chosen. Fetuses may be selected because they do not appear to be as well developed or have smaller gestational sacs than others. Two fetuses who share a placenta (identical twins) may be selected because they are more likely to have problems, or a fetus with a known or suspected birth defect may be selected for reduction. When there is no reason for choosing a specific fetus, selection may depend on the fetus' location in the uterus and the accessibility.

Reduction is sometimes considered an abortion, although technically it is not since the fetus or fetuses are not removed from the uterus. And, the intention is that the pregnancy continues. However, many people feel that reduction is, in essence, an abortion because it is the planned death of a fetus.

WHO IS A CANDIDATE?

Currently, multifetal pregnancy reduction is usually recommended for very high multiple pregnancies because of the extreme risks for preterm birth and long-term disabilities in these babies. Reducing triplets is more controversial, because the likelihood of a better outcome must be balanced with the psychologic effects and the risk of the procedure. Most doctors do not recommend reduction of multiples to less than twins, because reducing to a single baby does not appear to improve outcomes any more than reducing to twins.

In about half of all early multiple pregnancies, including those not yet diagnosed, there can be a spontaneous loss or miscarriage of one or more multiples. This natural loss is called the "vanishing twin" phenomenon. Generally, the rate of natural loss is higher with more fetuses in the pregnancy, and is as high as 45 percent for triplets. A natural loss occurring before the end of the first trimester eliminates the need for reduction, and some parents feel this is God or nature's way of making their decision.

THE PROCEDURE

Multifetal pregnancy reduction is usually performed late in the first trimester, between about ten and thirteen weeks of pregnancy. The couple receives extensive counseling that describes the procedure, its risks, and possible outcomes, and they must sign a consent. Before the procedure, the woman receives a sedative and antibiotics. Her husband or support person is encouraged to be at her side. Ultrasound is used to locate all of the fetuses, and the woman's abdomen is cleaned and draped with sterile towels. Using ultrasound as a guide, the doctor inserts a needle through her abdomen and into the uterus to the chest or abdomen of a fetus. A lethal medication, usually potassium chloride, is then injected into the fetus. When the fetal heartbeat stops, usually very quickly, the fetus has died. Any fluid is drawn out from around the fetus and the needle is removed. The entire procedure takes a few minutes. Many couples choose not to watch the ultrasound screen during the procedure; however, the heartbeats of the remaining fetuses are shown to the parents on ultrasound before they leave. There are other methods of doing this procedure that are not used as much today, such as inserting a needle through the mother's cervix or through her bladder instead of through her abdomen.

Following the procedure, the woman goes home to rest for a couple of days. Some women experience cramping or spotting or leak amniotic fluid. A follow-up ultrasound usually is done a day or so after the reduction procedure to confirm the death of the reduced fetuses and the heartbeats of those remaining. Over the following weeks and months of pregnancy, the reduced fetuses are absorbed into the tissues of the uterus. There is no visible evidence of reduction at the birth of the remaining babies; however, microscopic studies can show remnants of the reduced fetuses.

RISKS AND COMPLICATIONS

There are physical risks associated with this procedure, as well as residual effects on the remaining fetuses and pregnancy. Infection for the mother and remaining fetuses can occur. The risk of losing the entire pregnancy after reduction is about 6 to 7 percent. Generally, the chance for pregnancy loss after reduction increases with a high number of fetuses at the start of pregnancy. If there are connecting blood vessels in a shared placenta of identical twins, reduction of one fetus can be life threatening for the other. There is the possibility of reducing a normal fetus and leaving an abnormal one because reduction is often done before testing for abnormalities. Also, there are no guarantees that a reduced pregnancy will be problem free. Some studies have shown that, even with reduction, the likelihood of pregnancy complications remains high. For example, a woman with a quadruplet pregnancy reduced to twins still has a greater risk of delivering early than a woman with a nonreduced twin pregnancy. This is more likely when many fetuses are reduced. There is also evidence that the babies remaining after reduction tend to be smaller and have growth problems in pregnancy.

> When we first found out we were having quadruplets, we were so excited. Then our bubble burst. We heard about all the terrible consequences that could happen with early birth.

DECISION MAKING

Making a decision about whether reduction is in the best interest of babies and parents is difficult for all involved. The decision is complicated because many parents already have "fallen in love" with all of their babies. With early ultrasound exams, parents can see these tiny babies move and recognize their human characteristics. In one report, some couples chose not to reduce when they learned their babies were normal following early diagnostic chromosome studies.

Was I being unfair and selfish to try to carry all four babies?

If you are faced with multifetal pregnancy reduction, you must consider your personal ethics and religious beliefs. Making a decision that is against your beliefs, whether religious or moral, could have long-term effects. Women who have reduction often feel loss and grief at the time of the procedure and again at the birth of their remaining babies. Some women are still grieving and feeling guilty and sad years after reduction, even though they believed the procedure was needed. Fathers, too, feel deep sadness and loss. Seeing the surviving babies can be a constant reminder of the loss. As a couple, you should talk openly to one another about what you each believe, and how you might feel if you do or don't go ahead with reduction. Don't be afraid to admit sadness and grieve together.

> After our triplets were born, I had such depression. All I
> could think about was "that" baby [that had been reduced]
> and how I could possibly have done this. I love my babies so
> much, and I can't say if they would have been as healthy if
> we had not done the reduction, so my feelings are still very
> mixed. We wonder if we should tell the triplets when they
> are older that they had a brother or sister. Our family knows,
> but they don't talk about it.

Many couples feel they cannot discuss reduction with family or friends because they are afraid of being judged. Often they are alone in trying to reach a decision. Some parents come to feel there was a bias on the part of their care providers about reduction, while others have felt they were bombarded with statistics but were not given direction on how to come to a decision. It may be helpful to have a consultation with a perinatologist. As a specialist in high-risk pregnancy, a perinatologist has experience in caring for multiple pregnancies and can help you foresee possible outcomes. An important question to ask your doctor is, "Will you support us and our decision if we decide not to reduce?" Because this is a permanent decision, you need to know that you have support and that you are not being judged in either case. It may be helpful to talk with parents who chose reduction as well as those who chose not to reduce. Also you can seek advice from your religious advisor or a psychological counselor. You may want to do some research on your own so you can see the studies yourself without feeling misled or pressured.

> We wanted someone to tell us what to do, but there was no one—*we* had to decide.

Infertility experts struggle with ways to help couples conceive healthy children without increasing physical risks and creating ethical dilemmas. Obviously, it would be best when advances in infertility technology can reach the point where couples do not have to make such decisions. However, you must do what you believe to be right for you and your babies using today's technologies, regardless of outside influences.

• • •

PART III

The Joys and Challenges of Giving Birth to Multiples

After all the waiting and worrying during pregnancy, it is often a relief when the time finally comes for your babies to be born. But your work isn't over. There is much ahead for you and your babies, whether they are born vaginally or by cesarean delivery.

Although giving birth is timeless—a natural process experienced by nearly all women—it may be a new experience for you. Moreover, interventions are usually needed to manage a multiple birth. So it is important to understand your options. Many women find that having a birth plan helps them communicate personal preferences to the health care team. A birth plan also helps women prepare for possible changing situations. Whether the birth plan is written or verbal, it must be flexible. If you are mentally and emotionally locked into a specific plan, you'll be disappointed if that plan doesn't work out. A sample birth plan for multiples can be found in Appendix C.

In 1996, several national maternal-infant organizations formed the Coalition for Improving Maternity Services (CIMS) and developed recommendations for mother-friendly birth care. While the CIMS initiative focuses primarily on low-risk, uncomplicated births, its goals for mother-friendly care are good starting points for discussion about multiple births. You may want to use the following questions adapted from the CIMS initiative*:

---

*Used with permission of the Coalition for Improving Maternity Services.

- Who can be with me during labor and birth? Does this change if there are complications?
- What happens during a typical labor and birth of multiples in your hospital?
- How do you allow for differences in culture and beliefs?
- Can I move around or walk during labor with multiples?
- How do you help the nurses, doctors, midwives, and specialists work and communicate with each other?
- What procedures and interventions are necessary for my care during labor?
- How do you help mothers stay as comfortable as possible, and what are my pain relief options?
- What if my babies are born early, or have special problems?
- What is your position on circumcision?
- How do you help mothers who want to breastfeed their babies?

In addition to these questions, you should ask about your doctor's experience with delivery of multiples, and how various birth situations will be handled. You should also know how to contact your doctor and where to go when your labor begins. If possible, take a tour of the maternity area, including the neonatal intensive care unit to help you feel more familiar with your surroundings. The chapters in this part of the book give you more information on the preceding questions and describe the process of labor and what you might expect in both vaginal and cesarean deliveries of multiples.

Chapter Fourteen

Planning for the Birth of Your Babies

When the time comes to go to the hospital, your mind will be on a thousand different things. It is easy to become anxious and flustered. Take a deep breath and collect yourself. It helps to do some advanced planning—know what to take to the hospital as well as where to go and how to get there. This is the time to benefit from the help and support of others, including dads, other family and friends, and professionals such as a doula and the hospital staff. Knowing what comfort and pain relief measures are available also helps you prepare for labor and birth. You'll also want to learn how your babies will be delivered and where the birth will take place.

WHAT TO BRING TO THE HOSPITAL

Have your bags packed and ready before you enter your third trimester of pregnancy. With multiples, you never know when you'll need to go to the hospital. Even if it's just a temporary stay, it helps to have your personal belongings with you. Table 14.1 lists some of the items you'll need or want during your hospital stay.

Table 14.1.   Suggested Items for the Hospital Stay

- Insurance card
- Small amount of cash, coins for vending machines and phones
- Your own pillow
- Socks (feet often get cold in labor)
- Personal stereo with headphones, and CDs or tapes of favorite music
- Leave jewelry and valuables at home.
- Two nightgowns (nursing type, if breastfeeding)
- Two bras (nursing type if breastfeeding)
- Robe and slippers
- Underwear
- Shampoo and hair dryer
- Brush and comb
- Deodorant, toothpaste, and toothbrush
- Make-up
- Going-home clothes for yourself. Don't expect to jump back into your skinny jeans. Instead, bring some comfortable, loose-fitting clothes or a maternity outfit.
- Baby clothes. You'll want to have going-home outfits as well as some soft sleepers your babies can wear in the hospital. Be sure to prewash any baby clothes. If your babies are sick or premature and need intensive care, they will not be able to wear clothes at first. Once the babies "graduate" to a less-intensive care area, many hospitals encourage parents to provide gowns and sleepers.

You'll also want to have some other items ready to be taken to the hospital. A camera, video camera, and fresh batteries are essential, but be sure you know the hospital's policy on photography in labor and delivery. Because of litigation, many hospitals restrict the use of video cameras during delivery. As a courtesy, ask the nurse and doctor for permission if you are including them in the filming. And be sure you have purchased a car seat for each baby. Practice securing them in the car ahead of time, and know how to latch the buckles and straps.

Have the phone numbers for your doctor near each phone in your home. Some women program their doctor's number into their phone's speed dial memory. Make a list of all the people you want to notify and give it to a family member or friend. Then when your babies are born, you make just one call, and that person can notify everyone else. Have a map or directions to the hospital with your bags. Many expectant parents like to make a test drive to learn the best way and to find alternative routes in case traffic is heavy. Be sure you know which hospital entrance to use. Some hospitals have women in labor enter through the emergency room, while others have a special maternity entrance. Some even have valet parking.

SUPPORT IN LABOR AND DELIVERY

For most births today, having people you love at your side is routine. And you need people near you who make you feel safe and secure. But don't feel obligated to entertain family and friends during your labor or to have them attend your delivery. Having too many people with you can be tiring and stressful. It may be better to limit visitors and avoid the added stress if you have complications. Even if your labor is uncomplicated, this is a special time as a couple. If you don't want visitors and have a hard time telling them, ask your nurse to help.

Dad

Sharing the miracle of birth is something no father-to-be should miss, and being part of the birth of multiples is even more special. Yet the birth experience can demand that dad fill unfamiliar roles—labor coach, support system, and new father all at the same time. And he can feel quite lost in all of the technology sometimes needed for the birth of multiples. Not knowing what to do or how to help, dad might feel that he's just in the way when things become complicated. However, the father-to-be is often the one consistent individual in this experience. Shift changes bring new nurses and possibly even a different doctor, but your husband is often with you the entire time and has the advantage of knowing you better than anyone.

Ahead of time, you should talk about how much he wants to participate. Some men want to be involved in every aspect, while others get squeamish at the thought of an IV. If you attended childbirth classes together, he probably learned what to expect and ways to be supportive. Labor is a chance for him to support you and be your advocate, expressing your needs and interests if you can't. And it's a time to be together as you share this incredible experience. During labor, if things get hectic or complications come up, ask your labor nurse for suggestions about specific ways he can help.

> I don't know what I would have done without my dear husband. He was truly amazing. He did everything right, he knew exactly what to say and do for me. I can't even express in words how wonderful he has been through everything from my pregnancy right up to now.

If you are a single mother, or if your babies' father is unavailable, you can still find support from other delivery specialists.

Doula

In recent years, an old method of birth support has come back into use. Many women are using the services of a doula, who is a supportive female (other than a friend or loved one) professionally trained to provide labor support. A doula does not function as a nurse or midwife, but teams with your babies' father to help support you and suggest comfort measures in labor. Most doulas work with women who want an unmedicated birth experience, but they can be very helpful during complicated labors and cesarean births. Many doulas also provide postpartum assistance as well, helping with recovery, baby care, and breastfeeding. Costs of doula services vary with the area of the country and the type and amount of services they provide. Look for a doula that is certified by Doulas of North America (DONA). Table 14.2 lists some of the issues you should discuss during an interview.

Hospital Staff

Whether or not you have a doula or other support persons, you have support from your nurses. You also have the attention and care of many health professionals throughout your entire labor and birth. Because it can take a small army of personnel to provide the specialized care needed for the birth of multiples, many couples are quite surprised at the number of people who come in and out during labor and delivery. If you feel your labor room has a revolving door, speak to your labor nurse and/or your doctor. They can help coordinate the timing of procedures and limit the number of interruptions.

Table 14.2.   Questions for a Prospective Doula

- What training have you had?
- Tell me (us) about your experience with birth—personally and as a doula.
- May we meet with you to discuss our birth plans and the role you will play in supporting me (us) through childbirth?
- May we call you with questions or concerns before and after the birth?
- What care providers have you worked with? In what hospitals have you attended births?
- When do you try to join women in labor? Do you come to our home or meet us at the hospital?
- Do you meet with me (us) after the birth to review the labor and answer questions?
- Do you work with one or more backup doulas (for times when you aren't available)? May we meet them?
- What is your fee? Is any part of your fee refundable if you do not attend the birth?
- Can you provide references? (And be certain to check them.)

Used with permission from Doulas of North America

Along with the expectant parents, the following hospital personnel usually attend an uncomplicated vaginal delivery of twins:

- Obstetrician and/or certified nurse-midwife
- Anesthesiologist or nurse anesthetist
- One or two labor and delivery nurses
- Pediatric nurse for each baby

A certified nurse-midwife attending a twin delivery always works with an obstetrician who is immediately available in case an emergency cesarean needs to be performed. For higher-order multiples or when there are complications such as prematurity, more care providers are needed. Often, there are teams from the neonatal intensive care unit (NICU) with a nurse and respiratory therapist for each baby. Another obstetrician and additional nurses are on standby in case a cesarean delivery is needed.

More personnel are needed for a cesarean birth, including two surgeons. Usually these doctors are members of your obstetric practice, but others might be called in for an emergency delivery. A scrub nurse is positioned near the doctors to assist with instruments, and one or more labor and delivery nurses circulate around the room. An anesthesiologist and often an anesthesia assistant monitor your vital signs and make sure your anesthesia is working properly. A nursery team is there for each baby. Depending on the status of your babies, the team may have nurses, respiratory therapists, and a neonatologist or pediatrician.

With all the personnel, equipment, and technical interventions that can surround the delivery of multiples, it is important that you don't feel lost in the shuffle. Some hospitals designate one nurse to be at your side throughout your labor and birth to help answer your questions and communicate your needs. This primary care nurse is also your advocate with the other members of the team. If you feel more comfortable with a certain nurse, request to have that nurse as your primary caregiver.

COMFORT IN LABOR AND BIRTH

No matter how your babies are born, there will be discomforts before, during, and after delivery. Pain in labor and delivery can be managed in many ways. The overall goal is to help you manage your pain with as few ill-effects as possible for you and your babies.

Options for Pain Relief

There are nondrug comfort measures as well as a number of medications and anesthesia. All of these have advantages and disadvantages. Most nondrug methods of pain relief are without danger. However, these methods aren't helpful if they create anxiety. Medications and anesthesia are effective at relieving pain, but they have side effects for you and your babies. Because most medications freely cross the placentas, they can build up in fetal tissues. How they affect your babies depends on the amount and how close to the time of delivery they are given.

Your health and the health of your babies must be considered when choosing any method of pain relief. Even if nondrug comfort measures are working well, certain medications or anesthesia might become necessary. Ask about the risks and benefits of each technique and medication. You can also talk with an anesthesiologist about the various anesthesia options. Tables 14.3 and 14.4 list common options for both nonmedicated and medicated pain relief during labor.

Epidural Anesthesia

Epidural anesthesia is administered through a small catheter placed in the epidural space outside of the spinal canal. It is the most frequently used anesthesia for births of multiples, and it has several advantages. It provides excellent pain relief for labor and vaginal delivery and allows you to be awake for a cesarean birth. Epidural anesthesia also allows some relaxation of your uterus if a baby has to be turned or delivered breech. Narcotic medications can be

Table14.3. Nonmedicated Pain Relief

Method	When Used	How Used	Effects on Mother and Possible Risks	Effects on Babies and Possible Risks
Massage	Throughout labor.	Hands of labor support person to stroke back, arms, legs of mother.	Relaxation. Potential for dislodging a blood clot in legs.	No ill effects known.
Back rubs, hot or cold packs	Throughout labor.	Massage, ice or warm packs to the lower back area.	Pain relief directly on back.	No ill effects known.
Relaxation techniques	Throughout labor and after.	Focus, detect, and release tension.	Relaxation of muscles and mind.	No ill effects known.
Breathing techniques	Throughout labor.	Focus on breathing and counting.	Focus directed away from pain.	No ill effects known.
Warm shower or bath	Throughout labor (as long as able to walk).	Stand or sit in shower or bath. Direct shower head or spout to back.	Relaxation. Relief directly at area of pain.	No ill effects known.
Changing positions	Throughout labor (as long as position is safe for babies and mother).	Walking, rocking in a rocking chair, sitting on a birth ball, squatting, leaning.	Position changes can help relieve pressure. Upright positions are best. Avoid the back-lying position. Some positions not possible if cause pressure on babies' umbilical cords.	Gravity and movement can help get babies into correct position for birth.

Table 14.4. Medicated Pain Relief

Method	When Used	How Used	Effects on Mother and Possible Risks	Effects on Babies and Possible Risks
Sedatives	Early labor. Often used with long labor.	Given as pill or injection. Examples: Seconal, Nembutal	Sleep, rest. Can make mother disoriented.	Sleepy. Weak suck.
Tranquilizers	Early and active labor.	Given as pill or injection. Examples: Atarax, Largon, Phenergan. Compazine	Help relieve anxiety and tension. Many of these drugs also work to decrease nausea. Often given with analgesics.	Decreased tone and suck.
Analgesics	Active and transition labor, pushing.	Given as injection. Examples: Demerol, Stadol, Nubain. Fentanyl, Morphine	Helps relieve pain. Can cause dizziness, sleepiness, nausea. Cervix may relax and dilate faster with Demerol.	Decreased respirations. Weak suck. Neuro-behavioral changes for 2–4 days.
Local	At crowning or after delivery.	Injection of anesthetic into the mothers' perineum.	Numbs the local area for the episiotomy or its repair or to repair spontaneous tears.	None.
Pudendal block	Must be given before crowning.	Injection into pudendal nerves at back of vagina.	Relieves pain around the vagina and rectum.	Rare depressant effects with large dosage.

Continued on next page.

Table 14.4. Continued

Method	When Used	How Used	Effects on Mother and Possible Risks	Effects on Babies and Possible Risks
Epidural	Labor, usually given after active labor begins. Also for cesarean delivery.	Placement of thin epidural catheter into epidural space just outside spinal canal. Catheter stays in place through-out labor and sometimes postpartum. Medication often delivered through a pump.	Relieves pain. Helps with relaxation. Allows mother to be awake for cesarean birth. Helps relax uterus for turning the second baby or a breech extraction. Decreases blood pressure. Can slow labor if given too early. Can increase pushing time. Increased maternal temperature in labor. Possibility of spinal headache, allergic reaction, total anesthesia, neurologic injury.	Drop in mother's blood pressure may slow babies' heart rates. Decreased muscle tone and breastfeed-ing difficulties. Increased maternal temperature can cause babies to need blood tests to rule out infection.
Walking epidural, combination spinal/epidural	Labor and vaginal or cesarean birth.	Same as above but uses injection of analgesic medication into spinal fluid and/or epidural catheter.	Same as epidural. Pain relief without numbness. May be able to walk during labor. May have itching and nausea from analgesic.	See above.

Spinal block	Analgesic medications used in spinal for labor and vaginal delivery. Numbing medications for cesarean delivery.	Medication is injected into the spinal fluid.	Immediate numbing of lower body, inability to move legs. Effects last for several hours. Major adverse effect is spinal headache caused by decrease in amount of spinal fluid.	If mother's heart rate drops, possible decrease in oxygen to babies.
General anesthesia	Emergency cesarean delivery.	IV anesthesia and muscle relaxants. Mother must breathe through endotracheal tube.	Mother unconscious (put to sleep) for delivery. Risk of aspiration of stomach contents.	Only small amounts of muscle relaxants cross placentas, but babies are affected by general anesthesia.

given through the epidural catheter to provide pain relief with less numbness, allowing women to have better control of their legs in labor—hence the description "walking epidural." Epidural catheters can also be left in for a day or so to provide pain relief after delivery or used for later surgery such as a postpartum tubal ligation.

An anesthesiologist usually places epidurals, although in some hospitals, it is done by an obstetrician or a nurse anesthetist. For the procedure, you either sit up or lie on your side with your back curved out—a little hard to do with a big belly! Your lower back is cleaned with an antiseptic solution. Then a small amount of numbing medication is injected with a tiny needle into the skin over your lower spine. Most women say this is the worst part of the epidural because it burns and stings for about fifteen seconds. Once your skin is numbed, a larger needle is inserted between your spinal bones into the epidural space just outside the spinal cord. You feel some pressure and occasionally some tingling down one leg. A thin, flexible catheter is inserted through the needle and into the epidural space. Usually a test dose of medication is given. Then the needle is removed, and the catheter is taped in place and connected to a pump with medication. You feel the full effect of the epidural within about fifteen minutes. Depending on the medication, your legs begin to feel heavy and clumsy. After you feel the epidural's full effect, let your nurse and the anesthesiologist know if you think the dosage is too strong. The medication can be changed or turned down to allow you better control when you are pushing.

The most common side effects of epidural anesthesia are a drop in your blood pressure and a rise in your body temperature. If you do get a fever, there is no way to know whether it is caused by infection or if it is a side effect of the epidural, so your babies may need diagnostic blood tests after they are born. A small number of women develop a spinal headache after delivery if the epidural needle also penetrated into the spinal canal or if they had a combined spinal/epidural procedure. Spinal headaches occur when spinal fluid pressure decreases as spinal fluid leaks out of the hole made by the spinal or epidural needle. These headaches occur only when you sit up and go away immediately when you lie flat. Spinal headaches can be treated using another epidural to place a clot of your own blood over the hole in the spinal covering. This epidural blood patch stops the leaking of fluid and allows the spinal fluid pressure to rebuild. The headaches often disappear dramatically.

DELIVERY DECISIONS

Many factors come into play in deciding how multiples are delivered. When, where, and how depend on your health, the health of your babies, their size, the number of weeks gestation, whether or not you have had a baby before, and the position of the babies and placentas. You have probably heard that you are more likely to have a cesarean birth than a woman with just one baby. While the actual numbers vary depending on your doctor and the practices of your area, somewhere between 50 percent and 70 percent of women carrying twins and nearly all with higher-order multiples will have a cesarean delivery. Yet, a vaginal birth is possible for many women with twins and even some with triplets.

> I had the most wonderful birth experience. My twins were born vaginally and everything went so smoothly. My girls were sixteen minutes apart and were perfectly healthy at thirty-eight weeks. It was an experience I wish everyone could have. I cried, they cried, and so did the nurses and doctor.

Sometimes the plan for delivery is clear. For example, having a placenta previa or a presenting baby in a breech position almost guarantees a cesarean birth. But sometimes everything is tentative right up to the time of delivery. It is important to be flexible and open to a number of options and possible changes. Remember, no matter what happens, the goals for your delivery are healthy babies and a healthy mother.

> My delivery room expectations were higher than they should have been. I expected certain things to take place and they didn't. But I was so relieved just to see my twins.

When Should Multiples Be Born?

Finding the right window of time for delivery can be complex. In all decisions, the main focus is the well-being of mother and babies. Research has found that the majority of multiple birth babies appear to have lower risks of health problems and fetal death when they are born slightly earlier than singletons. As you learned in Chapter Ten, multiple birth placentas begin to age earlier in pregnancy than do singleton placentas. Because this aging can reduce placental function and increase the babies' risks, slightly earlier delivery may actually be best for some babies. For many pregnancies, the optimal times for delivery are at thirty-five to thirty-eight weeks with twins, thirty-four to thirty-five weeks with triplets, and thirty-one to thirty-three weeks with quadruplets. Careful monitoring is important as pregnancies get closer to their due dates to identify a need for a change in plans. If complications place the health of the babies or mother at risk, there may be no choice in the timing of delivery—the babies must be born, whether or not they are ready.

Where Should Multiples Be Born?

An in-hospital birth is the safest option for multiples. Birthing centers located outside hospitals only accept women with low-risk pregnancies. Many of these birth centers are not equipped for cesarean deliveries and do not have the trained personnel needed for a high-risk birth. Home birth is never a wise choice for multiples, even twins; the risks are too high.

Ideally, multiples should be delivered where there is specialized obstetric and newborn care for high-risk mothers and babies. There are three levels of perinatal care facilities: basic, specialty, and subspecialty. Basic care facilities are able to provide care for healthy mothers and babies but do not have advanced care capabilities in-house. Specialty care facilities can care for healthy mothers and babies as well as some high-risk mothers and preterm babies. Most have NICUs capable of caring for babies who weigh more than 1,500 grams at birth and are more than thirty-two weeks gestation. Subspecialty care facilities, often called tertiary care centers, provide comprehensive, intensive perinatal services for mothers and babies at all risk levels. In these centers, perinatologists and other specialists are immediately available around the clock. Most are regional medical centers or teaching hospitals.

The American Academy of Pediatrics (AAP) and the American College of Obstetricians and Gynecologists (ACOG) recommend transporting a mother before her delivery to another hospital for specialty or subspecialty care if appropriate services and staff are not available. Babies born to women transported before delivery have better survival rates and lower risks of long-term problems than those who are transported after birth. This practice also helps keep mother and babies together. But being transferred to another hospital, possibly one far from your home, is stressful. It may mean that you are isolated from your husband, other children, and family. Try to remember that this is a temporary measure to help give your babies the best possible start.

In most hospitals, women with multiples experience labor in a room called an LDR (labor/delivery/recovery) or LDRP (labor/delivery/recovery/postpartum). Women are usually moved to an operating room to complete pushing and for the actual births of the babies. This is because of the increased chance of needing a cesarean delivery. Some doctors and hospitals allow twins to deliver in an LDR or LDRP if the chance of complications is low. However, if a problem occurs, precious time could be lost moving to an operating room for cesarean delivery. Don't be dismayed if your delivery must take place in the operating area. The curtains and pretty wallpaper found in most birthing rooms aren't as important as your babies' well-being.

> Our priority upon learning that we were having twins became the quality of the NICU, not the hospital furnishings. So the choice of a hospital that has LDRPs with nice furnishings, as opposed to a hospital that moves you around during labor/delivery/postpartum and is furnished more like a traditional hospital, is not so important.

How Are Multiples Delivered?

The babies' positions in your uterus play a major role in deciding the method of delivery. Although they can change position at any time, even during labor, most twins are fairly well settled by about thirty-two to thirty-four weeks. They just don't have enough room to turn. Higher-order multiples' positions are set even earlier. It's important to have an ultrasound performed during labor to find out exactly how each baby is positioned. Figure 14.1, page 215, illustrates the three most common positions for twins.

Vertex/Vertex

In the most common position, vertex/vertex, both babies have their heads down in the uterus. At delivery, about 42 percent of twins are in this position. When there are no other complications, twins that are vertex/vertex can usually be born vaginally.

Vertex/Nonvertex

The second most common position, vertex/nonvertex (not head-down), can make the delivery decision a bit more complicated. About 26 percent of twins are vertex/breech (buttocks or feet first), and about 11 percent of twins are vertex/transverse (crossways). Usually, the presenting baby can be delivered vaginally with-

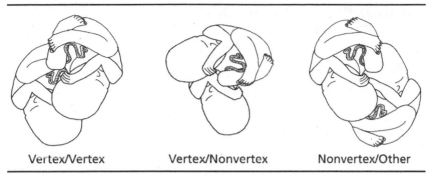

| Vertex/Vertex | Vertex/Nonvertex | Nonvertex/Other |

Figure 14.1   Common Fetal Positions for Twins

out problems. Several delivery options are possible when the second baby is nonvertex:

- Turn the baby to a head-down position (external cephalic version).
- Breech vaginal delivery
- Cesarean delivery for the nonvertex baby
- Cesarean delivery for both babies

You can read more about these options in Chapters Fifteen and Sixteen. Be sure to talk with your doctor as well as the other members of your obstetric care team to find out their experience and comfort levels with all of these procedures.

Nonvertex/Vertex or Nonvertex/Nonvertex

If the first baby is not in a vertex position, ACOG recommends delivery of both babies by cesarean. One reason is that the lack of room in the uterus makes turning the first baby inpossible. Another reason is the risk of a dangerous complication called "locking," when the first baby is breech and the second is vertex. This complication occurs when the babies' chins lock together as they enter the birth canal, preventing delivery of both babies. This is a life-threatening complication that can be avoided with cesarean birth.

Combined Vaginal/Cesarean Delivery

Some women are able to deliver the first baby vaginally, but the second must be delivered by cesarean. A combined vaginal/cesarean delivery is necessary if the remaining baby is in distress, or when there are complications such as placental abruption or cord prolapse. Although nearly every mother fears having this "double whammy," it only happens in about 3 to 4 percent of twin deliveries.

Higher-Order Multiples

Cesarean birth is usually the method of delivery for higher-order multiples. In the United States, over 90 percent of triplets and nearly all very high multiples are born by cesarean. However, a vaginal birth of triplets is possible in certain circumstances. Triplets can be in many different positions, but the most common combinations are vertex/breech/breech and vertex/vertex/breech. Most doctors have strict conditions for considering vaginal delivery of higher-order multiples. Usually, the babies must be at least thirty-three weeks gestation, the first baby in the vertex position, and all babies approximately the same weight. In some studies comparing vaginal and cesarean triplet deliveries, there do not appear to be any differences in the outcomes of the babies. However, other research has shown much higher risks, especially for the third-born baby in a vaginal delivery, including birth asphyxia and neonatal death.

Special Situations

Some conditions require a cesarean delivery even if your babies are in good positions for vaginal birth. Because of the very high risks for monoamniotic twins, cesarean delivery is usually recommended for these babies. Babies with birth defects and conjoined twins are nearly always delivered by cesarean. Very small babies who weigh less than 1,500 grams may be unable to withstand the stress of labor and are often delivered by cesarean. Women with active genital herpes lesions should deliver their babies by cesarean, so be sure to tell your doctor if you have a history of herpes. Even if you do not have a visible sore, you may have an active internal lesion that can be dangerous for babies born vaginally.

Emergency cesarean delivery is needed when the health of you or your babies is threatened. Situations that can require such urgent action include severe fetal distress, placental abruption, bleeding, eclampsia, and umbilical cord prolapse.

The next two chapters discuss what you may experience in a vaginal or cesarean birth. Keep an open mind about the possibility of having either type of delivery, and never allow the word "failure" to become a part of this experience. No matter how your babies are born, what really counts is helping them arrive safely into the world.

Chapter Fifteen

Labor and Vaginal Birth of Multiples

Many women with twins and even a few with triplets can have a vaginal delivery. If you and your babies are candidates for a vaginal birth, you must first go through the process of labor, the contraction work of your uterus that moves the babies into position for birth. Although it's a process that millions of women go through, it becomes unique when it is your own experience.

SIGNS OF LABOR

You might already be alert to the signs of labor simply because you have been watching for preterm labor throughout pregnancy. In fact, the signs of labor are much like those of preterm labor. Here are some of the signals that labor is near:

- Engagement occurs when the lowest baby's head drops down into your pelvis. With multiples, you may not notice a distinct change because the lowest baby often engages gradually during the last part of pregnancy.
- Nesting is a feeling or urge to get everything ready for your babies' "nest." Some women have a burst of energy and try

to clean everything at home from top to bottom. Don't overdo or you will tire yourself before labor even begins.

- Vaginal discharge usually increases, appearing clear or pink- or brown-tinged, with streaks of mucus and blood, called "bloody show." You might see the passing of your mucus plug, a thick clear/white glob that forms inside your cervix. In some women the plug passes gradually due to preterm contractions and cervical changes. Labor usually begins twenty-four to forty-eight hours after bloody show.

- Loose or frequent bowel movements accompanied by cramping are nature's way of helping your system get ready for labor and birth.

- Contractions increase and become stronger and more painful. They might be irregular at first, coming five minutes apart one time and then twenty minutes apart the next time. Even if they go away or seem to get better when you change positions, call your doctor.

- Leaking of watery fluid from your vagina (your "water breaks") is an important sign. This spontaneous, natural rupture of an amniotic sac may occur before labor begins, during labor, or not until delivery. Call your doctor at once and be prepared to go to the hospital if your water breaks. Be sure to tell your doctor the time your water broke, and describe its color. Amniotic fluid is normally clear and has a distinctive odor. If the fluid is brown or greenish, it usually means the baby has passed its first bowel movement, called *meconium*. Meconium in amniotic fluid can cause respiratory problems for babies if aspirated. Once your water breaks, there is no longer any protective barrier between that baby and bacteria in your vagina. You should not take a tub bath, wear a tampon, or have intercourse because of the risk of infection after your water breaks.

Call your doctor for specific instructions if you think you are in labor. Usually, you will be instructed to come to the hospital, even if your contractions are irregular. Unlike labor with a single-ton, when women often stay at home until their contractions are closer together or until their water breaks, labor with multiples needs to be followed closely. Complications are more likely, and monitoring can help identify them as soon as possible.

HOSPITAL ADMISSION

Depending on the hospital, you either go to a special maternity en-trance or to the emergency room. From there, you are admitted to the labor and delivery unit. Your husband usually needs to go to the admitting office to sign papers. This may take some time, but you're busy getting settled in labor and delivery. Some hospi-tals allow you to preregister, which helps streamline the admission process.

In the labor and delivery unit, nurses take your pulse and breathing rates, measure your blood pressure, and hook up an elec-tronic fetal monitor to check the babies' heart rates and your con-tractions. They also ask you about your pregnancy history. Often, your doctor has sent a brief overview of your pregnancy to the la-bor and delivery unit ahead of time, but be sure to let the nurses know about any recent problems. You then change into a hospital gown—a good idea because labor and birth can be messy and hos-pital gowns are easy to get on and off. You also have blood drawn and are asked to give a urine sample. A cervical exam is performed to find out how far in labor you are.

This is usually a good time to talk with your nurses about your birth plan and personal preferences for labor and delivery. For ex-ample, if you want to wait as long as possible before getting an epidural, let your nurses know ahead of time so they can work with you on breathing techniques and other coping measures. Be sure to ask about taking pictures. Some hospitals have strict policies for taking photographs and videotaping in labor and during deliv-ery. Also ask about having visitors and who can be with you for delivery. This policy may be different if you have a cesarean delivery. Be sure to let the nurses know in advance if you plan to breast-feed. They can help you feed your babies right after delivery, or arrange to have a breast pump ready if the babies cannot nurse.

PROCEDURES FOR THE BIRTH OF MULTIPLES

Because labor and birth with multiples can be complex, you may need certain procedures and interventions that seem high tech. Don't be frightened or intimidated by these. Their use does not necessarily mean something has gone wrong. Although some procedures are merely routine and may not be essential, others are preventive or are used to gain more information to help make decisions about your care. Learn about each procedure or technology, and talk with your doctor to find out which ones might be necessary and which ones aren't. Ask for explanations if you don't understand why a certain procedure is needed.

Enema
A large enema was once a routine procedure in early labor to help empty a woman's bowels and stimulate contractions. Today, most hospitals no longer use enemas routinely. However, a small enema such as a Fleet is helpful if you are constipated or your bowels are full. Although many women worry that they will pass a bowel movement while pushing, this is not something to be embarrassed about. It is a natural part of the birth process. Never use an enema without checking first with your doctor.

Shave Prep
Like enemas, shaving pubic hair used to be a routine procedure for laboring women. When studies found that pubic hair did not contribute to infection in vaginal deliveries, most care providers

stopped shaving. Occasionally, long hair around the vaginal opening may need to be trimmed for a vaginal delivery. Because a cesarean delivery is a sterile surgical procedure, clipping or shaving the hair on the upper part of your pubic area is necessary.

Antacids

Because of the increased chance of needing a cesarean delivery, you'll probably be given a special antacid during labor and before a cesarean delivery. Usually, a clear, citrus-flavored antacid such as sodium bicitrate is given about every six hours during labor to help prevent damage to your lungs in case you aspirate very acidic stomach fluids.

Intravenous Line/Fluids

Most women with multiples will have an intravenous line (IV) started when they are admitted to labor and delivery. IV fluids help prevent dehydration and are also given when an epidural anesthesia is used because of the side effect of low blood pressure. Medications such as Pitocin and analgesics can be given through the IV. An IV is also needed because of the greater chance of a cesarean birth and the possible need for a blood transfusion.

Fetal Heart Monitor

The rates and rhythms of fetal heartbeats are monitored to see how your babies are reacting to labor. Babies' heart rates can be monitored externally by placing transducers on your abdomen over the babies. Their heart rate patterns show on an electronic screen and print out on paper. Once your cervix dilates and the amniotic sac is ruptured, an internal fetal monitor (spiral electrode) can be placed directly on the scalp of the first baby. This gives a very clear reading of that baby's heart rate. External monitors continue to monitor the heartbeats of the other babies. Some monitoring equipment can only trace one baby per machine, while others can trace two or three fetal heart rates on the same device. You must stay in bed during monitoring, except for going to the bathroom. Intermittent monitoring, which only records fetal heartbeats for a few minutes each hour, is sometimes used with uncomplicated singleton pregnancies. Because of the higher risks with multiples, most doctors feel continuous fetal monitoring is safest.

Tocotransducer

At the same time the babies' heart rates are being traced, your uterine contractions are monitored using a *tocotransducer* placed on your abdomen over the fundus (upper part of the uterus). The monitor prints out patterns that show the length, frequency, and relative strength of contractions along with the fetal heart rates.

Intrauterine Pressure Catheter

This flexible catheter is inserted into your vagina through the cervical opening and into your uterus. The *intrauterine pressure catheter* (*IUPC*) has a transducer located in its tip to detect the strength of contractions. Another type of intrauterine catheter infuses sterile fluids into the uterus, which can increase low amniotic fluid levels, deliver antibiotics, or dilute thick meconium in the amniotic fluid. You must stay in bed with an IUPC.

Fetal Oxygen Saturation Monitor

This is a new technique approved in 2000 by the Federal Drug Administration (FDA). The *fetal oxygen saturation* (*FSaO$_2$*) *monitor* directly measures a baby's blood oxygen levels before birth. Fetal heart rate monitoring can only tell indirectly about fetal well-being because a baby's heart rate changes after blood oxygen levels decrease. In contrast, FSaO$_2$ monitoring can detect a drop in blood oxygen before the heart rate begins to slow. An FSaO$_2$ monitor measures oxygen using a sensor that is inserted into the uterus in a way similar to the IUPC. The sensor is placed against the presenting baby's cheek or temple. The other end of the sensor is connected to the monitor, where the reading is displayed. Once the first baby is delivered, it may or may not be possible to use the FSaO$_2$ monitor with the next baby.

Ultrasound

During labor, ultrasound is helpful in learning the position of each baby, the amount of amniotic fluid, and the location of the placentas and umbilical cords. Once the first baby is delivered vaginally, ultrasound monitors the second baby until birth. If the second baby needs to be turned or delivered breech, ultrasound helps guide the doctor in moving the baby into the right position.

Forceps

Forceps are long, spoon-shaped tongs that are placed along each side of the baby's head to assist with delivery. In years past, forceps were used to deliver babies in distress or change abnormal fetal positions because cesarean delivery was considered too great a risk. A complicated forceps delivery sometimes resulted in injury to the baby as well as the mother. Today, epidural anesthesia has improved the safety of cesarean delivery, so certain forceps deliveries are not necessary. Low or outlet forceps are still frequently used today, but these have much lower risks than other types. Low forceps are used when a baby needs help descending past the mother's pubic bone and out the birth canal. The doctor guides the baby's head using the forceps while the mother pushes. Forceps are more likely with epidural anesthesia because it can decrease pushing effectiveness. Talk with your doctors about the use of forceps and their experience with them.

Vacuum-Assisted Delivery

Another method to aid delivery is called *vacuum-assisted delivery*. The vacuum device has a soft, molded cup that is placed on the presenting baby's head and attached to a suction pump. Suction is applied to help move the baby down through the pelvis. In 1998, the FDA issued a warning about use of vacuum-assisted delivery devices. The advisory indicated that improper use of this device places babies at risk for serious complications, including death due to subgaleal hematoma and intracranial hemorrhage (bleeding inside the skull). Because of these risks, It's a good idea to talk with your doctors about their use of these devices and their experiences with vacuum-assisted delivery.

Episiotomy

An *episiotomy* is a surgical incision made at the bottom of the vagina to enlarge the opening for the birth of a baby. Although episiotomies are often done routinely, they are not always necessary. An episiotomy can help if your baby is in distress and must be delivered quickly, a forceps or breech delivery is required, or your baby is large enough to cause tearing. You might need an episiotomy to deliver a fragile preterm baby because the procedure decreases the pressure on the baby's head from your perineum (area from vagina to rectum). An episiotomy is done just as your baby's head begins to stretch your perineum. The incision is usually straight down or slightly to the side and is about one-half to one inch long. If you have an epidural, you will not feel the incision being made. With an unmedicated birth, you have a sort of "natural anesthesia" caused by the stretching of the perineum. Placing stitches to repair an episiotomy after delivery requires a local anesthetic if you have not received any other anesthesia.

Urinary Catheter

This is a tube inserted through the urethra and into the bladder to drain urine. With epidural anesthesia, you usually are catheterized several times during labor because you lose the sensation and muscle control needed to urinate. When your bladder gets full, the catheter is inserted, the urine is drained, and then the catheter is removed. During cesarean delivery, the catheter stays in to keep the bladder empty so it does not get in the way during surgery. The catheter is removed once you can get up and walk to the bathroom, usually the day after surgery.

LABOR

Labor is the work of your uterus and the changes in your body as it prepares for the birth of your babies. These are the four stages of labor:

- Stage 1—onset of labor until complete cervical dilatation
- Stage 2—pushing and delivery of the babies
- Stage 3—delivery of the placentas
- Stage 4—the first hour of recovery

The progress and timing of labor through these four stages is called a *labor curve*. Labor curves of multiple pregnancies are often different from labor curves of singleton pregnancies. With twins, Stage 1 is often one to two hours shorter. This reduction can be a result of multiples being smaller or preterm labor, which can cause early cervical dilatation and effacement. About half of women with multiples have already dilated 3 centimeters when they go to the hospital in labor. For a first pregnancy, expect Stage 1 to last about eight to ten hours. Stage 2 is usually longer with multiples because more than one baby must be pushed out and delivered. If you have had a vaginal birth before, your labor will likely be shorter. Remember, every labor is different, so don't watch the clock too closely and try not to let yourself get locked into rigid time frames.

Your progress in labor is evaluated using several factors:

- *Dilatation* refers to how wide your cervix opens and is measured in centimeters, from 0 to 10 centimeters.
- *Effacement* refers to the thickness and length of your cervix and is expressed as a percentage. For example, a cervix that is shortened to half its normal length and thickness is said to be 50 percent effaced.
- *Station* refers to the location of the lowest baby's head compared to the bones of your pelvis. Station is measured

from minus four to plus four, with zero station being midway through the birth canal.

Stage 1—Onset Until Complete Cervical Dilatation

During this stage of labor, you have a nurse with you nearly all the time. In most hospitals, your nurse examines your cervix, monitors your babies' heart rates, and keeps you informed about what is happening. Your doctor checks in regularly for updates on your progress and to perform any necessary exams and procedures. Most doctors stay with you once you are close to the time of delivery.

Early Labor—Dilatation from 0 to 3 Centimeters

Early labor is the easiest time for most women. You are likely to feel only mild discomfort with contractions and be excited and talkative during this time. Because of the increased risk for cesarean delivery with multiples, you may not be allowed to drink or eat during labor. Ice chips are usually permitted. Early labor contractions usually last thirty to forty-five seconds and are irregular at first. The early phase of labor for first pregnancies lasts about six to eight hours. However, if you already have some cervical changes or if you have had a prior vaginal birth, the time may be less.

Active Labor—Dilatation from 4 to 7 Centimeters

This stage usually lasts about three to four hours. Contractions get stronger, often lasting forty-five seconds to one minute, and become more regular. Women often become very focused on labor and involved in the medical aspects during this time. Epidural anesthesia can usually be started once your cervix is at least 3 to 4 centimeters dilated or your contractions are regular. Your doctor may perform an amniotomy (breaking the amniotic sac) of the presenting baby if there is a need to see the color of the amniotic fluid or if more accurate fetal monitoring is needed. To do this, the doctor uses special plastic hook to make a hole in the amniotic membrane. This is painless, but you can hear a pop and feel a gush of warm amniotic fluid flowing from your vagina. Your nurse changes the pads on your bed and makes you comfortable afterwards. Once the lowest baby's amniotic sac is ruptured and your cervix is dilated a few centimeters, a scalp electrode is often applied for internal fetal monitoring.

Your uterus can become so large and distended that it can't contract efficiently and can even stop contracting. A medication called Pitocin is often used to help create and strengthen contractions. Pitocin is a synthetic form of oxytocin, the natural contraction hormone produced by your pituitary gland. Pitocin is given through an IV and the amount is carefully controlled, usually with a pump. For some women an intrauterine pressure catheter helps measure the strength of contractions when Pitocin is used. This helps determine the amount of medication using a more accurate assessment of uterine contractions.

The positions of the babies can also affect labor. If the presenting baby is not in the proper position to move down into the pelvis, there may not be enough pressure on the cervix to make it dilate. Sometimes, your position can be changed to help the baby move into a better position. If not, you might need a cesarean delivery.

About one-third of women experience back labor, when they feel their labor contractions and pain in their backs. This is due to the position of the babies. Usually, a baby faces toward your back. If a baby is facing forward instead, contractions cause the baby's head to press on nerves in your lower back. Back labor is hard, but changing your position or using pain relief measures can help with the discomfort. Stay off your back, and try leaning forward or lying on your side. Movement, such as rocking or swaying, can also help. Sometimes these techniques can also help the baby rotate. However, this may not work when other babies are crowding the space. Some practitioners use a technique called a sterile water block to relieve back labor pain. Tiny amounts of sterile water are injected under the skin at various points on the woman's back.

Transitional Labor—Dilation from 8 to 10 Centimeters

This is the most difficult part of labor, but it is usually the shortest, lasting only about an hour, or just a few contractions. During this time, your cervix dilates from 8 to 10 centimeters, or "complete." Transition contractions are often very intense (lasting sixty to ninety seconds), and occur as often as every two to three minutes. Many women experience nausea and vomiting during transition. Another common experience is hot or cold flashes or trembling limbs. It isn't clear why these "shakes" occur, but you might have them after birth as well. Your nurses are ready with warm blankets to help you cope with the shakes.

As the first baby moves further down into your pelvis, you will feel pressure in your rectum and the urge to push. You can experience this strong urge even with epidural anesthesia. When you feel the need to push, tell your nurse. If your cervix is completely dilated, you can begin pushing. If your cervix is not ready, you need to pant or blow with your contractions instead of pushing. This usually lasts just a few contractions until your cervix is ready. Transition is tough, and you need a lot of support, but it helps to know that the time to push is near.

> It was my second pregnancy, but I was shocked at how fast my labor went, the first 4 to 5 centimeters in less than an hour and a half. Forty-five minutes later I told the nurses, "I think I have to push." They quickly checked me again. I was fully dilated!

Stage 2—Pushing and Delivery of the Babies

Once your cervix is completely dilated (10 centimeters), you begin Stage 2 of labor—pushing and the birth of your babies. Pushing is a very gratifying part of labor because you now have more control and can actively participate in the birth process. If this is your first pregnancy, expect to push about one to two hours or more. Pushing time is usually less for women who have had a prior vaginal delivery. Because of its numbing effect, heavily dosed epidural anesthesia can make pushing more difficult. For this reason, your epidural dosage may need to be turned down or even off during pushing. If this is necessary, don't be anxious about feeling pain. It takes a while for the pain sensation to return. During that time, you might find you have more control of your pelvic area and can push better.

Gravity is an important force in the pushing process. Ask your nurses and doctor to help you move into an effective pushing position that is safe for your babies. Depending on the type of anesthesia, you can try sitting up, squatting, kneeling, or lying on your side, but avoid lying on your back. This is usually ineffective, and it can decrease the blood supply to your placentas. Some positions are not possible with multiples because there is a greater chance that one baby can compress another baby's umbilical cord. Your babies' heart rates are monitored carefully to make sure they are doing well through this second labor stage.

Push only with contractions or urges. As you bear down, picture in your mind the path that the baby must take through your pelvis and the birth canal. The baby's head must move down under the pubic bone and make a curve forward—a sort of J-shape. Avoid holding your breath for long periods. Some women find it easier to groan out loud as they push. You may feel totally exhausted with pushing, but most women get a second wind that renews their energy and determination.

Birth

Babies go through an amazing series of maneuvers as they make their way through the mother's pelvis and birth canal. As the first baby's head moves nearer to the vaginal opening, ask for a mirror so you can see the first glimpses of your baby as it crowns. What an incentive to push! Usually, the baby's head emerges facing toward your back. Then you see the baby's head turn to one side to allow the shoulders to pass through the widest part of your pelvis. The baby's nose and mouth are suctioned at this point or right after birth. The rest of the baby's body slips out easily after the shoulders.

You usually hear the beautiful music of your first baby's cries within a few moments of birth. Sometimes the first cries are strong and loud. Other times they are weaker, especially if your babies are premature. The umbilical cord is clamped in two places close to the baby and then cut between the clamps. Dad might want to cut the cord as his part in the birth. Let your nurse and doctor know ahead of time if he wants to do this.

The baby is usually dried, wrapped with warm blankets, and placed on your abdomen. Often a small knitted cap is placed on your baby because a newborn loses a significant amount of heat through its head. If all is well, you can hold your new baby. Try putting the baby directly against your bare skin, covered snugly with a blanket to keep away drafts, and your body heat will help keep the baby warm.

Often with multiples, the nursery team needs to do a thorough assessment for any problems before you can hold the baby. Sometimes a little suctioning or extra oxygen is all that is needed. Sick and premature babies often must to go to the NICU immediately after delivery. This can be upsetting, but try not to worry, and recognize that your babies are in good hands. Usually, you have a chance to see and touch them before the nursery team takes them to the NICU.

Immediately after delivery, each baby receives two identification bracelets: one for the wrist and one for the ankle. The bracelets are numbered and labeled with your name and the baby's sex, date, time of birth, and birth order—Baby A, B, C, and so on. These bracelets correspond to a bracelet you wear throughout your hospital stay. Your bracelet is used to check your identity when you go to the nursery or when your babies are brought to you. Some hospitals also provide a second adult band for dad.

The Second Baby

Once the neonatal team takes over the care of the first baby, all the attention of the obstetric team turns to the second baby. The extra space in your uterus gives the second baby room to move and turn, so the fetal heart monitor must be readjusted and the baby's position checked with ultrasound. If the second baby has moved to a nonvertex position, such as breech or transverse, it can change the plan for delivery. There are three possible options: two vaginal delivery techniques and cesarean delivery.

External cephalic version is a technique to turn the baby from a nonvertex position to a vertex position. Using her or his hands, the doctor pushes on the outside of the mother's abdomen, to rotate the baby's head forward and down into the pelvis. Once the baby is in a vertex position, the mother can begin pushing to deliver the baby vaginally.

Breech delivery is needed if the second baby is positioned with its buttocks or feet first. The baby's legs can be tucked under or extended straight in the breech position. A vaginal breech delivery is usually possible when there is not a large difference in the weight of the two babies, and when the second baby weighs more than 1,500 grams (3¼ pounds) and less than 3,600 grams (7½ pounds). The second baby is delivered buttocks first or feet first, often with the help of forceps. Another method of breech delivery is called breech extraction. This is often used with very small babies using the doctor's hand to support the baby's body and head through the birth canal.

Epidural anesthesia is usually recommended for version and breech deliveries. It is important for the mother's uterus to be relaxed for these procedures, and epidural anesthesia helps accomplish this. Also, these procedures are uncomfortable for the mother. Such deliveries should be done in an operating room so that the equipment and personnel are ready if an emergency cesarean is needed.

Both external cephalic version and breech delivery can be very effective, allowing the second twin to be born vaginally. However, they require special medical skills and monitoring. These procedures also involve risks that make an emergency cesarean delivery more likely. The umbilical cord of the second baby can prolapse (fall down) through the cervix or get compressed between the baby and the uterus, reducing blood flow and oxygen to the baby. Also, the placenta of the second baby may begin to prematurely separate (placental abruption) from the wall of the uterus, causing bleeding and reducing oxygen to the baby. There is also the chance of the second baby changing to a position that cannot be managed with a version or breech delivery.

If external cephalic version or breech delivery of the second baby is not possible, or if the baby is in distress, a cesarean birth may be necessary. This combined delivery is not very common, but does happen. Some doctors prefer cesarean delivery of both babies rather than attempting a version or breech delivery or having to do a combined vaginal and cesarean delivery. Be sure to talk with your doctor in advance about what is possible for you.

Time Between Births

Your uterus can become quiet for a while and your cervix may begin to close after the birth of the first baby. If contractions stop or are very slow, Pitocin is often used to help restart contractions. Once the second baby moves lower, the pressure helps to reopen your cervix. If you are delivering triplets, the third baby's birth is managed in a similar way. You must push each subsequent baby out, but it does not take as much time because the first baby paves the way for the others.

The average length of time between the births of babies in a vaginal delivery is between fifteen and thirty minutes. Many doctors feel that as long as the remaining babies are doing well, there is no reason to rush the delivery. However, monitoring the other babies is critically important because of the increased risks during this time. These risks include cord compression, cord prolapse (falling down through the cervix), and placental abruption (separating from the uterus). These situations can decrease the amount of oxygen going to the babies and increase the need for an emergency cesarean delivery.

> At thirty-seven and one-half weeks I went into labor on my own. Both of my babies were vertex and I was looking forward to a vaginal delivery. My membranes had ruptured and as I was sitting on the bedpan to empty my bladder, the first baby's cord was out. They immediately rushed me into the operating room and put me under general anesthesia. Within just minutes they had delivered my precious babies, both healthy. I can't imagine what might have happened if I had not been in a hospital with qualified, trained nurses and doctors.

Stage 3—Delivery of the Placentas

Once your babies are born, the placentas are ready to be delivered. You might be so busy with your new babies that you won't be aware when your placentas are delivered. Within about five to ten minutes of the birth of the last baby, the placentas begin to separate from the uterine wall. Often the doctor pulls gently on the umbilical cords to help the separation occur. Each placenta is examined to make sure no fragments are left inside. Sometimes it is necessary for the doctor to examine the inside of the uterus using his or her hand. This is not a comfortable procedure, but it's not painful if you have epidural anesthesia. Your placentas are usually be sent to the pathology department for examination. Questions about chorionicity can often be answered by microscopic examination of the placentas.

LABOR INDUCTION

If a woman does not go into labor on her own or testing shows that her babies' health warrants delivery, her labor may be induced. *Labor induction* can often "jumpstart" the natural labor process.

Depending on the readiness of the woman's cervix, labor can be induced several ways. Usually, a hormone called prostaglandin, that helps ripen the cervix, is applied directly to the cervix, given by mouth, or given by IV.

Because preterm contractions are so common in multiple pregnancy, a woman's cervix may already be ready for labor. Pitocin, a synthetic form of oxytocin, stimulates uterine contractions and can help trigger natural labor. Pitocin is given IV using a pump to carefully control the level of medication. Some women begin labor on their own, but because multiples can overstretch the uterus, contractions may be ineffective. Pitocin can also be used to increase the strength and frequency of contractions, called *labor augmentation*.

Another method of labor induction is *amniotomy*, the artificial rupture of the amniotic sac. This procedure may be used if the doctor needs to check the amniotic fluid for meconium, or if more accurate fetal monitoring is needed. Once the amniotic sac is ruptured, a fetal electrode can be applied directly to the head of the presenting baby.

Labor induction or augmentation may or may not be successful. Complications can include failed induction when the cervix does not ripen or dilate; uterine hyperstimulation; or umbilical cord prolapse when the cord passes through the cervix ahead of the baby. Cesarean delivery may be needed if induction is unsuccessful or there is fetal distress.

WHAT ABOUT VAGINAL BIRTH
AFTER CESAREAN?

Vaginal birth after cesarean (VBAC) is sometimes offered to women who have had a cesarean birth with a previous pregnancy. There is continuing debate over the use of VBAC with singleton pregnancy, and even more discussion over its use with multiple pregnancy.

The benefits of having a successful VBAC include fewer blood transfusions, fewer postpartum infections, shorter hospital stays, and possibly reduced costs when compared with a cesarean delivery. The major risk of VBAC is rupturing of the uterus—a life-threatening complication for both babies and mother. If this happens, babies can be injured or die from lack of oxygen before an emergency delivery can be completed. For some women, treatment for a uterine rupture is a hysterectomy. Infection in mother and babies is another possible complication of VBAC.

More research is needed to find out if VBAC is appropriate for twins and higher-order multiples; however, many doctors feel that the risks for uterine rupture in a VBAC are higher because the uterus is more distended with the added stress of more than one baby. Talk with your doctor about the pros and cons of VBAC and whether it is appropriate for you.

CORD BLOOD BANKING

Another option at birth that has come about in recent years is cord blood banking. This is the collection and storage of a baby's umbilical cord blood for future medical use. Blood that remains in the umbilical cord and placenta after birth is withdrawn using a syringe. The blood is then placed in special containers and shipped to a cord blood banking facility.

Cord blood banking is sometimes considered "biological insurance." This blood is rich in stem cells, which are special cells capable of developing into other types of immune system and blood-making cells. Stem cell transplantation is used in the treatment of certain types of cancer, including leukemia. Transplanted cells must very closely match the cancer patient's genetic makeup, and stem cells from his or her own cord blood is a 100 percent match. For identical twins, the match would also be 100 percent. There is also a high probability of a match for the mother and about a 50 percent chance of a match with a fraternal twin or other sibling. The likelihood of a person ever needing a stem cell transplant from cord blood ranges from 1 in 1,000 to 1 in 200,000.

Parents can choose to store their babies' cord blood for personal use or donate the blood to a public bank. Private cord blood banks charge a fee at the time of deposit as well as annual storage fees. Initial costs for private cord blood banking range from about $300 to more than $1,000, with yearly fees ranging from $50 to $100. Occasionally, medical insurance covers these costs when there is a known need for the family's use of stem cell transplantation. Public banks store cord blood at no cost to the donor, but the donor and family give up all rights to its use.

Currently, the American Academy of Pediatrics (AAP) considers cord blood banking investigational and does not recommend private banking of cord blood unless there is a family member with a current or potential need for stem cell transplantation. Also, the AAP does not recommend cord blood collection in complicated deliveries. If the cord is clamped too soon after birth to collect the blood, the baby might not receive enough placental blood and become anemic.

Talk with your doctor about cord blood banking. If you choose to bank or donate your babies' cord blood, you will need to register with a bank at the beginning of your third trimester. Many hospitals also require you to give written permission before you go into labor.

Chapter Sixteen
Cesarean Birth of Multiples

As many as half of twins and nearly all higher-order multiples are born by cesarean delivery. The need for a cesarean birth depends on your condition, your babies' conditions, or both. Sometimes you know in advance because of the babies' positions or because certain medical conditions make vaginal birth dangerous. Such planned births have the advantage of being conveniently scheduled and are without the anxiety of an emergency procedure. However, you should be prepared for the possibility of a cesarean birth even if you are a candidate for vaginal delivery. Cesarean delivery can become necessary after an unsuccessful labor, or because a complication develops during labor. But it doesn't have to be a scary experience. Being prepared for the possibility makes it easier if it does happen. You may feel a little disappointed if you aren't able to deliver your babies vaginally, but having a cesarean birth is not a failure. Don't think of cesarean birth as unnatural. Instead, think of it as just a different way to have your babies. Whatever way your babies are delivered, what's important is that they enter the world as safely as possible.

> I have a hard time saying "I gave birth" because it was surgery. But they were born healthy—and that's really all that matters.

PREPARING FOR A
CESAREAN DELIVERY

Just as with a vaginal delivery, you need to go through the admission process at the hospital, but if your surgery is scheduled, your admission location might not be the same as it would be if you arrived at the hospital in the middle of the night in labor. Once the paperwork is done, your nurses take a brief history, check your vital signs, and draw blood. Because a blood transfusion is more likely with surgery, your blood must be typed and checked for antibodies that might make transfusion dangerous. You also need to sign a consent giving your permission for surgery and anesthesia. The consent forms also ask for permission to care for you as needed in an emergency.

In most hospitals, cesarean deliveries are performed in operating rooms in the labor and delivery area. Some hospitals use the regular operating rooms, which means you are transported to another area of the hospital. Once you are in the operating area, you are "prepped" for surgery. An IV is started in your arm and your lower abdomen near your pubic bone is shaved. This helps make the area as clean as possible and prevents your hair from being pulled by adhesive bandages after surgery. Your abdomen is cleaned with an antiseptic; sometimes this involves scrubbing the area for several minutes or simply "painting" on an antiseptic. A catheter is inserted to keep your bladder empty during surgery. Usually you can wear glasses, but you need to take out contact lenses, and possibly remove dentures and nail polish. (These are precautions for any surgery. Lenses and dentures can become dislodged and nail polish blocks the observation of oxygen levels that can be observed at your fingertips.)

Regional anesthesias such as an epidural or spinal block are usually recommended for cesarean birth because they allow you to be awake for the birth of your babies. Regional anesthesia provides complete loss of sensation from your breasts down. In an emergency, general anesthesia (making you unconscious) may be necessary. In some hospitals, you receive your anesthesia in a holding area before being moved to the operating room. Otherwise, the anesthesiologist puts in the epidural or spinal just before surgery begins. Don't worry about feeling pain. The anesthesiologist checks you carefully to make sure the anesthesia is at the right level and that you are comfortable. You may have one last ultrasound exam to verify the babies' locations before surgery.

IN THE OPERATING ROOM

For a cesarean delivery, you lie flat on a narrow operating table with belts secured across your legs to keep you from rolling off. Fetal monitors are kept on for as long as possible until the actual surgery is started. Each of your arms is extended to the side, and you have a blood pressure cuff, an IV, and a small clip over one finger to monitor your oxygen levels. Sterile paper or cloth coverings are draped over your abdomen and legs, and a small vertical screen is placed across your chest. This prevents you from viewing the actual surgery but allows you to see your babies as they are lifted out of your abdomen. Usually you are given a small amount of oxygen through a mask or short tubes called nasal cannula that fit inside your nostrils.

> It is a very strange thing to be so out of control—you're strapped down and can't see anything. You have to place your trust in others.

Your husband can be with you for most cesarean deliveries. He wears a surgical scrub suit, along with a hat, shoe covers, and a mask. Once he is dressed and everything is ready, he joins you in the operating room. Usually, he sits close to your head so he can tell you what is happening and comfort you. Before and during the surgery, he should stay seated and not touch any of the equipment or drapes, as this could contaminate the sterile area. Be sure to ask in advance about using cameras or video equipment during the procedure. Some hospitals have rules regarding their use because of electrical safety and liability issues.

The operating room is filled with equipment for you and your babies. It can be a little unsettling to look around the room and see so many medical devices, not mention the unfamiliar faces under hats and masks, and some with plastic shields over their faces. It's even hard to recognize people you know. And being the only one lying down can make you feel quite vulnerable. But it's reassuring to hear familiar voices of your doctors, nurses, and husband as they talk to you and each other throughout the surgery. Don't be afraid to talk to them and ask questions. You can also ask them to describe what is happening during surgery.

> I cried from the time I was brought into the operating room . . . the anesthesiologist had to keep wiping tears as they rolled into my ears! But I wasn't scared, they were tears of joy, tears of anticipation, and tears of relief. I was finally going to see my babies.

The Procedure

Once everyone is ready, things happen quickly. The skin incision for a cesarean is usually made low across the upper pubic area. This "bikini cut" is about 4 or 5 inches wide. The next major incision is on your uterus, usually made transverse (crosswise) across the lower part just above your cervix, as shown in Figure 16.1. This type of incision makes it possible to have a vaginal delivery with a future pregnancy, called a VBAC. Sometimes a transverse incision must be widened for a difficult delivery. In an emergency, the incision may need to be vertical. VBAC is not recommended after having a vertical incision because the uterus does not heal in a way to withstand labor contractions. If your babies are very preterm, a vertical incision may be needed because the lower uterus is not fully developed.

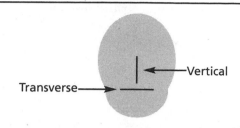

Figure 16.1   Cesarean Incisions

During your surgery, you feel no pain, but you do feel some tugging and pulling, similar to the sensation of having dental work done with your mouth numbed. You may feel heaviness or pressure as the doctors push on your abdomen to reposition a baby closer to the incision for delivery. Many women also feel some nausea during this time. So if you feel very ill, tell the anesthesiologist, and a dose of medicine in your IV can quickly relieve the nausea.

It only takes about five minutes or less from the time the first incision is made until your first baby is born. The doctor's hand helps the first baby through the opening. Usually just one minute apart, each baby is lifted out of your uterus, and the umbilical cord is clamped and cut. The baby is handed immediately to a nursery nurse or doctor and placed on a warming bed. You hear your babies' cries as they are dried and warmed. Just as with a vaginal delivery, they are evaluated and given any necessary oxygen or suction.

Who Is Who?

During your pregnancy, your babies are often identified by their positions in your uterus as seen on ultrasound. The presenting baby is labeled A, the next is B, and so on. At delivery, the babies are identified by the order in which they are born. The first-born is A, the next is B, and so on. The birth order is usually the same as the pregnancy order, but not always. For example, triplets labeled A, B, and C before birth may be delivered A first, then C, and then B. So be sure to ask which one came first, second, and so on.

It was really weird seeing these babies just appear. I could
hardly believe they were coming from me!

If all is well with your babies, each one is brought to you while
you are still on the operating table. Ask the anesthesiologist to help
you free one hand so you can touch your new babies.

Your doctor now begins the cesarean repair. The placentas
are removed first and the inside of your uterus is checked for any
remaining placental fragments. To inspect for bleeding, and to
examine the other tissues, your uterus is usually lifted through your
incision. Then the repair process begins. Each layer of uterus, muscle, tissue, and skin is sewn back together. The outside layer of
skin is closed using a buried suture stitch or with skin staples. The
entire procedure takes about forty-five minutes, and then you begin your recovery.

Chapter Seventeen

Your Recovery and Postpartum Care

Recovering from the birth of your babies involves more than the few short days you will be in the hospital. Recovery and postpartum is often called the fourth trimester—the final three months of your pregnancy experience.

Your health during pregnancy, the type of delivery, and any difficulties that occur postpartum can affect your body's return to its nonpregnant state. You need much of the nutritional stores built up during pregnancy for repair and healing, as well as for breastfeeding and producing milk. Pregnancy complications can influence your recovery. For example, limited activity or bed rest in pregnancy can cause your muscles to atrophy and sap your energy level, making it harder to regain your stamina. The type of delivery you had also affects your recovery. Vaginal birth is tiring and physically stressful—labor is a very descriptive word! After an uncomplicated vaginal delivery, it usually takes about two to three weeks to regain your strength. Cesarean delivery involves cutting and repair of tissues, so healing and a complete recovery usually takes a full six weeks. Blood loss after either type of delivery can lead to anemia and may make you feel drained and sluggish.

THE FIRST HOURS OF RECOVERY

In the first few hours after birth, your body makes major adjustments to no longer being pregnant. These include hormone changes, blood loss, and your body's response to the physical work of birth.

After a vaginal delivery, you may be moved back to the labor/delivery/recovery room; after a cesarean birth, you may go to a separate surgical recovery area. In either case, you are watched carefully for signs of *hemorrhage* (uncontrolled bleeding).

Hemorrhage is the most likely postpartum complication after a twin delivery and occurs in as many as one-third of mothers of higher-order multiples. When several placentas have detached, there are large wounds left in the uterus, and these wounds bleed. Your nurses monitor your blood pressure and heart rate and massage your uterus to keep it firm and contracted. Just as putting pressure on a cut stops bleeding, contracting of uterine muscles helps control the amount of blood loss from the placental sites. You are also given medications, such as Pitocin, methergine, or Hemabate, to help control bleeding. If your blood loss is excessive, you may need a blood transfusion. In rare situations, hemorrhage can occur due to abnormal blood clotting or because a placenta does not detach properly. If this happens, and the bleeding cannot be stopped, a hysterectomy (surgery to remove the uterus) may be necessary.

The immediate recovery period is the ideal time to start the breastfeeding process. You can breastfeed healthy babies or use a breast pump if they can't nurse in the first few hours after delivery. This early stimulation of your breasts makes your uterus contract and helps minimize bleeding. And by breastfeeding or pumping right away, your babies benefit from the first milk, called *colostrum,* which is rich in immunities. In addition, pumping or having a baby nurse at your breast helps your body begin the cycle of producing milk—so important to the success of breastfeeding.

Having a difficult delivery or other complications doesn't

mean you can't breastfeed or pump. While you're likely to be very tired from delivery or dazed from anesthesia, there are only rare situations when your condition prevents breastfeeding. If you want to breastfeed your babies, but are too weak to hold them on your own, your husband or nurse can help position them one at a time at your breast. Likewise, if you are unable to pump by yourself, there is no reason others can't start the pumping process on your behalf. For more information on breastfeeding and pumping, see Chapter Twenty-Two.

YOUR CARE IN THE HOSPITAL

Once your immediate recovery time is over, you begin the rest of your hospital stay. In hospitals with labor/delivery/recovery/postpartum rooms, you can remain in the same room. Otherwise, you are moved to a separate postpartum unit, often on a different floor. When possible, request a private room or a room without a roommate. You'll appreciate the extra space with your extra babies! Some hospitals even have suites or extra-large rooms with a sitting area and a sofa bed.

Nurses continue to check your vital signs (pulse, blood pressure, temperature) as well as your bleeding for the remainder of your hospital stay. You are still at risk for hemorrhage during this time, so they continue to check and massage your uterus to make sure it stays firm and contracted. This can be quite uncomfortable, and you may find it helpful to massage your uterus yourself. Ask your nurse to show you how.

As soon as any anesthesia wears off and you are stable, it is important to get up and move. Even after a cesarean delivery, many women are able to be up and walking within the first twelve hours. Getting out of bed the first time is tough, and you may feel like you are a hundred years old. Your nurses must help you get up the first few times, for safety reasons. Take it slowly. Start by sitting on the edge of your bed, and then stand and take a few steps. Most women find that relaxation and breathing techniques are helpful. But it gets easier each time you get up. Soon you are going back and forth to the bathroom, and even walking the hallways.

You receive instructions about the care of your perineum, called "peri-care." This is necessary for both vaginal and cesarean deliveries. It involves good handwashing and rinsing your perineum from front to back with plain water or an antiseptic solution. This process is tedious—you must do it every time you change a pad or go to the bathroom—but it's important to prevent infection and help with healing.

MANAGING PAIN AFTER BIRTH

Although few women deny there is pain with labor and birth, many are surprised at the amount of discomfort afterward. After a vaginal delivery, your perineum is swollen and tender from the tissues being stretched. You may also have stitches from the repair of an episiotomy or tear. Hemorrhoids can develop or worsen with pushing and birth. For all these discomforts, ice is the immediate treatment. Whether it is a fancy cold pack or simply a hospital glove filled with ice, cold helps reduce swelling and feels great! Over the next few days, try a sitz bath—sitting in a tub or basin with either warm or cold water—to relieve your discomfort. Some women find that directing a gentle flow with a shower massage also helps.

After a cesarean birth, you have a significant amount of pain. After all, you've just had major surgery. You may be quite alert or very groggy, depending on the type of anesthesia and medications you received. The effects of epidurals begin to fade in two to three hours and are usually gone completely by five or six hours. You might not feel much pain at first. However, do take the pain medication offered to you, as taking it in advance helps reduce the severity of the pain when it peaks.

There are several options for postpartum pain medication. After a vaginal delivery, you may be given ibuprofen (Advil or

Motrin), or another analgesic. After a cesarean delivery, stronger pain medications are needed. In some hospitals, your epidural is continued for a day or so, using narcotics or other medications in the epidural catheter for pain relief. Other hospitals use IV pain medications, sometimes using a pump with a dosing button you can press when you need more relief. Once you are over the initial severe pain, after about forty-eight hours, a pill form of pain medication is usually sufficient. But don't scrimp on your medication if you are hurting. You need to feel comfortable enough to move around, and you'll make a faster recovery in the long run.

Don't be afraid to take pain medication if you are breastfeeding or pumping. You can't enjoy your babies if you are in pain. Generally, only about 1 to 2 percent of the mother's dose of most medications is detectable in breast milk. Morphine and most narcotics are usually considered safe for nursing mothers.

OTHER DISCOMFORTS

You may have pain in places you don't expect. With surgery, and especially general anesthesia, your gastrointestinal tract goes into slow motion. Gas can build up in your abdomen causing pain that is sometimes worse than the other postpartum discomforts. Unfortunately, there isn't much to make the gas go away. Walking can help, and you should avoid gas-forming foods such as carbonated beverages and apple juice. Getting your gastrointestinal system working again also means having a bowel movement—something new mothers often dread because of hemorrhoids or stitches. Most routine postpartum orders include a stool-softening medication. You can also try an old standby, prune juice, but do not use laxatives or enemas without a doctor's order.

Another surprising discomfort is swelling. Especially after experiencing a long labor or receiving IV fluids, many women find their feet, ankles, and sometimes their whole legs become enormous with swelling. This can be painful and make it harder to move and walk. It can take several days to a week for your body to clear the extra fluid.

If you were on bed rest for an extended period during pregnancy, your body needs time to regain muscle strength and stamina. You'll find that you tire easily with simple tasks. Just getting out of bed and going to the bathroom can be exhausting. It's easy to become frustrated when your mind and emotions tell you to get up and going, but your body can't.

> I thought I would be able to jump out of bed as soon as my babies were born. Boy was I surprised. Just three weeks of bed rest really took it out of me. Once I realized I had to take it slow and pace myself, things were easier.

YOUR BODY ISN'T PREGNANT ANYMORE

> The first time I stood up after delivery, all the organs that had been squished tightly up in my chest for months suddenly plummeted to the bottom of the cavern in my stomach. My stomach muscles had separated from pregnancy, so everything just sort of spilled forward and I could feel them hanging and sloshing around.

Although your body is usually healed by about six weeks, it can take a full three months to completely return to your nonpregnant state. The following sections describe some of the changes your body makes as you recover from birth.

Uterus

After birth, your uterus continues to contract. These contractions, called after-pains, can be painful, too. You may feel these after-pains when breastfeeding or pumping, and they are especially noticeable if you have had a baby before. Postpartum contractions are part of a process called involution, helping your uterus to shrink back to its nonpregnant size. Each day, the size of your uterus decreases by about a finger's width. You may be able to see your feet for the first time in months! By six weeks, your uterus has returned to the size it was before pregnancy.

Bleeding and Vaginal Discharge

When placentas detach from the wall of the uterus, they leave an open wound. Right after birth, this wound bleeds, and you may pass large clots of blood. Many women also have increased bleeding during the second week after delivery as the uterus sloughs off tissue. As the healing process continues, the bleeding slows and changes to a dark reddish-brown color, then to a whitish-yellow color. This discharge, called *lochia,* drains from your uterus and into your vagina. Over the next three to six weeks, you need to wear sanitary pads, but do not use tampons.

Watch for a change in this discharge, increased bleeding, pain, fever, or a foul odor. Sometimes a small piece of placenta remains attached to the uterus and later detaches, causing bleeding. Another complication is an infection in the uterine lining, called *endometritis.* It is more likely after cesarean delivery and is the most common cause of postpartum fever. Endometritis can make you very sick and it must be treated with antibiotics. Be sure to call your doctor if you have concerns about the amount or character of your lochia, or if you have fever.

Breasts

Throughout pregnancy, your breasts were getting ready for this time. Your nipples and areolas (the darkened area around the nipple) have enlarged, and the milk ducts are filled with colostrum. The tiny bumps around the areola, called Montgomery glands, now secrete a protective substance that lubricates your nipple. Between the second and sixth day after delivery, your milk "comes in" and fills your breasts. This results from hormonal changes and the extra blood and lymphatic fluids your body produces to help with milk production. You know when your milk comes in because your breasts greatly increase in size and feel full and heavy. Continue breastfeeding each baby at least eight times each day. If you are pumping, this should continue regularly as well. You begin to see changes in the amount and color as the colostrum changes to pure breast milk.

Sometimes so much milk fills your breasts that they become engorged, and overfull breasts can become so hardened that babies cannot nurse. This can be very uncomfortable, and some women may even have a slight fever. To help your milk let down and relieve some of the pressure, place warm compresses on your breasts or take a hot shower. You may need to hand express some of the milk if you are so engorged that your babies cannot get a good latch to nurse. Sometimes the engorgement is so severe that you need to relieve the swelling with cold compresses. Place ice packs wrapped in a cloth inside your bra for about twenty to thirty minutes every two to three hours until the engorgement improves. Regular breastfeeding or pumping helps establish a milk production pattern and reduces further engorgement.

If you are not breastfeeding or pumping, you should minimize stimulation of your breasts, which can increase milk production. Be sure to wear a well-fitting bra at all times. Some women find that binding their chests and using ice packs helps when their milk comes in. Cold compresses also work to reduce milk production. Keep the compresses inside your bra, changing them every few hours until the swelling goes down, usually by seventy-two hours. Medications to "dry up" your milk are no longer recommended because of their adverse side effects.

You should also watch for signs of a breast infection called *mastitis*. This occurs when a blocked milk duct becomes inflamed and infected, causing breast tenderness and redness. Mothers with mastitis can also have flu-like symptoms with fever, chills, and aches. Antibiotics are needed to treat mastitis, and you should continue breastfeeding or pumping unless instructed otherwise by your doctor. Breast massage and warm compresses can help clear the blocked duct and relieve pain.

Circulation and Kidney Function

As your body begins to eliminate the extra fluid acquired during pregnancy, you begin to urinate frequently. Many women also lose fluid through sweating, sometimes to the point that their nightgowns or bed sheets are wet. Even though your body is eliminating fluid, you should continue to drink plenty of fluids to help keep your kidneys and urinary tract working smoothly. Urinary tract infections are more likely after prolonged pushing or difficult vaginal deliveries. Urinary catheters also increase the chances of infection. Signs of urinary tract infection include fever, difficulty urinating, passing only small amounts of urine, dark or concentrated urine, pain or burning, and a foul odor. Be sure to call your doctor if you are having any of these symptoms.

Weight Loss and Muscle Tone

With the birth of your babies, you automatically lose the weight of each baby, placentas, amniotic fluid, body fluids, and blood. This can add up to as much as 15 to 20 pounds with twins. Most women find they lose the remainder of their pregnancy weight slowly over the next few months. However, if you are breastfeeding or pumping, expect to retain about 5 to 10 pounds in breast tissue, breast milk, and fat stores.

Even with weight loss, your body may not go immediately back to its nonpregnant shape. Remember, it took your entire pregnancy to stretch your abdominal muscles and skin. Some women regain the tone of their skin and muscles without any problem. Others have extremely stretched and flabby "twin skin" despite exercise and weight loss. Diastasis recti, the separation of abdominal muscles, is a common problem for multiple birth mothers. This may or may not heal back together on its own. Do not begin any kind of abdominal crunches, sit ups, or leg lifts until your doctor has given you permission.

Most women can start the following postpartum exercises the day of delivery:

- Kegel exercises: Contract the muscles of your perineum and pelvic floor, and hold for twenty seconds. Do this after urinating and several times each day.
- Abdominal tightening: Tighten your abdominal muscles for five to ten seconds while breathing normally. Repeat several times a day. After a cesarean, you can also do this as you get up out of bed or sit down.
- Foot and leg exercises: Rotate your feet in circles and flex and stretch your calves by slowly pointing your toes up and down.

POSTPARTUM BLUES AND DEPRESSION

After delivery, you may find yourself on an emotional and physical roller coaster. You have had major hormonal shifts, and you may be physically exhausted from giving birth. All of the excitement and anticipation of the months of pregnancy have come to a sudden end, and motherhood has arrived, whether or not you are ready. With multiples, there is often additional stress. A difficult pregnancy or delivery can be physically and emotionally draining, and your babies may have arrived early or need special care. Your body's fluid volume drops by about 50 percent after having twins, and you are likely to be anemic from the demands of pregnancy and blood loss after delivery. With all these changes, it isn't surprising that your emotions are in turmoil.

> After my babies came home after three weeks in the NICU,
> I was so happy they were OK and that we were all finally

home together. That wore off way too soon. Don't get me wrong, I love my babies and feel truly blessed; but I became depressed. I guess it was because of the weeks on bed rest and quitting my job and staying home. I cried a lot and never went out. I felt guilty for even going to the grocery store. I was really mixed up. I realized with the advice of other mothers from our twins club that Daddy can and will handle them a few hours.

The care of two babies was all-consuming, and I was not prepared for it. There were days when I was angry, even resentful for having twins, exhausted and disillusioned all at once. I couldn't wait for them to sleep so I could be alone with no one wanting or needing me.

After delivering my twin boys, I realized I had challenges, both physical and emotional, that even my experiences with my first set of twins hadn't prepared me for. My steady, predictable life with my four-year-old daughters was forever changed with my new responsibilities, and I mourned that loss. I went through a teary-eyed postpartum depression that was enhanced by the physical strains of breastfeeding, healing from a c-section, and sleep deprivation.

Baby Blues

There can be differences in the amount and deepness of the emotional upset mothers experience. It is estimated that 80 percent of women experience some amount of *postpartum* or *baby blues*—the happy, weepy, emotional ups and downs that often follow a birth. Usually, the blues begin in the first few days after delivery and last a week or two. Postpartum blues are characterized by episodes of crying, moodiness, irritability, difficulty sleeping, and anxiety. Many women also have some ambivalent feelings about their new role and feel guilty for having negative thoughts. It isn't clear why the blues happen, but they can be a surprise to mothers who are unprepared. If you're having these feelings in the first few days or weeks, remember that it's a natural, common response to everything you have experienced.

Postpartum Depression

Although baby blues are very common, a few mothers may experience a deeper form of the blues called *postpartum depression*. This condition develops out of unresolved postpartum blues or occurs separately in later weeks or months. Postpartum depression is more intense than the blues. The emotional lows are lower and the physical symptoms are more extreme. A mother sometimes feels ashamed that she cannot cope and overwhelmed because her life is beyond her control. A worrisome sign is when she is no longer interested in the care of herself or her babies.

Postpartum depression is a serious problem that needs professional attention. When a mother is in trouble, she is unable to recognize or meet her needs. Her husband, other family members, and friends must take action on her behalf by getting prompt medical attention. Medication, attendance at postpartum depression support groups, and counseling are very effective treatments to help a mother regain her emotional strength and place in the family.

Here are some signs and symptoms of postpartum depression:

- Continuation of baby blues after two weeks, or strong feelings of depression and anger that begin to surface one to two months after childbirth.
- Feelings of sadness, depression, or hopelessness that increase and interfere with a mother's normal functioning.
- Uncontrollable crying or irritability.
- Lack of interest or inability to care for herself or her babies, or excessive worry and anxiety.
- Inability to sleep even when exhausted, or sleeping all the time.
- Changes in appetite, either increased or decreased.
- Anxiety or panic attacks that can include a fear of being alone with the babies.

- Fear of harming herself or her babies. These feelings are very scary, but they are almost never acted out.

BIRTH CONTROL

Although another pregnancy is probably the last thing on a woman's mind after delivery, it is important to think about birth control. Many women who needed infertility medications or technology such as in vitro fertilization to conceive often don't see a need for birth control. To their complete surprise, they may become pregnant "on their own." A pregnancy that closely follows another is hard on your body and is more likely to have complications. Moreover, with several babies to care for, an unplanned pregnancy can be difficult.

Various birth control options are available, and you can discuss them at your postpartum check-up. Don't rely completely on breastfeeding as a means of birth control; although it does help decrease the chances of pregnancy, it is not a dependable method. You may want to consider permanent birth control methods, such as a tubal ligation, if the birth of your multiples completes your family. This can usually be done at the same time as a cesarean delivery or one to two days after a vaginal delivery. You must sign a consent form for tubal ligation, and some couples are hesitant to undertake a permanent method of birth control if their babies are sick or very premature. This is understandable and you may want to wait until a later date to do this.

TIPS FOR COPING

Coping with the emotional roller coaster of new motherhood takes time and effort. Here are some ways to help you manage some of the difficulties you may face:

- Acknowledge that you will have emotional ups and downs. You don't have to apologize for being weepy or moody.
- Get as much rest as you possibly can. Wear your nightgown in the hospital and at home for the first week or so. It will be a good reminder for you and others of your need for rest.
- Set realistic expectations for your physical recovery. Especially after a cesarean delivery or long-term pregnancy bed rest, you need to give yourself plenty of time to regain your physical strength.
- Keep up your own nutrition by eating well and drinking plenty of fluids. Healthy eating is as important now as it was during pregnancy.
- Take everything a bit slower, and eliminate extra stress in your life. Don't feel you must entertain visitors in the hospital or at home.
- Have plenty of help arranged when you get home. Make sure everyone knows your only jobs are to feed your babies and yourself and to rest. Someone else must do all the other jobs. Learn to accept and ask for help.
- As soon as you are able, get out of the house for a few minutes each day. A simple walk to the mailbox or to meet your older children at the school bus stop can help you feel refreshed. Later, take a short drive in the car or go to a friend's house for a break. Just like being on bed rest, staying in the house can feel like jail time if you let it.
- Talk or meet with other mothers of multiples. Locate a multiples club, and hook up with a telephone pal. You'll find tremendous support from those who have "been there."

• • •

PART IV

The Joys and Challenges of Multiple Babies

Your babies are here! Does it seem like a dream? For many women, especially those who have had a difficult pregnancy and birth, the reality can take a while to sink in. It may be that you only had a brief glimpse of your babies before they were whisked off to the NICU. But even when your babies are in your arms, it is often hard to believe it has really, finally happened. And it's natural to feel a wide range of emotions—relief, anxiety, happiness, concern—as you begin to realize the incredible task ahead.

Much will be happening to all of you during your stay in the hospital. It will be hectic, wonderful, and frustrating. Just as your body undergoes tremendous physical changes after birth, your babies make major adjustments as well. The next chapters will cover the care of your babies in the hospital, including the special needs of sick and premature babies. For all of you, this is a time for more than just physical healing. It is also a process of emotional adjustment and the transition to parenthood.

> I already had two children and thought I knew what to expect, but twins . . . this was so different.

> For us, ignorance was bliss. We had no idea how hard taking care of newborn twins would be. But since we had nothing to compare our struggle to, we just plodded along with each new and exciting phase of development and found each one more fun than the last.

Chapter Eighteen

Well-Baby Care
in the Hospital

There are many physical and emotional challenges for your babies in the first few days of life. During their hospital stay, they undergo several necessary tests and procedures. At the same time, you are getting to know your babies and helping them adjust to their new world.

THE FIRST HOURS FOR YOUR BABIES

If your babies are healthy, they are usually able to stay with you after delivery. In many hospitals, the routine assessments and treatments for healthy newborns can be done right at your bedside. Usually, babies born by cesarean are observed in a transition nursery before they can come back to you in the recovery area or postpartum unit. Sick or premature babies go to the NICU.

> I got to see my babies for a couple of minutes. Even though they were thirty-six weeks, they had to be checked out in the transition nursery. They came to my room a couple of hours later.

In the first hours after birth, healthy babies go through a marvelous alert phase. They open their eyes, look around, suck their fists, and are ready to take their first feeding. Newborn babies have a keen instinct to find their mother's breasts. Observations of babies who were placed on their mothers' tummies right after birth show them scooting, rooting, searching, and finally, on their own, locating and attaching to mother's nipples. This behavior is not as likely when mothers have had heavily medicated deliveries or when babies are sick, but it is wonderful evidence of babies' instinctive needs. If your babies must go to a transition nursery temporarily after delivery, make sure the staff knows that you want them brought back as soon as they are stable.

After these first hours, babies switch into a sleepy phase. It is their way of recovering from the stimulation of birth. For about the next twelve hours, they are not easily roused to nurse or to waken. Between feedings, allow them to sleep in your arms or together in the same crib. This is a good time for you to rest and begin taking in everything that has happened. Most women are totally exhausted after the past day's events, but they have a hard time coming down off of this emotional "high."

NEWBORN APPEARANCE AND CHARACTERISTICS

Many parents are surprised at how their babies look—nothing at all like they had imagined. They are often covered in the wonderful goo of birth—blood, amniotic fluid, and vernix (a white, greasy protective coating). Newborn babies are not always pretty, but they are beautiful little beings to you. Table 18.1 lists the common characteristics of newborn babies; and because many multiples are born preterm, it includes a brief description of how premature babies can differ.

Table 18.1.   Physical Characteristics of Newborns

	Term Newborns	Premature Newborns
Head Shape	Elongated or cone-shaped from moulding by mother's birth canal. Overall swelling may be present as well as some bruising. Cesarean birth babies often have more rounded heads. Two fontanelles (soft spots) on top of head will close by about 6 months of age.	May not have moulding if very small. Skull is soft and will flatten somewhat from positioning.
Cephalhematoma	Collection of blood under scalp that appears as a bump in first few days. Often caused by bruising from pelvic bones or forceps.	Same.
Hair	May have full head of hair or be bald. May lose much of hair in first weeks.	Same, amount depends on how premature.
Eyes	Small hemorrhages (broken blood vessels) in whites of eyes due to pressure during delivery. May be cross-eyed because of immature eye muscles. Eyes are sensitive to light. May not produce tears when crying. Able to see best at distance of 8–10 inches. Eyes can be irritated and drain from eye medication given at birth.	Same. Extremely premature babies may not open eyes. Others are unable to protect eyes from lights and open them indiscriminately.
Ears	Ears are soft but flexible. Cartilage is present. Hearing sharpens in first few days. Sensitive to loud noises and comforted by soft voices. Able to recognize mother's voice.	Cartilage may not be fully developed. Ears are soft and fold easily. Hearing is sensitive to loud and constant environmental noises.

Continued on next page.

Table 18.1. Continued

	Term Newborns	Premature Newborns
Skin	Overall blotchiness or redness. Hands and feet appear blue from immature circulation. Lanugo (fine body hair) often present, and disappears in first few weeks. Milia (tiny whiteheads) often seen on nose, chin, and forehead are due to immature oil glands. Late gestational age babies may have dry, cracked skin, especially on hands and feet.	Skin more transparent due to insufficient fat stores. Very red, even bluish tint at times. May have lots of lanugo. Extremely premature babies may not have any lanugo.
Breasts	Breasts may be swollen, especially in girls, due to mother's hormones.	Breasts and nipples flat.
Genitals	Both boys' and girls' genitals appear swollen. Girls may have some clear to white secretions from vagina due to mother's hormones.	Genitals of both appear immature. Boys' scrotums are small and rounded, and testicles may not be descended or move in and out of scrotum. Girls' clitoris and labia are enlarged.
Sucking reflexes	Sucking may be strong. Able to coordinate sucking with swallowing and breathing. Stimulation of rooting reflex (turning to a stroked cheek) helps elicit opening of mouth for feeding.	No coordinated suck/swallow/breathe reflex until about 34 weeks gestation. Suck reflex alone is usually present (babies do this before birth as well).
Other body reflexes	Fingers curl around your finger when placed in babies' palm (grasp reflex). Little head control due to weak neck muscles. May be able to turn head from side to side. When startled, arms and legs thrown out with fingers splayed.	Many reflexes do not develop until late pregnancy. Premature babies may show varying degrees of each reflex. Generally less muscle tone, unable to make large body movements such as head turning.

NEWBORN PROCEDURES
AND TREATMENTS

Once your babies are born, their health is monitored in many ways. Certain medications and procedures are needed for all newborn babies. If your babies are healthy and stable, their weights, measurements, medications, and first baths can usually be done right at your bedside. In fact, some of these procedures can be delayed for the first hour, giving you a special time for attachment and bonding. Talk with your nurses about how to make the most of this time with your babies. If they are premature or need close attention, or were delivered by cesarean, these procedures and assessments are usually done in a special care nursery or NICU.

Apgar Score
The Apgar is a numerical scoring system developed nearly fifty years ago to help assess the status of a baby right after birth. Five areas of a baby's status are evaluated: color, heart rate, breathing rate, reflexes, and muscle tone. An Apgar score is assigned at both one and five minutes after birth. Out of a possible total score of ten, most healthy babies score between seven and nine at five minutes of age. A lower score means a baby needs immediate care and intervention.

Gestational Assessment
This is a method of evaluating a baby's physical maturity and comparing it with the length of the pregnancy. This assessment is especially helpful if the dates of a pregnancy are uncertain. For example, a very small baby may actually be more mature than it appears by size. Instead of being premature, the baby may be small for gestational age (SGA). This distinction is important in the kind of care babies receive and in anticipating any problems. The Dubowitz/Ballard Exam for Gestational Age evaluates reflexes, skin texture, motor function, and reflexes. The physical maturity

part of the exam is done in the first two hours of birth. The neuromuscular maturity exam is completed within twenty-four hours after delivery. Cranial ultrasound is sometimes used to look at the development of structures within the baby's brain and is another method of estimating gestational age.

INITIAL NEWBORN CARE

Babies' temperature, heart rate, and respiratory rate are all monitored carefully after delivery and throughout their hospital stay. In addition, your babies have a physical assessment to screen for any problems. The nursery team does the initial screening, and your pediatrician or the neonatologist at the hospital performs a complete physical examination of all body systems.

Vitamin K Injection
Newborn babies normally have low levels of vitamin K, an essential component of blood clotting produced by intestinal bacteria. Because of the risk of a serious bleeding problem called *hemorrhagic disease of the newborn* (*HDN*), most babies receive an injection of vitamin K. It is given in the upper thigh in the first few hours after birth.

Eye Prophylaxis
This is a medication given as drops or ointment in babies' eyes within one hour after birth. Eye prophylaxis is required by law to prevent infection from undetected gonorrhea or chlamydia infection in the mother's body. Antibiotic eye medications such as tetracycline or erythromycin are used in most hospitals. Another preparation called silver nitrate is sometimes use but is very irritating to babies' eyes.

Weighing
Babies are weighed shortly after birth and each day they are in the hospital. Most hospitals use the metric scale to report babies' weights, and it can be confusing for many in the United States who

are accustomed to pounds and ounces. You can use Table 18.2 to help you convert pounds and ounces to grams. For example, 4 pounds 3 ounces equals 1,899 grams.

Bathing

The first baby bath doesn't have to be given immediately. Babies must regain a normal temperature after delivery and be physically stable. And unless a baby is really messy, whole-body bathing may not be necessary. Simply wiping the face, head, and body with warm water on cotton sponges may be enough. Babies with lots of blood and meconium do need careful cleansing and drying if there are risks for infection with microorganisms such as hepatitis B, herpes simplex, and HIV.

Cord Care

When a baby's umbilical cord is cut at birth, a clamp is placed on the short end near the baby's abdomen. To prevent infection, an antimicrobial agent is often painted on the cord. Alcohol is sometimes used to help the cord stump dry and eventually detach, but it is probably not effective in preventing infection. Sometimes the cord is simply allowed to air dry.

Newborn Screening

Various screenings and tests are performed on newborn babies depending on state requirements. In all 50 states, all babies will have a blood test for two metabolic disorders: phenylketonuria (PKU) and hypothyroidism. Babies with PKU lack an essential enzyme to metabolize a specific protein. Early diagnosis and treatment of this disorder is important in preventing serious lifelong problems. Congenital hypothyroidism can occur when a baby does not make enough thyroid hormone. If untreated, hypothyroidism can lead to mental retardation, neurologic and growth problems, and deafness. It is easily treated with thyroid medication. Most metabolic screening tests cannot be performed until babies have received at least twenty-four hours of breast milk or formula. Your

Table 18.2. Converting Pounds and Ounces to Grams

Ounces	Pounds													
	0	1	2	3	4	5	6	7	8	9	10	11	12'	13
0	0	454	907	1361	1814	2268	2722	3175	3629	4082	4536	4990	5443	5897
1	28	482	936	1389	1843	2296	2750	3203	3657	4111	4564	5018	5471	5925
2	57	510	964	1417	1871	2325	2778	3232	3685	4139	4593	5046	5500	5953
3	85	539	992	1446	1899	2353	2807	3260	3714	4167	4621	5075	5528	5982
4	113	567	1021	1474	1928	2381	2835	3289	3742	4196	4649	5103	5557	6010
5	142	595	1049	1503	1956	2410	2863	3317	3770	4224	4678	5131	5585	6038
6	170	624	1077	1531	1984	2438	2892	3345	3799	4252	4706	5160	5613	6067
7	198	652	1106	1559	2013	2466	2920	3374	3827	4281	4734	5188	5642	6095
8	227	680	1134	1588	2041	2495	2948	3402	3856	4309	4763	5216	5670	6123
9	255	709	1162	1616	2070	2523	2977	3430	3884	4337	4791	5245	5698	6152
10	283	737	1191	1644	2098	2551	3005	3459	3912	4366	4819	5273	5727	6180
11	312	765	1219	1673	2126	2580	3033	3487	3941	4394	4848	5301	5755	6209
12	340	794	1247	1701	2155	2608	3062	3515	3969	4423	4876	5330	5783	6237
13	369	822	1276	1729	2183	2637	3090	3544	3997	4451	4904	5358	5812	6265
14	397	850	1304	1758	2211	2665	3118	3572	4026	4479	4933	5386	5840	6294
15	425	879	1332	1786	2240	2693	3147	3600	4054	4508	4961	5415	5868	6322

1 lb. = 453.59237 grams; 1 oz. = 28.349523 grams; 1000 grams = 1 Kg.

babies may need to be tested at a follow-up visit if you are discharged before this time.

Other tests are performed depending on state requirements and if your babies are at risk. For example, when parents carry the genetic code for sickle cell disease, a common inherited disorder in African Americans, their babies may be at risk for this problem.

Blood Glucose Testing

Blood glucose (sugar) testing is often needed for small or very large babies, babies of diabetic mothers, or when a baby shows signs of low blood glucose such as trembling or jitteriness. Early feeding or possibly IV glucose may be needed.

Hepatitis B Vaccine

Hepatitis B is a standard childhood vaccine. The first dose is given to newborn babies to help prevent the liver inflammation that can result from exposure to hepatitis B.

Circumcision

This is an elective surgical procedure to remove the foreskin of a male baby's penis. For centuries, circumcision has been performed as a cultural and religious tradition and in recent history as a routine procedure for many babies. In March 1999, the AAP issued recommendations for circumcision based on analysis of all available medical literature on circumcision. The recommendations state that circumcision is not essential to a child's well-being at birth, although it does have some potential medical benefits. The AAP encourages parents to discuss the benefits and risks of circumcision with their pediatrician and then make an informed decision about what is in the best interest of their child. The AAP policy also states that analgesia is safe and effective in reducing the pain associated with circumcision and should be provided for the procedure. Analgesic methods include EMLA cream (a topical mixture of local anesthetics), dorsal penile nerve block, and subcutaneous ring block. In most hospitals, obstetricians perform circumcisions. Discuss circumcision with your doctor to get accurate information about how the procedure is done and the pain relief options that are available. Premature babies may not be able to be circumcised until later if their health is unstable or if they are too small.

Hearing Screening

The Joint Committee on Infant Hearing endorses the goal of universal detection of infants with hearing loss as early as possible. All babies with hearing loss should be identified before three months of age and receive intervention by six months of age. Hearing tests can be easily performed on newborn babies and are standard practice in many hospitals.

Chapter Nineteen

Your Babies in Intensive Care

If your babies are born early or have any difficulties at birth, they will be cared for in a neonatal intensive care unit (NICU). This is a specialized nursery with trained staff and equipment for the care of sick and premature babies. Some hospitals call their NICU a high-risk or special care nursery. As many as 50 to 60 percent of multiple birth babies go to the NICU for some amount of care. Sometimes all babies are admitted, and sometimes just one needs intensive care for a specific problem.

> I had pregnancy diabetes and a cesarean at thirty-six weeks. Even though my twins weighed 5½ pounds each, they had to go to the NICU because of low blood sugar. As a nurse, I had worked in an NICU, but it was a different ball game when I saw *my* babies lying on those beds.

The NICU is an intimidating place. The sights and sounds can be upsetting, especially if you have never seen very sick or tiny babies. Many parents have found that taking a prenatal tour of their hospital's NICU is helpful. They say they feel more prepared if their babies need to be in the NICU and are reassured that this highly specialized care is available. And it helps to learn about the kind of care that is available and to understand the purpose and function of some of the technologies.

My husband and I did not make it a priority to tour the NICU and we should have. I guess I was just in denial.

My sons were born early, and I was rather naïve. I was shocked that their neonatologist wanted them in the special care nursery. I never even entertained the idea that they wouldn't come home with me.

WHO WILL CARE FOR YOUR BABIES?

Specially trained professionals care for sick or premature babies. These are some of the care providers in a typical NICU:

- Neonatologist: A pediatrician with additional training in the care of high risk newborns. Most NICUs are under the direction of a neonatologist who is on the medical school faculty or in a private practice hospital. If your hospital is a teaching facility, doctors-in-training such as neonatal fellows, residents, and interns also provide care. Other physician specialists may be called in as consultants for medical or surgical complications.
- Neonatal nurse: One or more nurses will provide your babies' direct care around the clock. In many hospitals, nurses must go through a special orientation and training to work in the NICU.
- Neonatal nurse practitioner: A registered nurse with additional education in the care and management of sick and premature babies. They are trained to perform certain specialized procedures.
- Case manager: Often a registered nurse, the case manager helps coordinate babies' care among the various care providers. Case managers often help plan for babies' dis-

charges and coordinate services with social workers and home health agencies.

- Respiratory technician: Therapists trained to assist in the care of babies with breathing problems using respiratory equipment, such as ventilators and oxygen systems.
- Occupational therapists: Professionals trained in managing and providing developmental care for sick and premature babies. Many have Neonatal Individualized Developmental Care Assessment Program (NIDCAP) training. See Chapter Twenty for more information about developmental care.
- Certified lactation consultant: Specially trained and certified to help women with breastfeeding. Some large NICUs have lactation consultants who work exclusively with families whose babies are in intensive care. They can assist with pumping and storage of breast milk and with breastfeeding when babies are ready.
- Social worker: Help families with nonhealth-related concerns, such as finding lodging near the hospital, transportation, and accessing governmental and community services such as Social Security benefits. Social workers also provide emotional support and counseling.

HEALTH AND SURVIVAL OF PREMATURE BABIES

Premature babies are not simply small adults, nor are they small, full-term babies. As the word *premature* implies, they are born before many of their organ systems have completely matured and developed. And because their bodies are not completely able to function on their own, premature babies are more likely to require special care. In general, the earlier babies are born, the greater the chance of complications. Because of the tremendous technologic advances in the field of neonatology, babies now survive and have better long-term outcomes at earlier gestations.

Regardless of how early babies are born, the odds of survival depend on how healthy they are at birth, their birth weights, and how they respond to treatment. Their chances also greatly depend on the quality of neonatal care they receive. This is why it is important that premature babies are cared for in a hospital that has an NICU.

Survival statistics for premature babies vary from hospital to hospital, region to region, and country to country. The most premature babies, born before or at twenty-three weeks, are at the threshold of viability, meaning that in spite of the best treatment, survival is barely possible. Babies born at this gestation have only about a 10 to 30 percent chance of survival, and nearly all have significant long-term neurologic or developmental handicaps. Babies born after twenty-three weeks have much better chances. Every day means a 2 or 3 percent improvement in the odds for these tiny babies. Those born at twenty-four to twenty-five weeks have between a 50 and 90 percent chance of surviving. With just one more week, at twenty-six weeks gestation, the chances of survival increase to between 70 and 90 percent. After thirty weeks, survival odds are usually greater than 95 percent.

There are also differences among individual babies. For example, in a set of premature boy/girl twins, the girl has a statistically better chance than the boy, all other things being equal. There are also variations in survival and outcomes with race. Given the same set of problems, African American premature babies generally tend to do better than white babies.

> My triplets were so different. My daughter was strong even
> though she was the smallest. The two boys were classic cases
> of WWM—"wimpy white males." They took longer to re-

spond to treatments and gained weight slower. They just couldn't get it together as fast as she did.

PHYSICAL NEEDS OF PREMATURE BABIES

Premature babies have basic needs for warmth, oxygenation, nourishment, and growth, as well as completing their development. Because babies no longer have the dark, confining, cushioned environment of the uterus, the NICU environment needs to be as similar as possible.

Warmth

Premature babies do not have adequate fat stores to stay warm. Unlike larger babies and those born at full term, wrapping them in blankets is not enough. Without constant warm air around them, premature babies easily become chilled and use up calories and oxygen they need for growth.

In the NICU, open beds are used for the sickest babies and those who need constant attention and care. The open top and sides of the bed allow quick access to the baby if a problem occurs. A radiant overhead heater keeps the baby warm and is regulated by a temperature monitor attached to the baby. Incubators or *isolettes* are beds designed as clear plastic boxes with arm openings for parents and care providers to reach through. They are used for babies who are more stable, such as premature babies who are not sick but cannot stay warm in a regular crib.

Oxygen

Inside your uterus, babies receive oxygen from your blood passed through the placentas. Their lungs are not ready to breathe oxygen until about thirty-four weeks gestation. Until this time, their lungs do not produce enough surfactant—a substance that allows lung tissues to expand and contract easily when breathing. When babies are born preterm, the lack of surfactant causes one of the most common complications—*respiratory distress syndrome* (*RDS*), also called hyaline membrane disease (HMD). RDS is treatable, often with the help of a mechanical ventilator or respirator. An endotracheal tube (ET tube) is placed through the baby's mouth or nose into the trachea and connected to a ventilator. These machines do the work of breathing for babies, allowing them to rest and strengthen. Additional oxygen is usually needed as well. Some babies with RDS need a high frequency ventilator, which delivers hundreds of tiny puffs of air very rapidly. Many babies also are helped by the use of artificial surfactant. This treatment helps shorten the amount of time spent on the ventilator.

Most cases of RDS get worse in the first few days but improve with treatment. Severe or long-term RDS can lead to the development of *bronchopulmonary dysplasia* (*BPD*), or chronic lung disease (CLD), in which the lung tissues become hardened and have difficulty moving air. Some babies with CLD require long-term care on ventilators and can require oxygen at home after discharge.

Another treatment used for respiratory care is *continuous positive airway pressure* (*CPAP*). Through a respiratory machine, a continuous flow of air helps small airways in the lungs stay open. CPAP can be given through an ET tube or small tubes placed in the baby's nose.

Some babies do not need help breathing but simply need a higher concentration of oxygen than is in normal room air (21 percent). These babies may need an oxygen hood or nasal prongs. Babies with respiratory problems will often have an oxygen monitor that reads the amount of blood oxygen through the skin. This small sensor is wrapped around a baby's toe or finger or placed on the abdomen and back. The reading is transmitted to a monitor. Blood oxygen levels help determine the need for extra oxygen or other respiratory care.

Babies with respiratory problems can have some areas in their lungs that are thinner and weaker than other areas. This makes them vulnerable to actually "blowing a hole" in their lungs. The lungs can collapse as air accumulates outside them; a condition called a *pneumothorax*. When this happens, chest tubes are inserted through the baby's side to remove the air surrounding the lung. This helps re-expand the lung.

Apnea is another common problem in premature babies. With apnea, breathing stops, causing the baby's heart rate to decrease (bradycardia). Because apnea is often caused by neurologic immaturity, these apnea and bradycardia (A&B) episodes are most common in babies born before thirty weeks gestation. Most babies grow out of A&B as their brain function matures. In the NICU, all premature babies are monitored with heart and respiratory monitors. Alarms sound when breathing and heart rates drop below a preset level. Most babies with apnea simply need gentle stimulation to help them "remember to breathe." Others may need medication or CPAP.

Nourishment

Premature babies have great needs for nourishment because their bodies are growing at a very fast rate. And until they reach about thirty-four weeks gestation, they cannot coordinate the suck/swallow/breathe mechanism needed to feed from the breast or bottle. This means that many premature babies first receive nourishment from IV fluids, then from milk through a feeding tube.

An umbilical artery or vein catheter is often used to deliver fluids and medications to premature babies. The catheter is inserted into blood vessels in the baby's umbilical cord stump. These catheters also allow blood to be drawn without having to stick the baby in other places. For very sick babies, additional IVs are needed and may be placed in the hands, feet, or scalp.

Milk feedings are usually delayed until a baby's respiratory status is stabilized. Poor oxygenation can contribute to the development of necrotizing enterocolitis (NEC), a serious intestinal problem discussed later in this chapter. The risk of NEC is linked to feedings, but it occurs less often when babies receive breast milk feedings. Usually, milk feedings begin very slowly through a feeding tube that goes from the baby's nose or mouth into the stomach.

Breast milk is the ideal food for premature babies because it contains immunities that help protect against infection. In the first month or so, preterm breast milk also has other benefits. It is higher in protein and fat and it also contains more of certain minerals than full-term milk. These components are especially important in brain and neurologic development. Another advantage of breast milk for premature babies is that the lactose is broken down and used more easily than the lactose in formula. Also, breast milk is used for energy and digested very efficiently. Because preterm breast milk does not provide sufficient calcium and phosphorus to meet the needs of some extremely premature babies, human milk fortifiers are sometimes added. Many premature babies also receive vitamin supplements because they have greater needs than full-term infants. Except in rare instances, breast milk (with fortification when necessary) is the best food for your babies.

Until your babies are able to breastfeed, you need to pump your breasts to provide milk for them. With multiple babies, you can share you milk among them. However, when one baby is much sicker than others, most parents and doctors recommend giving only breast milk to that baby and sharing any extra among the others, making up the difference with formula. Fresh breast milk is best, but if your babies are not yet ready for feedings, you can freeze your milk. Although cold temperatures, time, exposure to light, and reheating can alter some of the qualities of breast milk, these effects are minimal. Even banked donor breast milk, which is heat pasteurized, is far better than formula. Chapter Twenty-Two has more information on pumping breast milk and breastfeeding.

COMMON HEALTH PROBLEMS
OF PREMATURE BABIES

As discussed in the previous section, RDS is the most common complication in premature babies. About one-third of twins and a larger proportion of higher-order multiples develop RDS. Here are some of the other challenges for premature babies, their parents, and their health care providers.

Infection

Because premature babies are born before they receive many of the immunities from their mother, they are less able to fight infection. Although many infections—bacterial, viral, and fungal—can be treated with antibiotics and other medications, some strains of germs are very resistant to medications. Frequent and thorough hand washing is vital in infection control. NICU personnel do an initial scrub with antiseptic soap at the beginning of work and wash before and after handling a baby or equipment. Parents also need to do similar scrubs when they visit. Although your babies shared your uterus, they don't need to share any infections they might acquire in the hospital. Also be careful to wash your hands between babies. If you have a cold or other illness, including a fever blister or cold sore, be sure to tell the nurses and doctors. You may need to wear a mask or wait until you are better before being with your babies to protect them as much as possible.

Anemia

Anemia is quite common in premature babies. In the first few weeks, babies are unable to make lots of new red blood cells and the cells they do have break down quickly. Premature babies also need frequent blood tests, which further reduce the amount of red blood cells. Babies need a blood transfusion if anemia is severe.

Hyperbilirubinemia

High levels of *bilirubin,* a chemical that results from the breakdown of blood, can build up in the baby's body. This leads to *jaundice,* a yellow discoloration of the skin and eyes. Mild jaundice is common in full-term babies, but it is much more likely in premature babies. Because very high levels of bilirubin can cause brain damage, premature babies are treated using special lights that help the body eliminate bilirubin. Blood transfusions are sometimes needed for severe jaundice.

Patent Ductus Arteriosus

Patient ductus arteriosus (PDA) is a condition in which a fetal blood vessel connecting the main pulmonary artery of the lung and the aorta of the fetal heart does not close off at birth. This allows too much blood to flow to the baby's lungs and can lead to breathing problems and heart failure. About one-fourth of babies born at twenty-seven to twenty-nine weeks gestation and over half of babies born before twenty-seven weeks develop PDA. Diagnosis of PDA is made by echocardiography, which shows the actual shunting of blood flow. PDA is often successfully treated with a medication called indomethacin. However, if drug therapy fails, surgery may be required to close the ductus.

Retinopathy of Prematurity

With *retinopathy of prematurity (ROP)* there is scarring and abnormal growth of the blood vessels in the retina of a baby's eye. Although changes in oxygen levels can contribute to ROP, the cause is unknown. ROP occurs in about 14 percent of babies weighing 1,250 to 1,500 grams, and in over half of babies weighing less than 1,000 grams. Mild eye damage sometimes results in a baby needing to wear glasses. However, severe ROP can cause blindness. Premature babies need eye exams to monitor for ROP. There are new treatments being studied that have shown encouraging results.

Necrotizing Enterocolitis

Although the exact cause of *necrotizing enterocolitis* (*NEC*) is unknown, prematurity is the greatest risk factor. This is an inflammation that damages part of the baby's bowel. NEC appears to be associated with infection, feedings, and poor gastrointestinal blood flow. The onset of the disease is usually three to ten days after birth and lasts ten to fourteen days. Exclusive breast milk feedings and breast milk supplementation are associated with a lower incidence of NEC.

Intraventricular Hemorrhage (IVH)

Intraventricular hemorrhage (*IVH*) refers to bleeding into the fluid-filled cavities (ventricles) of the brain. It can also refer to bleeding around these ventricles. Such bleeding is common in premature babies because tiny blood vessels inside the brain are very fragile and can easily rupture. The smallest and sickest babies have the greatest risks for developing IVH. It is diagnosed using cranial ultrasound to view inside the brain through the fontanelles (soft spots). Almost all bleeding occurs in the first four or five days of life. IVH is classified from Grade I to Grade IV, with Grade IV being the most serious. Grades I and II are most common and do not usually cause brain injury or long-term problems. However, the risks are higher with Grades III and IV. Babies can have brain injury or develop *hydrocephalous,* a condition in which fluid cannot drain from the ventricles.

Periventricular Leukomalacia

With *periventricular leukomalacia* (*PVL*), a softening of the white matter of the brain occurs near the ventricles because of damage and death of brain tissue. It is not fully understood why PVL occurs, but it is thought to be related to poor blood flow in the baby's brain either during pregnancy, birth, or in the first few days of life. PVL is a serious complication. It is the most frequent identifiable cause of cerebral palsy in children born prematurely. The highest incidence appears to be in babies born at twenty-seven to thirty weeks gestation and in those who had infections or prolonged membrane rupture.

> My babies were so tiny, funny-colored and skinny when they were born at twenty-seven weeks. Even though it was clear they were at great risk, in some ways I submerged in my mind all the possible problems.

It can be distressing to read about these complications. No parents ever want such things to happen to their babies. But when problems occur, it is important to be knowledgeable and prepared. New technologies and treatments are developing every day, giving babies better chances for survival and healthy outcomes.

Chapter Twenty

Specialized Care for Babies

Medically managing sick and premature babies requires more than just physical care. With the growth of technology, the neonatal intensive care unit (NICU) environment has become increasingly stressful. Babies are exposed to bright lights, loud noises, painful or uncomfortable procedures, and hard surfaces—quite the opposite of the safe, dark, warm comfort of their mother's body.

It has been reported that the average NICU baby has more than 130 direct care providers per stay. During a twenty-four-hour period, the average NICU baby is handled over 80 times for medical purposes, disturbed more than 130 times for nonmedical reasons, and achieves and maintains only fifteen minutes of deep sleep. This continual stress and overstimulation can make it harder for babies to mature, develop, and get better.

DEVELOPMENTAL CARE

To counter these problems, many NICUs are adopting the Neonatal Individual Development Care Assessment Program (NIDCAP). The foundation of *developmental care* is the assessment of a baby's individual behavioral signals and ability to cope with excessive stimulation. Based on these evaluations, care providers change the environment and treatment strategies for that baby to reduce negative factors and provide greater opportunities for the baby's development. Treatments and procedures can either be done at less stressful times, or babies can be given individualized comfort measures and support to cope when stimulation is necessary.

Studies have found developmental care can have a great impact on a baby's health, including these benefits:

- Shorter hospital stays
- Fewer days on assisted ventilation
- Decreased rate of complications such as intraventricular hemorrhage, bronchopulmonary dysplasia, and retinopathy of prematurity
- Decreased need for sedation
- Faster weight gain
- Shortened time until direct breastfeeding
- Improved parent-infant bonding

Signs of Comfort and Stress

An important part of developmental care is recognizing babies' signals about what is comforting and what is stressful. As a parent, you are especially in tune with the nonverbal language of your babies. Table 20.1 outlines signals to watch for.

Modifying Babies' Care

Many aspects of babies' care can be changed to best meet their needs. Many NICUs already use developmental care that includes positioning, handling, nonnutritive sucking, and adapting the baby's environment. Other NICUs are beginning to implement these changes. Parents are encouraged to learn developmental care techniques and work with the NICU staff as they care for their babies.

Positioning

Positioning aids and soft bumpers can help a baby snuggle into a physically and emotionally comforting cocoon. Placed in positions that mimic the confining environment of the uterus, babies feel contained and secure. For example, when lying with arms and legs

Table 20.1.	Signs of Stress and Stability in the Newborn	
	Signs of Stress	*Signs of Stability*
Physiologic	Color changes	Stable color
	Change in breathing pattern	Regular breathing pattern
	Change in heart rate	Consistent heart rate
Motor	Extension or limpness of arms/legs	Flexed and/or tucked position
	Sagging cheeks and chin	Hands on face
	Hiccupping, gagging	Hand(s) to mouth or in mouth
	Yawning	Sucking and/or swallowing
	Looking away or hyperalertness	Smiling, relaxed brow
	Squirming	Even tone and posture
	Frantic, disorganized activity	Clear sleep states

spread in different directions, babies can feel vulnerable, stressed, and uncomfortable. A better position is with babies on their sides, with arms and legs closer to the center of their bodies, or on their tummies. (Note: This is a safe position in the NICU because babies are constantly monitored. At home, you should lay your babies on their backs to decrease the risk for SIDS.)

Body containment keeps babies' bodies snuggled within supportive boundaries, increasing feelings of security and self-control and decreasing stress. Babies who are contained tend to be calmer, require less medication, and gain weight more rapidly. Remember, these babies should still be in the uterus, so boundaries provide support similar to the mother's uterus, placenta, and abdominal walls.

Correct body positioning can also improve eye coordination and prevent postural deformities that can occur in premature babies. It is important for babies' bodies to be in proper alignment. Babies lying on their backs, with legs spread like a frog's, are not supported in the same plane as their bodies. Diapers that do not fit properly and are too big can also cause the frog-leg misalignment.

Handling

Excessive and frequent handling is physically and emotionally stressful for premature babies. One study found that 75 percent of low oxygen episodes happened during handling by nursery personnel. Frequent handling also disturbs sleep, which can lead to weight loss and stress. Handling of premature babies should be individualized and timed appropriately. Care providers can reduce a baby's stress when they are able to identify that baby's unique signals and respond appropriately, allow the baby to have undisturbed rest periods, and provide "time-outs" for the baby to reorganize during stressful procedures. When procedures such as drawing blood are necessary, a baby can be swaddled and given an appropriately sized pacifier to suck on for self-comforting. Other support includes keeping lights away from the baby's eyes, reducing noise and conversation around the bed, and holding and comforting the baby after the procedure. When possible, procedures should be delayed until a time when the baby is better able to handle the stress.

Nonnutritive sucking

Babies have a great need to suck, not just for nourishment, but for nonfood reasons as well. Before birth, each fetus sucks and swallows an average of one liter of amniotic fluid daily. This helps develop a coordinated sucking pattern by the time a baby is full term. Babies born prematurely miss out on this sucking practice.

The use of nonnutritive sucking has been well researched. Premature babies given pacifiers develop the most effective sucking patterns. But it is important to have a correctly sized and designed pacifier that allows the baby's mouth to develop and mature normally. If a pacifier is too big or too short, the baby learns abnormal tongue movements that cause difficulties later when the baby is learning to feed. Research has found that premature babies who are able to suck on such pacifiers during tube feedings have improved release of enzymes and hormone levels for gastrointestinal function, and improved insulin secretion and glucose utilization. Other reports found that babies who were allowed nonnutritive sucking during tube feedings were more successful at later breast and bottle feedings. Babies were also more contented and returned to sleep more easily.

An ideal place for nonnutritive sucking is at your breast. Initially, your babies can simply smell, touch, and nuzzle. Later they can progress to actual sucking when they are more mature and able to coordinate sucking and swallowing. Tube feedings can be timed to coincide with these sessions so that the babies begin to associate nourishment with the sucking and sensations at your breast. Eventually, the babies can progress to sucking for nourishment.

Light and Sound
Because lighting in most NICUs is continuous, bright, and fluorescent, there is growing concern about the consequences of long-term exposure for premature babies, who may spend weeks or months in an NICU. Researchers believe that continuous light can result in hormonal changes, variations in biological rhythms, and sleep deprivation during the NICU stay. Possible consequences of bright light in the NICU include disorganization of sleep and wake states, visual impairment, changes in growth hormones, biorhythm disruption, and breakdown of multivitamins in IV feeding solutions.

There are often no day/night patterns of light in the NICU. The impact of this is not fully known, although it may drain babies' limited energy and cause further stress. Many NICUs are now changing from twenty-four hours of bright fluorescent lights to a cycle of light and dark. Some have established mandatory nap times when all babies are undisturbed and the room is darkened for periods of time. Premature babies who have day/night patterns tend to sleep longer, feed more effectively, and gain weight faster. This also helps them synchronize their behavioral and hormonal rhythms with the external environment.

Noise is a major source of stress for premature babies. The vast amount of equipment in the NICU—including incubators, oxygen-monitoring devices, ventilators, intravenous (IV) pumps, monitor alarms, and telephones—causes much of the noise. Staff activities, including laughter, conversation, and the closing of doors, garbage lids, incubator ports, and drawers all add to the commotion. Sound levels in the NICU have been documented to range from 50 to 90 decibels, with peaks as high as 120 decibels. Excessive noise can damage delicate hearing structures and cause harmful effects including low oxygen, increased intracranial pressure, increased blood pressure, apnea, and bradycardia. Premature babies experience hearing loss at a rate of 13 percent compared with 2 percent in term infants. Testing is recommended for all babies before three months of age. Because of the risks for hearing problems, many NICUs are working to create quieter environments.

Steps You Can Take

Here are some things that you can do or ask the NICU staff to do to help decrease environmental stress for premature and sick babies. These techniques can also help once your premature babies go home.

- Decrease room lights or darken the incubator with a padded cover, and decrease the background room noise.
- Speak softly to your babies before and during care, and handle them slowly, smoothly, and gently.
- Help your babies maintain a tucked or flexed position using boundaries and containment.
- Watch for your babies' cues and signals during treatments, procedures, and position changes.
- Keep babies in boundary devices and provide extra hands during difficult and uncomfortable procedures.
- Provide two-person, care-giving techniques whenever possible. You can often be the second person.
- Organize caregiving and procedures. Watch for signs of stress and provide "time-outs" as needed.
- When possible, don't interrupt babies' sleep for procedures, and watch for sleep/wake cycles.

- Individualize care so that handling and treatments are timed to the babies and not the NICU.
- Learn and communicate your babies' cues.
- Keep a check on activities such as talking and laughing, opening and closing doors, drawers, and incubator ports; also manipulating equipment, and removing water from ventilator tubing.
- Respond quickly to monitor alarms or crying infants.

KANGAROO CARE

Parents and babies need one another's touch, yet the technology of the NICU often keeps parents and babies apart. A technique called Kangaroo Care holds a dual promise: helping babies recover from the effects of their prematurity and helping parents empower themselves and bond with their infants. Kangaroo Care is holding an NICU baby skin-to-skin (usually between the mother's breasts) to provide close human contact. The concept originated in Colombia in the late 1970s and has been adopted worldwide because of the benefits for premature babies. With Kangaroo Care, premature and sick newborns appear to relax and become content from the touch of their parents' skin. Parents also benefit because they are allowed to play an active role in the recovery of their babies.

The Benefits of Kangaroo Care
Numerous studies have shown that Kangaroo Care offers premature babies and their parents many physical and emotional benefits. Among those for babies are:

- Stable heart rate
- More regular breathing
- Improved distribution of oxygen throughout the body
- Prevention of cold stress

- Longer periods of sleep
- Faster weight gain
- Reduction of purposeless activity that burns calories at the expense of growth and health
- Decreased crying
- Longer periods of alertness
- Opportunities to breastfeed and benefits from breast milk.
- Earlier bonding
- Increased likelihood of being discharged from the hospital sooner

Among those for parents are:

- Deeper feeling of closeness to their infants
- Confidence about monitoring their babies' health
- Feeling that "it's about time" that they're allowed to have this contact
- A sense of confidence that their baby is well cared for and will survive
- Feeling in control
- Increased breastfeeding and milk production

Kangaroo Care can be used with nearly all babies. Most hospitals encourage Kangaroo Care for babies who weigh over 1,000 grams, have stable vital signs and stable respiratory conditions, and can maintain their temperature during routine care. If they are stable and have the doctor's approval, babies on ventilators and those weighing less than 1,000 grams might be given Kangaroo Care. However, it is not advised for babies who have severe respiratory illness, chest tubes, or who are medically unstable.

Using the principles of developmental care, Kangaroo Care can be timed with feedings. It improves babies' digestion, and breastfeeding mothers who kangaroo tend to have a better milk supply. These benefits are apparent even when Kangaroo Care occurs for only a few minutes each day.

How to Kangaroo

With multiples, you can kangaroo with one baby at a time or two together. However, this is a wonderful opportunity to get to know your babies individually. Let dad kangaroo one while you kangaroo another. The nurses can help move your babies from the bed to your arms. Babies are held upright, skin-to-skin, and chest-to-chest. Lying on the mother or father's chest, the baby feels warmth, hears heartbeat sounds, calms, snuggles, and falls asleep. Some babies may try to nurse. Kangaroo Care usually lasts for one hour, but there are no maximum time limits as long as the baby is stable. The following are some guidelines for Kangaroo Care:

- The baby's temperature is taken and must be within normal range.
- You need to be in a warm, draft-free area and be seated comfortably. A recliner chair is ideal. If a rocking chair or straight back chair is used, pillows and a footstool are needed. Privacy screens are also recommended.
- The baby is dressed in a diaper only. A hat is recommended for very small babies. You should wear a front-opening shirt or gown and remove your bra.
- There is no time limitation as long as the baby is stable or until a procedure is required.

CO-BEDDING OF MULTIPLES

An outgrowth of developmental care is something that mothers of multiples have been doing throughout history—putting their babies together in the same bed. The concept of co-bedding uses the principles of developmental care to help babies feel secure. Just as all babies need the comfort of their mother after birth, it is natural for multiples to need the continued sensations of their co-multiples. Co-bedding is based on the premise that a multiple birth baby's life outside the uterus is enhanced by continued physical contact with the other multiples.

Mutual relationships and interactions between multiples occur throughout pregnancy. Before birth, multiples show similar patterns of sleep and wake states, and they tend to have movement and heart rate increases at the same time. Multiples have been observed on ultrasound interacting with their co-multiples in the uterus—they touch, embrace, and lovingly bat and push each other around. Co-bedding helps recreate this environment after birth.

There appear to be other advantages to co-bedding premature multiples. Cuddling them together in one bed prompts healing and helps babies cope with environmental stress. Co-bedding allows care giving and feeding of multiples to be timed together. This may synchronize babies' circadian rhythms and sleep/wake patterns. Studies have also found that when multiples are co-bedded, they tend to settle more quickly, stay warmer, and begin to feed earlier and better.

In various reports, multiples have been observed while co-bedded. The babies showed a variety of movements directed at each other: moving closer, touching, hugging, rooting, sucking on each other, and smiling.

Mothers have reported their babies were more restless when they were separated and interpreted this as signs that they missed and were looking for the other babies. Mothers sensed that babies liked to touch and hug each other. They also observed that when one baby was picked up, the other one appeared to notice it immediately, even if they were asleep. Mothers also reported differences in their babies' sleep/wake states depending on whether or not they had physical contact with their co-multiples. Babies who were co-bedded tended to wake up together and were awake at the same time. After care giving and feeding, they calmed down and fell asleep more easily when they could feel the presence of the other baby. Without physical contact, they were more irritable and cried more. Mothers felt their babies displayed temperaments and personalities as they interacted with each other. In one report, when babies were alone for stressful procedures, they each "complained" more than when they were together.

Guidelines for Co-Bedding Multiples

Putting babies together in the same bed in an NICU is not as simple as doing it at home. Equipment, monitors, and caregiving must be kept organized and separate. The following are some general guidelines for using co-bedding in the NICU. Your hospital may have other requirements or guidelines.

- Twins and higher-order multiples located in the same NICU can be put together after they all become stable. All must be weaned from the ventilator but can receive oxygen through nasal cannula.
- IVs, tube feeding, heart, oxygen, and apnea monitors, and phototherapy are usually permitted.
- All equipment, clothing, and chart forms must be color-coded to match each multiple, and hospital identification bands must be on at all times.
- Babies are placed side-by-side in the same bed. They can either be facing each other or facing the other one's back (as long as they are all in the fetal position.) Babies can be placed in the same positions they were in during pregnancy.
- One blanket is lightly swaddled around the babies. Each baby is able to freely reach his own face with his hands, as well as the face or body of his co-multiple.
- Multiples can be co-bedded until they are ready for discharge.
- A baby who becomes unstable must be separated.

The goals of co-bedding are to show improvement in heart rate, respiratory rate, oxygen requirements, physical growth and development, and motor development. As a result, it can decrease the length and costs of hospitalization. Co-bedding is designed to enhance parent-infant bonding, ease the transition to home, and provide consistency of care. However, this is a new practice with little published research to support or negate its use. Risks are unknown at this time, although infection might be a potential risk. Talk with your babies' care providers about using co-bedding. If your babies don't like it, they'll let you know by their cues and body signals. If they do, you will have given your babies another comfort in an often distressing environment.

BEING YOUR BABIES' ADVOCATE

Many believe that family-centered, developmentally supportive care will be the standard of care for all NICUs in the future. Although many hospitals are already adopting this approach, some have not. You can be your babies' advocate, helping secure for them the best options in care. If developmental care, Kangaroo Care, and co-bedding are new concepts for the NICU staff of your hospital, you can help educate them about the benefits. Remember, you are the nurturer, caregiver, and essential decision maker for your babies. So you may need to make specific requests such as establishing a day/night schedule or using co-bedding. Form a working relationship with your nurses. Some of them may already be working to help bring about these care strategies. Find out if your hospital conducts developmental care committee meetings, and request to attend or be on the agenda to discuss specific issues. Other options are to have discussions with the NICU medical director, nursing director, or social worker. Be prepared for some resistance. These practices can mean more work for the personnel caring for your babies. However, once they recognize the benefits, they often become great supporters of your efforts. And your efforts may help other parents as well.

YOUR EMOTIONS WHEN
YOUR BABIES ARE IN THE NICU

The experience of premature birth and having your babies need intensive care can be overwhelming. It's a shock to realize your pregnancy is over and you are now the parent of two, three, or more babies. You are elated and want to celebrate the birth of your babies. But your joy is overshadowed by worry and fear because they are so tiny and sick. The procedures your babies are having can be scary, and you worry what may happen to them and if they will be healthy. It is frustrating to not have the physical stamina to spend time with them and it often makes you feel helpless. Many parents feel disappointed that their babies don't look anything like they had envisioned, even if they had seen premature babies before. Some mothers feel deeply the loss of a "normal" pregnancy and birth experience. It is natural to feel angry toward yourself and others, and guilty about something you should have done or not done to stop this from happening.

> I needed the time my babies were in the NICU to recover from my surgery and blood pressure problems.

> Emotionally I was a mess—it made me crazy not being able to take my babies home for two and one-half weeks. For me physically, it did not even enter my mind that I was in pain.

> It was actually good that my twins came home separately so we could find out what it was like with one baby before having to juggle two. Still, it was great to have them both home, with no more daily trips to the hospital.

Parents handle all these feelings in many different ways. Some are able to express them openly, while others keep them inside. You may be hesitant to become too close to your babies, not wanting to let yourself fall in love with them if they might not survive. Some parents delay giving their babies names and don't want to tell others about the birth. These feelings and reactions are normal, and you aren't crazy. They are very real, natural responses to having a sick or premature baby.

Don't feel that you are alone. Wonderful support systems are available for parents of babies in NICUs. Some hospitals have ongoing support groups for parents. The Internet also has many resources, including forums, chat rooms, and e-mail lists for parents of multiples and premature babies. Use these resources to draw strength from others who have been through this experience.

Here are some ideas to help you during the time your babies are in the NICU or special care nursery.

- Pay attention to your own health, and don't feel you must be at your babies' sides twenty-four hours a day. Your babies need a healthy, rested mother. Eat well, sleep, and regain your strength. This is especially important if you are pumping breast milk for your babies. Milk production is physically demanding, and your body is trying to recover from pregnancy and birth as well.
- Recognize that your feelings about this experience are expected and normal. Disappointment, fear, anxiety, and guilt are often mixed with joy, love, and concern. Talk with other parents with babies in the NICU. You'll find you aren't the only one with these feelings and worries.
- Allow yourself to love your babies. Give them names, and don't hold yourself back from them. You'll soon find yourself worrying about one, rejoicing about another, and loving them all.
- Don't be afraid to ask questions about your babies' care, and learn all you can about their health needs and prob-

lems. Ask your nurses and doctors to explain complex problems in terms you can understand.

- Work with your babies' health care team to develop an individualized care plan, share in its implementation, and revise it as necessary.

- Participate as much as possible in your babies' care. Find out the times and schedules for feedings, baths, and when your babies are most alert and awake. Make sure your babies' nurses know when you will be coming.

- Request developmental strategies such as Kangaroo Care and co-bedding. Don't be confrontational, but be assertive if these have never been done before. Explain the benefits, and ask for a trial run—the results can be surprising.

- Give yourself permission to feel disappointed, helpless, or incompetent when you can't figure out what your babies want or need. Your babies may not know either. Feel happy and proud when you can read your babies. The important thing is that you are trying to understand what your babies are telling you.

- It is natural to feel a loss of control when your babies' health is dependent on technology and skills you can't provide. You may feel jealous of the nurses and doctors in the NICU. While professionals often become attached to the babies they care for on a daily basis, this doesn't mean your babies belong to them. Rather, they are temporary caretakers. Remember that these babies are yours—they are intimately connected to you, no matter how long they are in the hospital.

- Meet with the NICU social worker. Social Security benefits related to newborn disability are available for certain low birth weight and very low birth weight babies. Social workers can also help you find reduced-cost lodging near the hospital after you are discharged and can coordinate home health services when your babies go home.

- If your babies are discharged separately, don't feel guilty about spending more time with the baby or babies that go home. Their needs are immediate and cannot be met by anyone else but you and your family. Everyone knows that you can't be in two places at once. Be assured that the baby or babies still in the hospital have attention and care twenty-four hours a day.

- Before your babies are discharged, request at least one night's stay at the hospital with your babies. Some hospitals have parenting rooms located near the nursery just for this purpose. This gives you an opportunity to care for your babies on your own, with the reassurance of having the NICU staff nearby for questions.

Chapter Twenty-One

Getting to Know Your Babies

> After my C-section, they wheeled my daughter's crib next to
> my bed. She was just lying there, quiet. I said something to
> my husband and she immediately jerked her head toward
> me. I just broke into tears. She really knew me.

There is little to compare with the complex emotions that accompany birth. The planning and dreaming are over, and reality has arrived, packaged in two, three, or more little beings that are totally dependent on you. You now have the tasks of getting to know your babies and meeting their individual needs while handling the physical recovery that comes after multiple pregnancy and birth. Learning to manage all this is complicated but not impossible. This chapter discusses some of the emotional challenges you may experience as you get to know your new babies.

TIME WITH YOUR BABIES IN
THE HOSPITAL—ROOMING-IN

There is much to learn before you go home from the hospital. The best way to learn is hands-on—spending time with your babies with the help of your nurses and other health professionals. Many hospitals are using a combined mother-baby care system, in which one nurse is responsible for the care of a mother and her babies. Other hospitals have a postpartum nurse assigned to the mother and a nursery nurse assigned to her babies. The mother-baby care model is ideal because it offers a consistent source for care and information. Your nurse helps you learn baby care skills such as diapering, bathing, cord and circumcision care, and feeding. Typically, your nurse asks you to complete a checklist of basic skills before you go home.

Most hospitals have a policy of rooming-in for healthy babies. With *full rooming-in* your babies are with you twenty-four hours a day. *Partial rooming-in* allow you to be with your babies as much as you wish, but they can also be cared for in the hospital nursery. Rooming-in is good practice for what to expect at home, but it can be overwhelming when babies are all crying at once. Your nurses will not be able to stay with you all the time to help. So be sure that you have a family member or friend with you during the day and night if you room-in.

BONDING

One of the important tasks of new motherhood is getting to know your babies through the process of *bonding*. While entire books have been written to describe the complexities of mother-infant relationships, bonding isn't a big mystery. It is simply how parents and babies fall in love with each other. Unfortunately, there is much misunderstanding about the how, when, and what of bonding. For example, one myth says that you cannot bond if you don't see and hold your babies right after birth. Another myth says your babies won't know you if they are taken to the NICU or to another hospital. Such false information has caused many parents to lose hope and confidence and feel they have missed out on an important part of parenting. Here are some truths about bonding:

- Bonding is a process through which you come to love your babies and they to love you. Bonding is when parents become committed by a flow of concern and affection toward their babies. It is a two-way relationship that develops out of the affection and interactions between parents and their babies.

- There is no time limit on bonding, and it doesn't start with any one specific event. Bonding begins during pregnancy when you fall in love with the idea of being pregnant, with the sight of your babies on ultrasound, and with your dreams of what they will be like. This continues to develop with the growth of your belly and the feel of your babies' kicks and their movements. After delivery, your love is strengthened when you and your babies touch, gaze eye-to-eye, and respond to each other.

- There is no one way or method of relating to your babies that makes bonding and attachment happen. There are no tests to say you have or have not bonded. Your feelings for your babies can develop slowly or immediately. You may not have a deep gush of emotion when you see or hold your babies. Rather than feeling an instantaneous bond with them, your feeling of closeness to your babies might take time to develop—days, weeks, or months. Parents develop feelings and interact with each baby in unique ways—mothers respond differently from fathers and from other mothers. Your feelings for your babies are your own, and they are valid.

- Separation from your babies does not prevent bonding and attachment. You feel lost and sad if your babies cannot stay with you after birth, but be assured that they won't "forget" you, the sound of your voice, or your smell and touch.

Building Relationships with Multiple Babies

Having multiples doesn't change the basic processes of bonding. But you do have to go about getting to know each of your multiple babies a bit differently. Humans are able to establish a relationship with only one person at a time. So having more than one baby at a time means the process can take a little longer. You might bond to the set of multiples first with your feelings and concerns focused on the well-being of the unit rather than the individuals. It isn't until you can direct your attention toward each baby that you can begin to form individual relationships, even if it means you have only a few minutes with each one.

Recognizing differences in babies is an important part of forming these relationships. Fraternal multiples have obvious differences. They not only look different but usually have different temperaments, personalities, and body rhythms as well. So it is easy to see them as unique individuals. When babies are all the same sex and look or behave very much alike, it's more challenging to find differences. You have to look harder for unique traits that make each baby a separate and distinct individual.

As parents begin to establish relationships with their babies, they often find that their feelings switch back and forth between the babies for several days or weeks. This flip-flopping of feelings is a natural response. You simply need to focus on one baby at a time to get to know each one. This doesn't mean you don't love the other baby or babies. Rather, it can be a necessary part of learning each baby's unique needs and personality.

> I felt guilty because I really wanted to hold and cuddle my twin daughter by herself. I loved my son, but I needed to be with her. After a few days, the whole thing reversed, and I wanted him.

The first couple of weeks with the babies, exhausted from
lack of sleep and physical demands on my body, I lived from
one feeding to the next, not particularly wanting to hold the
babies. I thought I needed to decide who would be held and
when and I felt guilty for the one who wasn't being cuddled,
so I'd rotate them until we were all too tired.

Relationship Difficulties

Getting to know more than one baby at a time can be affected by
many factors. When one baby is hospitalized or is sicker than the
others, it can be harder to sort out your feelings. Sick babies may
be less responsive to a parent's voice or unable to make eye contact,
making it harder for parents to connect with them. You may feel
closer to the one that you can hold, breastfeed, or take home from
the hospital. Or you may find yourself holding back your feelings
when you fear a baby will not survive. These feelings are natural responses to situations beyond your control.

Occasionally, a parent develops strong preferences for one
multiple over another. These may be occasional feelings or a long-
term partiality. It is important to recognize these feelings and
make a special effort to overcome them. Make opportunities to
spend time with any less-preferred baby, picking up that one first
or feeding separately from the others. Preferential attachment can
be harmful to the emotional and physical needs of the babies.
You should seek professional counseling if you find yourself unable to overcome this situation.

Naming Your Babies

Naming your babies gives each of them their own identity and can
help you see them as distinct individuals, separate from you and
separate from each other. With the advances of ultrasound and prenatal testing, many parents learn the sexes of their babies and name
them before they are born. Others prefer to wait until after delivery to choose names that fit the babies' personalities. Rather than

choosing names that rhyme or sound similar, such as Carlene and Darlene, Christine and Christopher, or Donnie and Ronnie, consider names that reinforce each baby's individuality. Be aware that giving your children names with identical initials such as Jennifer Ann Smith and Jason Adam Smith can be confusing later. Another pitfall is the use of tags after the father's name such as Junior or III. It isn't wise to name one boy Junior, even if he was first born of the boys because it can create jealousy later on. Rather than focusing on the multiple birth factor, try to choose names that you like, that work well with your last name, and that sound good together. You will be calling their names a lot!

TIPS FOR BONDING IN THE HOSPITAL

With so much to learn, and postpartum hospital stays so short, you'll want to make every minute count. Here are some tips that can help in the first few days in the hospital and at home as you get to know your babies:

- If possible, have someone with you at all times in your hospital room. If you want to rest or go to the bathroom, you can relax, knowing that your babies' needs are met. Many hospitals also have a sleeper chair, pullout bed, or rollaway in the postpartum room. Dad or some other helper can use this to rest at night.
- Limit your visitors. Not only do visitors bring germs, but also they take up time that you can use for rest and getting to know your babies. Visitors can also interfere with breastfeeding or pumping routines. Tell visitors that you would love to see them after you go home (have them call first), as long as they bring a meal or agree to do a load of laundry!

- When possible, keep all your babies with you in your hospital room. When you aren't holding them, put them in one hospital crib together, or if they are big babies, roll the cribs next to each other. This is a reality check—you really did have multiples!
- If there is no established co-bedding policy for your hospital, you may need an order from your pediatrician for the babies to stay together when they go back to the nursery. If your babies are in the NICU or special care nursery, request that their beds be placed next to each other. Sharing the same incubator or crib is better. Chapter 20 has more information on the advantages of co-bedding.
- Identical multiples are easy to tell apart if they are different in size or if their heads or faces are shaped differently. But if you can't tell them apart, paint one twin's toenails with nail polish, or use several different colors for higher order multiples. Do this before you leave the hospital, while their identification bands are still secure. It won't take long before they look completely different to you.
- When possible, give yourself some time alone with each baby. Have someone else watch the other babies so you can have uninterrupted one-on-one time. Examine each baby from head to toe and look for unique characteristics such as birthmarks, curls of hair, or family traits such as the shape of hands or fingers. This time may be helpful as you both learn to breastfeed. You'll be able to learn each baby's unique feeding style and needs.
- Name your babies early, and use their names in your conversation as often as possible. Most hospitals are happy to write babies' names on the crib cards. It's much better than Twin A and Twin B. Get other family members and the hospital staff in the habit of calling them by name as well.
- From the very beginning, don't refer to your babies using labels such as "the fussy one" or "the smallest." These

names tend to stick. Avoid using phrases such as "the twins" or "the babies," and discourage others from these practices.

- Use a different color scheme for each baby, such as blue t-shirts for one baby, yellow for another, green for another. Color-coding is also useful when you have helpers at home, so they can easily tell who is who. Use each baby's name in association with the appropriate color, rather than just referring to the baby as "the one in blue."

- Let your babies "tell" you what they need. As you get to know each one, you'll learn their unique cues and signals, and you can meet each baby's individual needs with individual care. Some babies are simply fussier and need more attention than others. Just because you have to spend more time with one who needs it doesn't mean you are neglecting the others.

- Enjoy one-on-one time with each of your babies, but don't feel guilty when you have to do certain tasks with them as a group. For example, after each baby learns to nurse well, feeding them together is a real time-saver. Your babies don't know they are sharing you, but each does know the warmth, nurture, and love felt in your arms.

- At night, get as much sleep as you possibly can. Some mothers are more comfortable if their babies are with them, while others get more rest if babies are cared for in the hospital nursery. If yours go to the nursery, be sure to emphasize that you want your babies brought to you for all feedings in the night.

It may be a reality that you may not be able to leave your babies for days or weeks at a time. It's important to get a break, but do keep in mind . . . the newborn stage is exhausting, demanding, stressful . . . but it's not forever.

Chapter Twenty-Two

Feeding Multiple Babies— Creative Dining

How will you feed your babies? Breastfeeding? Bottle feeding? Both? It's a question on the minds of many parents. You're probably also wondering about the logistics of feeding more than one baby. How do you meet everyone's needs when each baby must be fed eight to twelve times every twenty-four hours. You have many feeding options, ranging from exclusive breastfeeding to bottle feeding formula, and many combinations in between. Each option has advantages and disadvantages. Become informed about each feeding method, and decide what is best for you and for your babies. You are not locked into any one option, and circumstances may arise that influence your decision. Feedings aren't simply for filling babies' tummies; they are an important part of the bonding process. Through feedings, whether breast or bottle, babies begin socialization, learning to trust the person who provides the food. With information, support, and encouragement, you can discover the best way to love and nourish your babies.

BREASTFEEDING

The most frequently asked question about feeding multiples is, "Can I breastfeed?" Not only is breastfeeding possible, but it is often a very practical answer to the needs of multiple birth mothers and babies. If you are planning to breastfeed your multiples, you'll join about half of mothers of twins and about three-fourths of mothers of higher-order multiples.

The basic technique of breastfeeding is no different whether you are nursing one or several babies. But there are some clear logistical differences. Holding two wiggling babies to nurse together, producing enough milk to meet several babies' needs, and the additional time necessary for feeding multiples are challenges mothers of singletons don't face. Despite this, many mothers of twins and higher-order multiples successfully breastfeed.

Breastfeeding involves much more than nutrition. It is a wonderful way of being intimately connected with your babies, whether any is able to nurse at your breast or receive pumped breast milk. Although it takes commitment, practice, and patience, nearly every mother can give her babies this special gift.

BENEFITS OF BREASTFEEDING

With few exceptions, breast milk is best. Human milk is perfectly matched for human babies and is superior to all other nutrition options. No formula or milk substitute can provide the nutrition, immunity protection, and developmental and emotional benefits of human milk. When you breastfeed or pump your milk, you are giving your babies a unique gift. Whether your babies are sick and premature or full-term and healthy, your milk is unmatched in its qualities and benefits.

The advantages of breastfeeding are well documented, and more are being recognized every year. The American Academy of Pediatrics (AAP) believes breastfeeding is the ideal method of feeding and nurturing babies and recognizes breastfeeding as primary in achieving optimal infant and child health, growth, and development. The AAP also encourages breastfeeding for at least one year.

The following two lists present some of the known benefits of breastfeeding.* Benefits to mother are:

Physical

- Women who breastfeed have less vaginal bleeding and less risk of hemorrhage (excessive bleeding) after birth. Breast-feeding causes the release of oxytocin, a hormone produced in the brain that makes the uterus contract. Uterine contractions limit the flow of blood from the uterus.
- Uterine contractions caused by oxytocin return the uterus to its nonpregnant size sooner.
- Milk production requires 500 to 1,000 calories a day. One-half of the calories come from body fat stored during pregnancy. The remaining calories come from foods eaten each day. Women who breastfeed lose pregnancy weight more easily than women who formula-feed. However, high calorie foods with no nutritional value should be avoided.
- Breastfeeding reduces the risk of breast cancer in young women. The longer you breastfeed, the lower your risk. Women who breastfeed two years or more have the most protection.
- Breastfeeding reduces the risk of uterine cancer. The risk is lowest in women who have breastfed recently and for longer periods of time. There is less protection after age fifty-five.
- Women who breastfeed are less likely to develop ovarian cancer.
- Breastfeeding improves bone density and reduces the risk of hip fractures in older women.

---

*Adapted with permission from *Breastfeeding, A Parent's Guide,* 7th edition, by Amy Spangler, 1999.

- Full or nearly full breastfeeding can reduce fertility and aid in child spacing. Babies are fully breastfed when no other liquids or solid foods are given. Babies are nearly fully breastfed when most feeds (more than 85 percent) are breastfeeds, and non-breast milk substitutes are given rarely.
- Breastfeeding requires no mixing, no measuring, and no cleanup, making nighttime feedings quick and easy.

Social

- Human milk is always available. It requires no sterilization or refrigeration.
- With a little practice, mothers can breastfeed two babies fairly discreetly. Mothers who are shy or easily embarrassed can choose a quiet place where they will not be disturbed.

Emotional

- Breastfeeding promotes a special relationship between a mother and babies, a closeness that comes with time and touch, a bond that lasts forever.
- Breastfeeding provides an opportunity for mothers to rest during the day, something every new mother needs.

Economic

- Parents who breastfeed save more than $400 per baby in infant feeding costs during the first year alone.
- Breastfed babies have fewer illnesses, fewer doctor visits, and fewer hospitalizations. As a result, parents who breast-feed have lower health care costs.
- Breastfed babies are healthier, even if they are in day care. As a result, parents working outside the home miss fewer days of work and lose less income.

And some of the known benefits to baby are:

Physical

- Human milk is nutritionally perfect for human infants. Human milk changes to meet the needs of a growing baby, something formula cannot do.
- Human milk is readily available and requires no preparation, sterilization, or refrigeration.
- Human milk is easily digested, so breastfed babies have less gas, colic, and spitting up.
- Human milk contains important nutrients as well as special protective factors. It is nature's way of safeguarding the immature newborn against infections.
- Breastfeeding lowers the risk of asthma, colic, food allergy, and eczema in infants with a family history of allergic disease.
- Breastfed babies have less diarrhea.
- Breastfed babies have fewer urinary tract infections.
- Breastfed babies have fewer respiratory infections.
- Breastfed babies have fewer ear infections.
- Breastfed babies are less likely to develop chronic bowel diseases, including ulcerative colitis, Crohn's disease, and celiac disease.
- Breastfed babies are less likely to develop insulin dependent diabetes mellitus (IDDM).
- Breastfed babies are less likely to develop some childhood cancers, including leukemia and lymphoma.
- Breastfeeding promotes nervous system development and increases intelligence quotient (IQ).
- Breastfeeding may reduce the risk of sudden infant death syndrome (SIDS), the leading cause of death in babies after one month of age.

Emotional

- Breastfeeding gives babies a chance to touch, smell, hear, see, taste, and know their mother from the first moment of birth.

Breastfeeding multiples offers even more benefits to mothers and babies. Because many multiples are born preterm, breast milk provides many of the immunities they would have received during the last part of pregnancy. Preterm colostrum (the milk produced in the first few days after birth) has nearly twice the amount of antibodies as term colostrum. Preterm milk is higher in protein than full-term milk and it is more easily digested than formula. These qualities make it perfectly suited for premature babies. And when your babies cannot yet nurse, pumping your milk for their tube feedings gives you a sense of purpose and a great deal of satisfaction. You are doing something for your babies that no one else can do. Breastfeeding and pumping also help with bonding, which can sometimes be more challenging with multiple babies. It provides closeness and one-on-one time with each baby, allowing you to get to know each one as an individual.

Breastfeeding also requires you to take rest breaks from your busy day. It's just not possible to wash dishes with two babies nursing at your breasts! You are forced to get off your feet and stop your activities—something you welcome in these hectic days.

Another advantage of breastfeeding is the time you can save. In addition to the instant availability of breast milk, the overall number of feeding times is reduced once babies nurse simultaneously. Nursing two babies together also has other advantages. When one baby is a weaker nurser than another, the stronger nurser stimulates the flow of breast milk so that the other baby doesn't have to work as hard. Simultaneous feedings also stimulate the release of prolactin, which increases the flow and production of breast milk.

Disadvantages of Breastfeeding

While mother's milk is clearly superior to all other alternatives, it is not without disadvantages. Mothers who breastfeed multiples don't get the rest in the first few weeks that they would when helpers feed their babies. Mothers often worry about being able to produce enough milk to meet all the babies' needs. Nursing two babies at the same time may feel unnatural, and some mothers find breast pumping distasteful. Another difficulty is that mothers of multiples can suffer from very sore nipples if one or more babies are not latching on correctly.

A Learned Technique

Breastfeeding is a very natural process, but the technique doesn't necessarily come naturally. Both mother and babies have to learn how. Over the ages, when extended families lived together or nearby, women could observe their mothers, sisters, aunts, and cousins breastfeeding. Today, families are much more isolated, and women don't have as many opportunities to learn from the breastfeeding experience of others. So it's a good idea to take a breastfeeding class during pregnancy to learn the basic mechanics and how the whole process works. It is also important to have your doctor or a certified lactation consultant examine your breasts and nipples before the birth to identify any potential difficulties.

Expectant fathers should attend class along with mothers. They can learn ways to help with breastfeeding, such as bringing babies to the mother, changing and burping, and encouraging mothers when they are tired or frustrated.

Commitment

Breastfeeding is a personal and family undertaking. One of the main reasons mothers give up on breastfeeding is lack of support from their families. Although you can succeed on your own, having your family standing behind you can make a great difference. This is especially important when you are recovering from a complicated pregnancy or a difficult delivery and you have limited energy reserves. Everyone, including you, must understand that your only responsibilities for the first few weeks are to rest, eat, and feed your babies. This means others must take on all the remaining duties in the home. Someone else must cook, clean, and care for older children. Many mothers create their own support networks with other mothers of multiples and La Leche League groups. Don't feel guilty about relying so heavily on others. You have two or more important little beings that are totally dependent on you!

> I was lucky enough to find incredible support from my husband, the kids' pediatrician, and a couple of close girlfriends. I'm still breastfeeding my girls at fourteen and one-half months. I realize that I'm in an extreme minority and I've found lots of reasons why women quit breastfeeding twins early or never even start . . . because I ran into ALL of them!

> I breastfed my twins until they weaned themselves—one at ten months and the other at eleven months. I was determined!

Making Milk

Your body uses a demand-and-supply system to produce adequate amounts of breast milk. The more milk that flows out of your breasts, either through nursing or pumping, the more milk your breasts produce. This is why most women can make enough milk for two or more babies. It's no coincidence that, on average, mothers of twins produce double the amount of milk produced by mothers of singletons. Your breasts respond to how well milk is moved out of your breasts. If babies need to nurse more frequently, and if you allow babies to nurse more often, your milk supply increases to meet their needs. The opposite is also true. Dropping a nursing or substituting a bottle feeding for a nursing makes your breasts think less milk is needed. The result is a decrease in milk production.

You can help your breasts make more milk if your babies are not strong nursers or you are trying to provide enough milk for higher-order multiples. Immediately after feedings, you can pump the remaining milk from your breasts. This "tricks" your body into thinking the babies are still nursing and it responds by producing more milk. Results are not always immediate. You might not see your milk supply increase for a day or two, and you might have to continue this process for several days. Be patient and persistent. Pregnancy or delivery complications, and delays in nursing or pumping in the first few days can slow the time when your milk "comes in." This usually occurs three to five days after birth, but it could take as long as seven to ten days. Don't give up, keep nursing and pumping.

Getting Started Breastfeeding

Ideally, babies begin breastfeeding within the first thirty to ninety minutes after birth, nuzzling at their mother's breasts. This coincides with a period of wide-awake alertness of most healthy babies in the first hours after birth. If your babies are born preterm or need special care, you may need to pump at first and start direct breastfeeding later.

Multiples born at term or near term can often breastfeed in the mother's recovery room. During labor, let your labor nurses know you want to breastfeed as soon as possible after delivery so they can plan to help you. If your babies need to go temporarily to the nursery for evaluation, let the nursery staff know you want to breastfeed. Request that they bring them back to you as quickly as possible.

Breastfeeding may seem awkward at first, but with practice, you and your babies learn how. Here are some steps to help you get started.

- Start with one baby at a time.
- Sit up straight with a bed pillow or nursing pillow in your lap.
- Place your baby across you so that his body is turned and squarely facing your breast.

- The football hold, with the baby's feet tucked under your arm, is helpful for small babies and after cesarean delivery.
- Snuggle his whole body in so that he is wrapped close to your body. You may need to tuck his lower arm out of the way so he can get closer.
- Cup your hand around your breast, with your palm and fingers below and your thumb above. This helps support your heavy breast and allows the baby to latch on more easily.
- Stroke your baby's cheek near his mouth. You'll see him open and root toward that side.
- When his mouth opens wide, draw your baby in toward you, guiding his head to your breast. Don't lean toward him. His mouth should be open wide to take in your whole nipple and a good part of the areola (dark area around the nipple).
- When the baby latches to the areola, the milk sinuses (where milk is stored beneath the areola) are compressed, and milk is released. Without a proper latch, you and your baby may become frustrated. In addition, your nipples are likely to become sore.
- As your baby nurses, look for his cheeks and jaws to move in rhythm, and listen for swallowing. Talk softly and soothingly to your baby as he nurses. It will help both of you relax.
- Each baby should spend at least ten minutes feeding on one breast, but allow each to remain latched until the baby lets go on his own.

Don't be frustrated or disappointed if your babies aren't ravenous nursers right away. They may not actually latch on at first. Try expressing a small amount of colostrum onto your nipple to help entice your babies with its smell and taste. Any type of baby/breast contact is helpful, whether it is the feel of your skin, smelling, tasting, or some suckling effort. Try again whenever your babies show signals that they are hungry, or at least every two to three hours.

Signs of hunger include increased alertness or activity, mouthing, bringing hands to face, or rooting. Crying is a late sign of hunger.

Rooming-in with your babies enhances the breastfeeding process. The babies are always with you, and you can nurse them frequently. It is also easier to observe their cues and signals. Sometimes you need to waken sleeping babies to make sure each baby nurses eight to twelve times a day. Because multiples tend to be smaller, their feedings need to be more frequent than those for larger babies. Your pediatrician can give you guidance on how often to feed your babies. In the first few days, totally breastfed newborns may wet two to four diapers each day and have three bowel movements. By the end of their first week, you'll know your babies are getting enough when each baby has at least seven wet diapers and three bowel movements in twenty-four hours.

Feeding Rotation

After feeding the first baby on one breast, start the second on your other breast. Repeat the feeding procedure described in the previous section with this baby. If you have triplets or more, after feeding the second one, you can feed your third baby half-time on one breast and half-time on the other. Or you can feed the third baby on the first breast. Rotate the babies at the next feeding so that the third baby starts first on the other breast. You may literally be feeding around the clock in the first days! Once your babies can feed together, you'll save time and be able to coordinate feedings more efficiently.

Breastfeeding Higher-Order Multiples

It is possible to produce enough milk for three or more babies, but it is a serious commitment for you and your family. Mothers have successfully provided enough breast milk for quadruplets through nursings and pumped milk. However, these mothers are either pumping or nursing babies nearly every hour of the day and night. There are several options for breastfeeding higher-order multiples. You can breastfeed two babies and bottle feed the others. Or nurse all of them and feed each a supplemental bottle afterwards. Some mothers pump their breast milk and divide it among their babies. Be sure to give them breast milk first, and offer formula afterward if necessary. Remember, no matter how many babies you have, breastfeeding doesn't have to be all or nothing.

A Typical Feeding in the First Few Days

The entire process of feeding one baby may take half an hour or more. Here's a typical scenario with a slightly premature baby or a sleepy term baby in the first few days:

- 10:00—Mother wakes baby: undresses, tickles toes, strokes body, puts warm, wet cloth to face as last ditch effort.
- 10:10—Baby finally awake, showing cues of hunger: hand to mouth, rooting, grunting. Baby put to breast, refuses to open mouth.
- 10:12—Mother strokes baby's cheek, coaxes, changes positions. Baby finally opens mouth and latches. Baby sucks at breast, swallowing is heard.
- 10:15—Baby falls asleep at breast. Mother tries to wake baby, burps baby, changes baby's diaper.
- 10:20—Baby now crying frantically.
- 10:23—Baby settles and begins nursing again.
- 10:27—Baby fusses and has bowel movement, continues nursing.
- 10:30—Baby falls back asleep. Mother burps baby, changes diaper with sticky meconium bowel movement.
- 10:35—Baby goes back to sleep.
- 10:40—Mother wakes second baby to feed and repeats cycle.
- 11:00—Mother pumps both breasts for ten minutes. These babies are just learning to breastfeed but are not nursing well enough or long enough to really get milk production going. So pumping after their feedings reminds the breasts that more milk is needed for the extra babies.

Troubleshooting

If your babies seem to be having difficulties nursing, there are often remedies. Sometimes it's as easy as learning how to keep your
babies from tucking in their lower lip when breastfeeding. Or
maybe your babies simply need extra time to get their sucking organized enough to nurse effectively. Sometimes it is more complicated, such as when a baby has a short frenulum (the thin, web-like
membrane under the tongue). An international board certified lactation consultant (IBCLC) is a wonderful resource for breastfeeding mothers. These certified professionals are often nurses who are
specially trained to help with breastfeeding. Most hospitals have
IBCLCs on staff, or you may need to locate one in private practice.
The IBCLC helps you with positioning and observes your babies
during a feeding to identify any problems.

Request that your babies not be given any supplements (water, glucose water, formula) unless there is a medical reason. Usually you should avoid using pacifiers when babies are still learning
to breastfeed. Like bottles, pacifiers are different from your nipples
in texture and shape, and they can contribute to "nipple confusion." In the early days, if your babies still need to suck after they
are fed, they may need more time at your breast. If you choose to
use a pacifier, try to wait until your babies are well grounded in
breastfeeding. The exceptions are premature babies who may need
sucking practice. Specially designed pacifiers are available that can
help them develop the skills that will make it easier for them to
nurse later on.

Simultaneous Nursing

Once you and your babies are comfortable breastfeeding one at a
time, you can start feeding them together, one on each breast.
Most mothers are ready to try this when at least one baby is latching well. Some discover feeding two babies at the same time works
well, while others find it difficult. You may or may not be ready to
do this when you leave the hospital, so it's a good idea to practice

several feeding positions. Your nurse or the lactation consultant can show you how to position your babies so they can both latch correctly.

The following guidelines will help you begin simultaneous nursing:

- Have a helper nearby for assistance and reassurance.
- Place each baby on the bed or sofa, one on each side of you. Be careful that they are not near the edge.
- Use a nursing pillow or cushions across your lap and under your arms. Specially designed nursing pillows for feeding twins have a wider surface to accommodate two babies. Make sure that the pillow has a strap that wraps around you to keep it from slipping.
- Pick up the strongest nurser and help her latch on and begin nursing.
- Lean over and scoop up the other baby with your hand and forearm, lifting her onto the pillow. Help this baby latch on to nurse.
- Use your hands to support each baby's body and head during feedings as well as to reposition them or move them to burp.

Feeding your babies together may seem awkward at first. You'll have to experiment with different positions as shown in Figure 22.1 and maneuvering to get them "hooked up" when you are by yourself. If they are not proficient nursers, they may come "unhooked," and you'll need to help them latch on again. Simultaneous nursing might work the first day, or it may be weeks or months before you or your babies are ready.

Simultaneous feeding means that both babies have to be awake at the same time. Identical twins often adapt to such a schedule more quickly than fraternal twins, as their body clocks seem to be more synchronized. Usually when one wakes and is hungry,

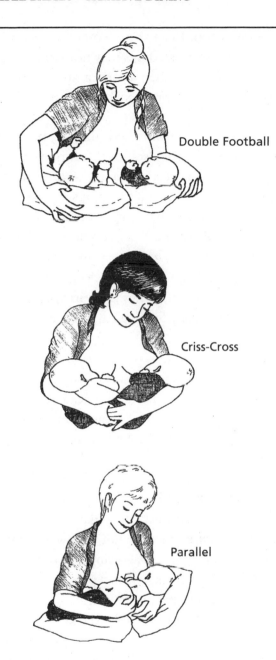

Double Football

Criss-Cross

Parallel

Figure 22.1   Simultaneous Breastfeeding Positions

the other one is, too. In any case, you may need to waken a sleeping baby. Simultaneous feedings may not work if one baby has very different feeding needs than another, such as when one is much smaller and has to eat more frequently. But this can change as the babies grow.

Once babies are established nursers, mothers find feeding them together is a creative solution for managing feedings. Having eight to twelve dual feedings a day certainly takes less time than sixteen to twenty-four separate feedings. However, some mothers have expressed concern that simultaneous feeding limits one-on-one time with their babies. Not every feeding has to be a joint experience. You can feed together at some feedings and separately at others. And remember, your babies don't know that they are sharing you. They do know that they are warm, loved, and nourished—important aspects of any feeding experience.

> Breastfeeding my twins was wonderful! I don't know how many people asked me, "How can you breastfeed *two* babies?" I can feed my son and daughter and write out checks to pay bills at the same time! Breastfeeding was easier, cheaper (free), and better for my children. Why would anyone not do it who can?

Premature or Sick Babies

If your babies are born early, they may or may not be able to directly breastfeed. Often they are not neurologically mature enough to coordinate sucking with swallowing and breathing. For these babies, and those who are sick, you can pump your milk using a breast pump and collect it. This pumped milk can then be tube fed to your babies. If they are not yet able to take feedings, you can freeze breast milk for later when they are ready. As you have already learned, preterm breast milk has protective antibodies and essential proteins not found in formula. However, both breast milk and formula may need to be fortified with certain nutrients for very small and premature babies.

Breast Pumping

Breast pumps come in several styles that work in different ways. The most effective are hospital-grade electric pumps that use a self-cycling piston action for removing milk from your breasts. These are available in most hospitals, or you can rent one from a lactation center or a rental station, such as a pharmacy. (See the resource list at the end of the book.) With these pumps, you can pump both breasts at the same time using a double-collection setup, also available at the hospital or rental station. Double pumping is more efficient than pumping one breast at a time. And pumping both breasts together for ten to twenty minutes increases the production of the hormone prolactin, which helps increase your milk production. However, single-sided pumping is more comfortable for some women at first. To do this, alternate breasts every five minutes until you have pumped both breasts for a total of ten minutes each. If you anticipate needing to pump for many weeks, you might want to consider purchasing your own electric pump. In the long run, it might be more cost-effective than renting. Contact your insurance company to find out if they reimburse for breast pump rental. This benefit is often available when babies are in the NICU.

Begin pumping your breasts as soon as possible after delivery, within five or six hours, if possible. This helps establish the hormonal stimulation for milk production and removes available milk to tell the breasts to make more. If you cannot begin pumping for several days because of your own health, don't give up. A long delay in starting to pump or breastfeed often means you have to work harder and that your milk supply may not be as great, especially at first. But it is not a prescription for failure. If you are too weak to use the pump yourself, your nurse or husband can help. Pump just as frequently as you would if your babies were breastfeeding— every two or three hours, or at least eight pumpings in twenty-four hours. It's okay to take a break at night, but don't go more than about five hours between pumpings or your milk supply will decrease. Some mothers feel inadequate if the amount of milk they are able to pump is small. There may only be a few ounces of colostrum in the first days. Once your milk comes in, you'll see a change in the quantity of your milk as you pump. Tiny babies often don't begin feedings right away, and they only need small amounts of milk. Several collected samples can be combined for one feeding if necessary. Find out if you can pump your milk at your babies' bedside. Once you are comfortable breastfeeding, try pumping one breast while you breastfeed one baby on the other. You'll need some help with the logistics of these techniques, but they can help. The emotional connection can stimulate the letdown of milk and help increase the amount of milk you pump.

Remember that every drop of your milk is a wonderful gift to your babies. Whatever amount you can give them is more than they would get if you weren't pumping. When there are several babies, you can divide your pumped milk among them and supplement with formula if necessary. When one baby is sicker than the others, parents often choose to give only breast milk to that baby.

Your babies may or may not be ready to be fed the colostrum and milk you pump, so the NICU will give you instructions for collecting, labeling, and storing your breast milk. At some point, babies must make the transition from being tube fed to breastfeeding or bottle feeding. This may be a slow process if babies were very premature. There are many techniques to help mothers and babies make this transition. Kangaroo Care, which is discussed in Chapter 20, is an effective way to help babies progress to breastfeeding. There are techniques and devices that can help with the transition, and an IBCLC or an experienced nurse should be able to determine if any of these might be helpful for your babies. The IBCLC can also provide wonderful support and advice as you and your babies make this transition.

A few babies, especially those who were very sick or premature, never make a successful change to complete breastfeeding. If this is the case, you can continue pumping your milk and bottle feeding for many weeks and months. Never feel that you or your babies have failed because direct breastfeeding did not work. Your milk, no matter how your babies receive it, is a precious gift.

> I tried for a week to breastfeed, with frequent hysterical calls to my lactation consultant for help. Recovering from a combined vaginal/cesarean delivery, I was simply too tired to keep it up. I was devastated, and I felt like I had let my babies down. A friend reminded me it was tough to nurse just one baby and not to feel guilty. So I started pumping and we fed our twins expressed milk plus formula for the first ten weeks. That way I felt like I had given them a decent start.

Taking Care of Yourself

After delivery, you might feel you should be totally focused on your babies and not on your own needs. But your body is working overtime, and your needs must be met. When you are pumping or breastfeeding, your body uses some of the reserves established during pregnancy for milk production. In addition, you must recover from pregnancy complications, bed rest, birth, surgery, or postpartum complications such as hemorrhage.

As you care for your babies, you must remember to take care of yourself, too. This means eating healthy meals and drinking plenty of fluids. You may need between 500 and 1000 extra calories each day to meet your needs while breastfeeding multiples. Don't worry about the calorie intake. You'll be amazed at how much you can eat and still lose weight. Many women find themselves getting hungry and thirsty during a feeding. Keep a well-stocked food and beverage center near where you feed your babies most frequently.

You'll also need rest. Many women feel a rush of excitement in the first few days and have a hard time "coming down" off this high. This elation is natural, but don't let it take over or let it wear you out. In the hospital and initially at home, set aside a specific time for visitors. This includes family members as well as friends and coworkers. Having visitors in and out all day long can be exhausting for you and can overstimulate your babies.

Conserve your energy. In the few precious hours and minutes between feedings, rest as much as possible. You may only get an hour of sleep here and there, but take advantage of every opportunity. Remember, your only responsibilities at first are to feed your babies and yourself, and to rest. Make sure that you have adequate help at home so that someone else does all other tasks. Have others bring your babies to you for feedings and change their diapers afterward. Your meals and snacks need to be prepared and brought to you. If you are using supplements, helpers can feed babies while you rest. Although this sounds like you are being lazy, remember that you are doing a tremendous job—making the best milk and feeding babies around the clock! And being forced to stay off your feet helps you recover from pregnancy and birth.

BOTTLE FEEDING MULTIPLES

Another option for many mothers of multiples is to bottle feed their babies. Bottle feeding includes feeding pumped breast milk or formula, or a combination of these. Bottle feeding, whether occasionally or for all feedings, does have its advantages—primarily that a mother can rest when others take over some feedings for her. Bottle feeding also allows mothers to see exactly how much milk each baby takes. However, like all feeding methods, there are disadvantages. Mothers of multiples who bottle feed often complain of the never-ending hassles of washing bottles and nipples and preparing formula. A big drawback is that formula does not provide babies with protective antibodies. In addition, it is more likely to be associated with milk intolerance and allergy. And the costs of formula can be overwhelming, especially if you are feeding several babies. Mothers who pump and then bottle feed breast milk to their babies are actually doing double the work. However, pumped breast milk is still a better alternative than formula, and it is often used for premature babies who have trouble making the transition to direct breastfeeding.

You can simultaneously hold and bottle feed two babies, although it takes coordination to juggle the bottles and keep the babies in the correct positions. Some mothers prop their babies on bed pillows or in infant seats directly in front of them or beside them. Another option is to hold and feed one baby while feeding the other in the infant seat. You'll need to rotate who gets held at each feeding. Other helpers can feed babies, too, but remember that feedings are your primary responsibility.

With three other children, their school activities, and other things going on, I felt bottle feeding was the way to go. What I found was that while others were feeding my babies, I was doing laundry and cleaning up the kitchen. That had to change.

If you choose to bottle feed your babies, keep in mind that there is more to feeding than filling your babies' tummies. Feeding is part of the bonding process and continues to be an important part of the emotional and social development of your babies. When you bottle feed, make sure that your babies are in your arms as much as possible, just as they would be with breastfeeding. For those times you feed babies in infant seats, try to spend some cuddle time after feedings. Babies need the closeness and intimacy that comes with being held and nurtured.

I could only feed my babies with them in their infant seats, facing me, with me holding their bottles. It seemed very cold and unmotherly. The few days I nursed aided in our bonding, but I think I missed out on some very sweet time with them.

Chapter Twenty-Three

Surviving the First Days at Home

What should we buy? How many diapers will we need? Can we use just one crib? What type of stroller is best? Do we need help when our babies come home? What kind of help should we have? Where do we find helpers? These are just a few of the many questions likely to be on your mind as you get ready for your new babies.

Actually, getting your home ready for your babies is simpler than you might expect. Newborn babies don't do much more than sleep and eat. So at first, you'll need the basics: a safe, warm place for them to sleep, simple clothing and diapers, and food—breast milk or formula. You'll also need a car seat for each baby and transportation via stroller or carrier. Much of the other equipment and gadgets in baby stores are helpful but not always essential right at first. Many parents wait to purchase more until they see what they really need.

THE NURSERY—YOUR BABIES' ROOM

The nursery is where you and your babies will spend a lot of time over the next weeks, months, and even years. Choose a room in your home that is convenient for you. If the nursery is not on the same level as your bedroom, consider converting another nearby room to a temporary nursery. You can also give each baby his or her own room, but initially you'll find it easier to care for them if they are together.

You might rest better and feel more secure if you sleep in the same room with your babies. Babies can sleep in the parents' room, or you can sleep on a spare bed, recliner, or mattress on the floor in the nursery. This can really save steps between feedings. On the other hand, babies are noisy, making grunts, snorts, whimpers, and scratching sounds even when asleep. Although they don't usually bother each other, the combined noises from several babies can keep you awake.

> We used our living room as a makeshift nursery until our babies were consistently sleeping four hours straight. I couldn't go up and down the stairs to them fifteen times a night. It also made it easier in the daytime. I didn't have to walk far from the kitchen or our bedroom.

Decorating your nursery is one of the most delightful parts of having babies! Most mothers find that choosing colors and designs, paint and wallpaper, bedding and curtains for the babies' room is a thoroughly enjoyable task. If you are on bed rest and can't get to the stores, have friends or store designers bring samples and swatches to you. Catalog and Internet shopping are also good ways to make your purchases without leaving home. Unless you are very sure of your babies' sexes, choose décor with a gender-neutral theme and colors. Bringing home a boy to share a pink room with bows and flowers might not be what you had in mind! Some parents decorate a room for twins using coordinating colors but different themes on each half of the room.

As you plan the arrangement of furniture, keep things simple and practical, especially when a room is small without a lot of space for furnishings. Arrange cribs where they are most easily accessible to you. Think about the logistics of baby care and moving from bed to bed, and then arrange them to save steps. You can place two cribs lengthwise on one wall, across from each other, or in an L-shape. Three cribs work well in a U-shape rather than lined up in a row. You can take advantage of space underneath the beds for storage of clothing, extra diapers, and bed linens. If cribs are placed close together, make sure that the rails will move without catching on another bed.

ESSENTIAL EQUIPMENT

Valuable sources for baby equipment and clothing are the garage sales sponsored by parents of multiples clubs and other organizations. You can often find a treasure of multiples-related items for a fraction of the new prices. Contact local clubs to find out when their next sale is planned.

Here are the basics you'll need in the first few weeks. If your budget is tight, focus on buying these items now and get other things as you need them.

Cribs
Your babies' beds are likely to be the most expensive equipment purchases you will make. One basic crib and mattress together can cost over $200. This doesn't count the sheets, mattress pads, and blankets that are needed. Designer cribs and those made for twins are quite expensive and are really no more functional than a standard design. Most newborn multiples can share one full-sized crib for several weeks or months, so don't feel pressured to buy all the beds at once. Many parents start with one crib and either borrow or purchase another later. However, if your home has more than one level, using one crib upstairs and one downstairs is a step-saver. Also, think about buying cribs that "grow" with your babies, such as those that convert into toddler or youth beds.

If you want your new babies to sleep in your bedroom, you can use one crib, a large cradle, or bassinets. Another option is to use a crib placed next to your bed. If you lower the rail, make sure that the mattress is at the same level as yours and that the crib is tightly connected to your bed. There should not be any space that might allow a baby to fall down through. One product especially designed for this purpose is the Arm's Reach Co-Sleeper. This is especially helpful for breastfeeding mothers because it places the babies close enough to reach without getting up.

Be sure that every crib, cradle, and bassinet meets current safety standards. Used cribs are responsible for about fifty infant deaths a year. If you borrow a crib or are planning to use a family heirloom, watch for safety hazards, such as faulty slats, too much space between slats (there should be no more than two inches), and lead-based paint used on the bed.

Bedding
Crib mattresses should be firm and well constructed. The mattress should fit snugly with less than two fingers' width between it and the bed. Baby mattresses have either foam or innerspring construction. Innerspring mattresses keep their shape longer and are more expensive. Foam mattresses are lighter, which makes changing crib bedding easier, but they do not have as long a life. Never use a soft cushion or pillow as a mattress. Excessively soft bedding is associated with sudden infant death syndrome (SIDS). Avoid using heavy blankets or quilts on your babies. Instead, use them as wall decorations or as floor mats for babies to lie on.

Clothing
Choosing clothing for your newborn babies is relatively easy. Except for visits to the pediatrician, your babies won't be going many places in the first few weeks and months. So they'll need the basics: sleepers and gowns, undershirts, socks, and diapers. Keep clothing simple. When you're changing each baby's clothes several times a day, you don't need extra hassles of buttons, ties, or complicated garments.

Generally, dress your babies in the same amount of clothing as you are wearing. If your babies are very small or premature, your pediatrician may advise you to keep the indoor temperature slightly warmer than normal, around seventy-two to seventy-four degrees. Babies also stay warmer if they wear hats or knit caps.

For warmth, layer each baby's clothing. Start with an under-shirt (the side-snap kind are easiest to get on) and add a sleeper or one-piece garment. Socks or booties are good for extra warmth, and if the temperature is very cold, you can add a blanket sleeper and a knit hat. A receiving blanket can be used to wrap or swaddle each baby.

Be sure to wash all garments and bedding before your babies use them. Premature babies have very delicate skin that can be irri-tated by garment dyes and finishes and soap residue. Use a mild de-tergent and run an extra rinse cycle on the washer. Also, be careful about using fabric softeners because these can also cause irritation.

Some babies may be too small to wear regular newborn size clothing. Some retail stores carry "preemie" garments as regular stock or can order them. Many baby clothing companies now of-fer premature sizes, including clothing that can be used while ba-bies are still in the hospital.

Diapers

You'll need at least 10 diapers for each baby, each day, in the first month or two. That's 20 a day and 140 a week for twins, or 30 a day and more than 200 a week for triplets. When the numbers of diapers add up, so do the costs. Most parents find that in the be-ginning, the brand of diaper doesn't matter as much as the cost, so buy the least expensive you can find. If your babies weigh less than five pounds when they come home, even the smallest new-born size diapers may be too large. Most large national retail stores in the United States carry premature size diapers. However, you may need to ask the store to order them for you. You can also order them from the manufacturer's distributor and have them delivered to your home. See the resources at the end of the book for information.

If you choose to use cloth diapers, consider using a diaper service. Although cloth diapers may cost less to use, there are added costs for diaper covers or pants. Unless you have unlimited household help, you won't have the time or energy to wash, dry, and fold the mountains of diapers your babies will use.

Some parents start buying disposable diapers during pregnancy and accumulate quite a stash by the time their babies are born. A diaper shower is also a great idea—each guest brings a package of diapers as a gift. Ask for a meal for the freezer, too!

Disposing of all the dirty disposable diapers is a big deal. Trash cans made specially for diapers—such as the Diaper Genie—are great, and the wide-opening styles can hold up to 180 newborn-size diapers. However, they take two hands to use—and your hands may be full! Many parents use simple step-on cans with a lid. Place a can by each diaper-changing area.

A changing table is a helpful addition to your nursery, but it doesn't have to be fancy. A pad on a bed or dresser also works fine. Remember to never leave a baby unattended on any table or bed. With a multilevel house, you need more than one changing area stocked with diapers, wipes, and extra clothing.

Car Seats

Each baby must have a car seat that is appropriately sized. A variety of styles are available, from basic bucket-style infant seats to full-size car seats that grow with your babies. Like cribs, car seats must meet government safety standards. When shopping, make sure that the car seats you select fit in your car. Some cars cannot accommodate three seats placed side by side. Never use a car seat in the front passenger seat with an airbag. Deployment of the airbag in an accident can be dangerous or fatal to infants and children. If you cannot fit all the babies in the back seat, and must place one in the front seat, have the passenger air bag disabled.

Infant-size car seats are designed for babies up to one year of age and weighing up to about 20 to 22 pounds. These are rear facing only and are the best fit for small babies. Some styles have a base that stays buckled in the car, allowing the seat to be used as a carrier. An advantage of these types of seats is that you don't have to disturb babies when moving them. However, many parents find it hard to handle two or more of these carriers when they are alone. If you are going to be on your own much of the time, consider transferring babies to a stroller rather than carrying their car seats.

Convertible car seats can accommodate babies from newborn to 20 pounds when rear facing and over 20 pounds when forward facing. Some full-size car seats are designed for older babies and can only be used forward facing. For small babies, avoid seats with shields or overhead trays because they can cause injury in an accident.

Because many multiples are premature and small, look for car seats that are adjustable. You may need to adjust the straps as well as the angle of the seat to keep babies from slouching. Shoulder straps must fit snugly down over the shoulders. You may need to tilt the seat back using a towel or small blanket tucked under the front base of the seat. Use a small blanket or rolled cloth diapers as padding under and on the sides of your babies for support. The American Academy of Pediatrics (AAP) recommends taking a tape measure when shopping and looking for car seats with less than 10 inches from the lowest shoulder straps to the seat, and less than 5½ inches from the crotch strap to the back. Five-point harness systems are a little more time-consuming to use, but these are safer and fit smaller babies better than the three-point systems.

Premature babies often have a car seat "test" done in the hospital before discharge. In this test, babies are observed while buckled in a car seat for changes in their oxygen levels, breathing, and heart rates. Babies who can't tolerate the semisitting position may need to use a safety rated car bed instead of a car seat. Cosco makes the Ultra Dream Ride, a car bed for babies up to 20 pounds and 26 inches long.

The AAP provides excellent information on car seats in their "Family Shopping Guide to Car Seats—Safety and Product Information." The guide is released each year and lists car seats by size, design, and manufacturer. It is available as a pamphlet by mail or on-line. The AAP also offers information about car safety for children with special needs, including premature infants, in their "Car Seat Shopping Guide for Children with Special Needs."

Strollers

A stroller is an efficient way to move all babies at once, and it can be a necessity when one parent has to transport babies alone. Many parents find they use their stroller every day, so it must be easy to use, sturdily built, and fit in your car trunk or storage area. Test how the stroller folds and unfolds. Can you do it with one hand? Also check the weight limits for the stroller. Will it hold your babies when they each weigh 25 pounds? Be sure that the seats recline flat for newborn babies. If the seats only partially recline, the babies cannot support themselves in an upright position and may slouch.

Strollers come in two basic styles: tandem and side-by-side. Each type has advantages and disadvantages. Most parents choose a stroller type that best suits their babies and lifestyle. Tandem strollers allow babies to be seated one in front of the other, either forward or opposite facing. They are often bigger and heavier than side-by-side models but are narrower. Some have large wheels that allow smooth rides and most have storage areas. Side-by-side strollers allow babies to be seated in a row. Some side-by-side models have independent seat movement while others are stationary. While most side-by-side models will fit through standard door openings, they don't work well in crowded stores.

Stroller prices vary from about $100 to more than $500. You will need a stroller for as long as three to five years, so invest in one that will last. Look for removable and washable coverings and a sturdy frame construction. Triplet and quadruplet strollers are especially expensive. The Triplet Connection and MOST (Mothers of Supertwins) offer discounts on strollers ordered through their organizations. Used strollers are also available through their networks of multiple birth families.

BABY SHOWERS FOR MULTIPLES

Nearly every woman looks forward to her baby shower. And baby showers for multiples are fun events for everyone involved. You might want to schedule your baby shower early in pregnancy—at around 28 weeks, especially if you are having triplets or more. If you are on bed rest, your party can take place at your home, while you lie comfortably on the sofa. Some moms have had their baby showers in the hospital! Or you can wait until after the babies are born. Twin or triplet shower invitations as well as baby announcements and thank you notes for multiples are now available.

Multiple gifts are always welcome at a multiples baby shower! And it's okay if you get lots of sleepers and booties—you can always use them. But don't hesitate to ask for the things you really need. Many stores have baby registries that allow you to request specific items and quantities. Some registries are available through the Internet, such as Target's Lullaby Club, eToy, or Babies R Us/Toys R Us. Even if you aren't registered, spread the word through friends and family. Many people like to combine funds for more expensive items. Here are some other ideas for gifts:

- Diapers and wipes
- Gift certificates for department and discount stores
- Gift certificate for a baby nurse
- Gift certificate to a portrait studio
- Housecleaning services
- Frozen meals

- Blank videotapes
- Camera film and coupons for developing
- Gifts of time (for laundry or babysitting, for example)
- Nursing gowns and clothing for you
- Twin breastfeeding pillow

GETTING HELP

If you feel some apprehension about taking your new babies home, you aren't alone. Most parents are acutely aware of the responsibility of being completely in charge of a new baby. When this responsibility is doubled or tripled with multiples, it can be overwhelming. The advice from those who have been there: Get help!!! Most parents have found they needed help for the first month to six weeks for twins and longer for triplets and other multiples.

In planning when your helpers should come, estimate the time your babies will arrive based on the average length of a multiple pregnancy: 35 to 38 weeks for twins, and 32 to 35 weeks for triplets. Most triplets and nearly all very high multiples stay in intensive care for several weeks. Schedule your helpers to come after the babies go home from the hospital.

So what kind of help do you need? Remember that your primary responsibility as a mother is to feed your babies and yourself, and to get as much rest as you can in the first few weeks. This means that others must assume all other household duties—cleaning, cooking, laundry, taking care of older children, and everything necessary to run your house. Some dads take several weeks of vacation time to help. Otherwise, a grandparent, sister, aunt, or friend might be the answer.

Most parents of twins don't need help twenty-four-hours a day, but an occasional break at night is nice. Because most parents find nights are the hardest, many take shifts so that one parent is only "on duty" for a few hours while the other sleeps. It is easier for breastfeeding mothers if someone else can change diapers and bring the babies to them for feedings both day and night. Parents of higher-order multiples often need feeding help around the clock.

You may want to use paid help if family or friends aren't available. A postpartum doula can be a great support for new mothers, helping with breastfeeding and baby care techniques. Home health agencies are a good resource for finding domestic helpers who cook, clean, and do laundry. Another source for paid help is by word of mouth among friends and other parents of multiples. Be sure to carefully check all references of your helpers.

It isn't usually necessary to hire a "baby nurse" unless one or more of your babies requires special care. Insurance helps pay for nursing care at home in some circumstances. Social Security benefits are also available for premature babies in certain situations. Check with the hospital social worker or your insurance case manager to find out if you are eligible for such benefits.

Whoever you use as helpers, make sure that everyone has a clear understanding of what needs to be done and who is responsible for what jobs. Keep a calendar posted for everyone that lists specific jobs—laundry, cooking, caring for other children, and so on. If helpers must take turns, try to schedule them in blocks of time, such as several days or a week at a time rather than alternating days. This will minimize the amount of disruption in your home since everyone will have their own ways of doing things. Above all, be patient with yourself, your babies, and those who come to help you. Give everyone plenty of time to adjust to the demands and joys of your new family.

Epilogue

Multiple pregnancy is demanding work, but the rewards are matchless. Your experiences over the next weeks and months will be unlike any other. There will be days of exceeding joy mixed with days of stress and worry. At times, you'll find your life completely unpredictable and uncontrollable. You'll need strength, support, and love from everyone around you—your husband, family, friends, and care providers. The actual experiences of multiple pregnancy and birth only last a few months, but the memories last a lifetime. Enjoy your pregnancy, and if difficulties come, don't let them defeat you. Work with your health care team to do all you can to have a healthy pregnancy and babies.

Here are some final words of encouragement to help you through your multiple pregnancy journey:

- Be excited about having multiples. This is an incredible experience that has so many rewards and blessings.
- Believe in yourself and your babies. Have faith that you can handle anything that comes along.
- Become informed. Although things may go just fine, your goal is to be knowledgeable in case they don't.
- Take advantage of the opportunities you have to make a difference in your care. Change things that can be changed and control things that can be controlled.

- Recognize that there are no guarantees and there are limits to what modern technology can do. Problems can happen despite everyone's best efforts.
- Let go of the things that are beyond your control, and don't allow negative influences to consume you.
- Maintain a positive attitude, and keep calm when faced with unexpected problems. A calm, collected approach will help you make the best decisions.
- Enjoy the specialness of your multiple pregnancy and the blessings of your multiple babies. The memories you create now will long be remembered in the years to come.

Declaration of Rights and Statement of Needs of Twins and Higher Order Multiples

adopted by the Council of Multiple Birth Organizations of the
International Society for Twin Studies May 1995

Introduction: The mission of the Council of Multiple Birth Organizations (COMBO) of the International Society for Twin Studies is to promote awareness of the special needs of multiple birth infants, children, and adults. The multi-national membership of COMBO has developed this Declaration of Rights and Statement of Needs of Twins and Higher Order Multiples as benchmarks by which to evaluate and stimulate the development of resources to meet their special needs.

DECLARATION OF RIGHTS

WHEREAS myths and superstitions about the origins of multiples have resulted in the culturally sanctioned banishment and/or infanticide of multiples in some countries:

I. Multiples and their families have a right to full protection, under the law, and freedom from discrimination of any kind.

WHEREAS the conception and care of multiples increase the health and psychosocial risks of their families, and whereas genetic factors, fertility drugs, and in vitro fertilization techniques are known to promote multifetal pregnancies:

II. Couples planning their families and/or seeking infertility treatment have a right to information and education about factors which influence the conception of multiples, the associated pregnancy risks and treatments, and facts regarding parenting multiples.

WHEREAS the zygosity of same sex multiples cannot be reliably determined by their appearances; and whereas 1) the heritability of dizygotic (two-egg) twinning increases the rate of conception of multiples; 2) the similar biology and inheritance of monozygotic (one-egg) multiples profoundly affect similarities in their development; 3) monozygotic multiples are blood and organ donors of choice for their co-multiples; and 4) the availability of the placenta and optimal conditions for determining zygosity are present at birth:

III.

A) Parents have a right to expect accurate recording of placentation and the diagnosis of the zygosity of the zygosity of same sex multiples at birth.

B) Older, same sex multiples of undetermined zygosity have a right to testing to ascertain their zygosity.

WHEREAS during World War II twins were incarcerated in Nazi concentration camps and submitted by force to experiments which caused disease or death:

IV. Any research incorporating multiples must be subordinated to the informed consent of the multiples and/or their parents and must comply with international codes of ethics governing human experimentation.

WHEREAS inadequate documentation, ignorance, and misconceptions regarding multiples and multiple birth increase the risk of misdiagnosis and/or inappropriate treatment of multiples:

V.

A) Multiple births and deaths must be accurately recorded.

B) Parents and multiples have a right to care by professionals who are knowledgeable regarding the management of multiple gestation and/or the lifelong special needs of multiples.

WHEREAS the bond between co-multiples is a vital aspect of their normal development:

VI. Co-multiples have the right to be placed together in foster care, adoptive families, and custody agreements.

STATEMENT OF NEEDS

Summary: Twins and higher order multiples have unique: conception, gestation and birth processes; health risks; impacts on the family system; developmental environments; and individuation processes. Therefore, in order to insure their optimal development, multiples and their families need access to health care, social services, and education which respect and address their differences from single born children.

WHEREAS twins and higher order multiple births are at high risk of low birth weight (<2,500 grams), and very low birth weight (< 1,500 grams), disability, and infant death:

I. Women who are expecting multiples have a need for:

A) education regarding the prevention and symptoms of preterm labor,

B) prenatal resources and care designed to avert the preterm birth of multiples, including:

1. diagnosis of a multiple pregnancy, ideally by the fifth month, which is communicated tactfully, with respect for the privacy of the parents;

2. nutrition counseling and dietary resources to support a weight gain of eighteen to twenty-seven kilos (forty to sixty pounds);

3. obstetrical care which follows protocols of best practice for multiple birth; and when the health of the mother or family circumstances warrant:

4. extended work leave;

5. bed rest support; and

6. child care for siblings.

WHEREAS breastfeeding provides optimal nutrition and nurture for preterm and full-term multiples; and whereas the process of breastfeeding and/or bottle feeding of multiples is complex and demanding:

II. Families expecting and rearing multiples need the following:

A) education regarding the nutritional, psychological, and financial benefits of breastfeeding for preterm and full-term infants;

B) encouragement and coaching in breastfeeding techniques;

C) education and coached practice in simultaneous bottle feeding of co-multiples; and,

D) adequate resources, support systems, and family work leave to facilitate the breastfeeding and/or bottle feeding process.

WHEREAS sixty percent of multiples are born before thirty-seven weeks gestation and/or at low birth weight and experience a high rate of hospitalization which endangers the bonding process and breastfeeding; and whereas newborn multiples are comforted by their fetal position together:

III. Families with medically fragile multiples need specialized education and assistance to promote and encourage bonding and breastfeeding. Hospital placement of medically fragile multiples and hospital protocols should facilitate family access, including co-multiples' access to each other.

WHEREAS multiple birth infants suffer elevated rates of birth defects and infant death:

IV. Families experiencing the disability and/or death of co-multiples need:

A) care and counseling by professionals who are sensitive to the dynamics of grief associated with disability and/or death in co-multiples; and

B) policies which facilitate appropriate mourning of a deceased multiple or multiples.

WHEREAS the unassisted care of newborn, infant, and toddler multiples elevates their families' risk of illness, substance abuse, child abuse, spouse abuse, divorce, and potential for child abuse:

V. Families caring for multiples need timely access to adequate services and resources in order to:

A) insure access to necessary quantities of infant and child clothing and equipment;

B) enable adequate parental rest and sleep;

C) facilitate healthy nutrition;

D) facilitate the care of siblings;

E) facilitate child safety;

F) facilitate transportation; and

G) facilitate pediatric care.

WHEREAS families with multiples have the unique challenge of promoting the healthy individuation process of each co-multiple and of encouraging and supporting a healthy relationship between the co-multiples; and, whereas the circumstance of multiple birth affects developmental patterns:

VI. Families expecting and rearing multiples need:

A) access to information and guidance in optimal parenting practices regarding the unique developmental aspects of multiple birth children, including the processes of: socialization, individuation, and language acquisition; and

B) access to appropriate testing, evaluation, and schooling for co-multiples with developmental delays and/or behavior problems.

WHEREAS twins and higher order multiples are the subjects of myths and legends and media exploitation which depict multiples as depersonalized stereotypes:

VII. Public education, with emphasis upon the training of professional health and family service providers, and educators, is needed to dispel mythology and disseminate the facts of multiple birth and the developmental processes in twins and higher order multiples.

WHEREAS twins and higher order multiples suffer discrimination from public ignorance about their biological makeup and inflexible policies which fail to accommodate their special needs:

VIII. Twins and higher order multiples need:

A) information and education about the biology of twinning; and

B) health care, education, counseling, and flexible public policies which address their unique developmental norms, individuation processes, and relationship. For example by permitting and/or fostering:

1. the treatment of medically fragile co-multiples in the same hospital;

2. the neonatal placement together of co-multiples in isolettes and cribs to extend the benefits of their fetal position together;

3. medical, developmental, and educational assessment and treatment which is respectful of the relationship between co-multiples;

4. the annual review of the classroom placement of co-multiples, and facilitation of their co-placement or separate placement according to the particular needs of each set of co-multiples;

5. the simultaneous participation of co-multiples on sports teams and other group activities;

6. specialized grief counseling for multiples at the death of a co-multiple;

7. counseling services addressing the special needs of adult multiples.

WHEREAS the participation by multiple birth infants, children, and adults as research subjects has made important contributions to scientific understanding of the heritability of disease, personality variables, and the relative influence of nature and nurture on human development; and, WHEREAS relatively little is known about optimal management of plural pregnancy and the unique developmental patterns of multiples:

IX. Scientists must be encouraged to investigate:

A) the optimal management of plural pregnancies;

B) norms for developmental processes which are affected by multiple birth such as: individuation, socialization, and language acquisition;

C) benchmarks of healthy psychological development, and relevant therapeutic interventions for multiples of all ages and at the death of a co-multiple.

Adopted by the Council of Multiple Birth Organizations (COMBO) (comprised of representatives of sixteen organizations from ten countries: Australia, Belgium, Canada, Germany, Indonesia, Japan, Sweden, Taipei, United Kingdom, United States) (COMBO) of the International Society for Twin Studies at the Eighth International Twin Congress, Richmond, Virginia. May 31, 1995.

Patricia Malmstrom, Chair
Council of Multiple Birth Organization

Endorsed by the Board of the International Society for Twin Studies, May 31, 1995.

Lindon Eaves, President
International Society for Twin Studies
DECLARATION OF RIGHTS AND STATEMENT OF NEEDS OF TWINS AND HIGHER ORDER MULTIPLES

Adopted at the Eighth International Twin Congress, Richmond, Virginia. May 31,1995 by the COUNCIL OF MULTIPLE BIRTH ORGANIZATIONS, International Society for Twin Studies.

ENDORSING ORGANIZATIONS and REPRESENTATIVES, MAY, 1995:

Country	Organization—Name
Australia	LaTrobe Twin Study—David Hay
	Australian Multiple Births Association—Maureen Copeland
Belgium	Association for Research in Multiple Births—Robert Derom
Canada	Parents of Multiple Births Association—Kim Johnson
China	Taipei Twins Association—Cheh Chang
Germany	ABC Club—Ute Grutzner
Indonesia	Twins Foundation—Seto Mulyadi
Japan	The Japanese Association of Twins' Mothers—Yukiko Amau
Sweden	The Swedish Twin Society—Margareta Olwe

U.K.   Twins and Multiple Births Association—Rachel Hudson,
            Audrey Sandbank
            Multiple Births Foundation—Elizabeth Bryan
U.S.A.   The Center for Loss in Multiple Birth—Jean Kollantai
            The Center for the Study of Multiple Birth—Donald Keith
            Illinois Mothers of Twins Clubs—Jean Herr
            National Organization of Mothers of Twins Clubs—
            Rebecca Moskwinski, Marion Meyer
            The Twins Foundation—Kay Cassill
            The Twin to Twin Transfusion Syndrome Foundation—
            Mary Slaman-Forsythe
            Twin Services, Inc.—Patricia Maxwell Malmstrom

http://kate.pc.helsinki.fi/twin/Rights.html
Reproduced with the permission of the Council of Multiple Birth Organizations of
International Society for Twin Studies.

The following sample menus will help you maintain the appropriate intake of calories and nutrients—for you and your babies.

Menu for Multiple Pregnancy

	SUNDAY	MONDAY	TUESDAY	WEDNESDAY	THURSDAY	FRIDAY	SATURDAY
	Breakfast	*Breakfast*	*Breakfast*	*Breakfast*	*Breakfast*	*Breakfast*	*Breakfast*
	½ Grapefruit ½ c Oatmeal 2 Tbsp. Raisins 1 slice Whole wheat toast w/ margarine and jam 1 c Milk	2 Scrambled eggs 1 English muffin 1 c Orange juice—calcium fortified	1 c Multigrain Cheerios with milk Bran muffin 1 c Grapefruit juice	2 Whole grain waffles with margarine and syrup 1 c Apple sauce 2 slices Canadian bacon 1 c Milk	½ c Grits 1 Egg 1 slice Toast with margarine and jam 1 c Orange juice—calcium fortified	Breakfast burrito 1 c Apple juice	Raisin bran cereal with milk 1 slice Cheese toast ¼ Cantaloupe
	Snack	*Snack*	*Snack*	*Snack*	*Snack*	*Snack*	*Snack*
	Banana Yogurt Oatmeal muffin	½ Peanut butter sandwich 1 c Milk	½ Bagel with cream cheese 1 c Strawberries	½ c Cottage cheese—calcium fortified Pear	½ c Trail mix (nuts sunflower seeds and raisins)	8 oz Yogurt with ¼ c Grapenuts cereal	Fruit smoothie
	Lunch	*Lunch*	*Lunch*	*Lunch*	*Lunch*	*Lunch*	*Lunch*
	Turkey/cheese Sandwich Apple slices Decaffeinated tea	Tuna melt Tossed salad 1 c Grapes 1 c Milk	1 c Beef vegetable soup Whole wheat roll 1 c Pineapple Chocolate chip cookies 1 c Milk	Pita pizzas Tossed salad with tomatoes and dressing 5 Vanilla wafers Decaffeinated tea	Ham sandwich on pumpernickel Carrot & celery sticks with ranch dressing 1 c 100% Fruit juice	Bagel roast beef sandwich Green grapes 1 c Milk	1 c Tomato soup Grilled cheese sandwich Granny Smith apple 1 c Milk

Snack	Snack	Snack	Snack	Snack	Snack	Snack
1 c Vegetable juice 2 oz Cheddar cheese 6 Triscuits	Mango 10 Pretzels	Fruit smoothie	6 Whole wheat crackers 1 Tbsp. Peanut butter	Strawberry/banana milkshake	2 oz Cheddar cheese 6 Triscuits 1 c Milk	½ Peanut butter/banana sandwich 1 c Milk

Dinner	Dinner	Dinner	Dinner	Dinner	Dinner	Dinner
Spinach salad with 3 oz Chicken and vinaigrette dressing ¼ c Wild rice ¼ Canteloupe 1 c 100% Fruit juice	Hamburger with 3 oz Ground round on whole wheat bun ½ c Baked beans 1 c Corn 1 c Decaffeinated tea	Seafood pasta 1 slice French bread Mixed field greens salad with tomatoes and dressing 1 c 100% Fruit juice	3 oz Teriyaki chicken breast 1 Loaded baked potato 1 c Collard greens 1 c milk	3 oz Grilled fish 1 c Wild rice Broccoli spears Vanilla pudding 1 c Milk	Spaghetti with meat sauce Salad with dressing Steamed vegetables—Zucchini, Squash, Onions, Snow Peas	3 oz Broiled salmon Baked sweet potato 1 c Green beans 1 c Milk

Snack	Snack	Snack	Snack	Snack	Snack	Snack
1 Tbsp. Peanut butter with 4 Graham crackers 1 c Milk	Raisin Bran cereal with milk	8 oz Flavored yogurt with ¼ c Bran	3 c Popcorn	1 c Frozen yogurt with raspberries on top	8 oz Vanilla yogurt with fresh or frozen blueberries	Banana Oatmeal cookies

Birth Plan for Multiples

My name is _____

My primary support person for this birth will be _____

_____

We are having: Twins ☐ Triplets ☐ Quadruplets ☐

Other ☐ _____

Our forty week due date is _____

We expect that our babies will be born (approx. date) _____

Our obstetrician/midwife is/are_____

_____

We do ☐ do not ☐ plan to use a doula during labor and birth.

We are planning to have a

☐ Vaginal delivery

☐ Cesarean delivery

☐ Unsure

We have consulted with the following specialists:

Perinatologist _____

Neonatologist _____

Other _____

We have attended or plan to attend the following classes: (check all that apply)

☐ Singleton birth preparation classes

☐ Multiple birth education classes

☐ Hospital tour

☐ Tour of NICU

☐ Breastfeeding classes

☐ Infant care classes

☐ Infant safety/CPR classes

☐ Other _____

We would like to record our birth:

☐ With still photographs

☐ With videotape

☐ We want to record our births from the mother's view.

☐ We want record our births from the doctor's view.

If I am a candidate for a vaginal delivery of my babies, I would like to: (check all that apply)

☐ Stay mobile as long as possible.

☐ Use no pain medication unless I specifically request it.

☐ Use nonmedication pain relief strategies such as hot/cold compresses, massage, focused relaxation, and breathing.

☐ Use pain medications only if other methods do not seem to be helping.

☐ Use pain medications as soon as pain is felt.

☐ Use epidural anesthesia if other methods are not helping.

☐ Use epidural anesthesia if needed for managing the birth of our babies.

☐ Use general anesthesia as an emergency measure vs. regional.

☐ Use alternative pushing and birthing positions that may help the babies move down.

I understand that certain interventions may be needed for the well-being of mother and babies. I am comfortable using the following interventions. Please discuss with me plans for using any others.

☐ Diet restricted to clear liquids or ice chips

☐ Intravenous fluids

☐ Contraction monitor, external

☐ Intrauterine pressure catheter

☐ Electronic fetal monitoring, external and internal

☐ Ultrasound

☐ Labor augmentation with oxytocin (Pitocin)

☐ Fetal oxygen saturation monitor

☐ Forceps

☐ Vacuum-assisted birth

☐ Episiotomy

When each of my babies is born, I want to:

☐ Have each of them placed on my abdomen immediately after birth.

☐ Have my husband/support person cut their umbilical cords.

☐ Have each baby stay with us the entire time unless they are medically unstable.

☐ Have them brought back to us from the nursery as quickly as possible.

☐ Breastfeed them within the first hour.

If a cesarean delivery is necessary, I want to:

☐ Use anesthesia that allows me to be awake and alert.

☐ Have my husband present the entire time.

☐ Have my babies brought to me to see, touch, and hold as quickly as possible.

If my babies will be born prematurely, I want to:

☐ Be transferred before delivery to a high-risk care center (if local hospital is not equipped with a Level III NICU)

☐ Meet with the neonatologist before delivery.

☐ See and touch them in the delivery room if they are medically stable.

☐ Have my husband go to the NICU with the babies.

☐ Have photographs made of the babies.

☐ Begin breast pumping in the first hour after delivery.

☐ Have my husband or nurse pump for me if I am not able to do so.

GLOSSARY

Abruption   Premature separation of part of the placenta from its attachment to the uterus.

Alpha fetoprotein (AFP)   A protein produced by the fetus present in amniotic fluid and detectable in the mother's blood. Fetuses with open neural tube defects produce increased amounts of AFP.

Amniocentesis   Procedure in which a small amount of amniotic fluid is removed from the amniotic sac surrounding the fetus for testing.

Amnion   The inner membrane surrounding the fetus.

Amniotic fluid   A liquid that surrounds the fetus during pregnancy, contained in the amniotic sac.

Amniotic sac   Membrane that contains the fetus and the amniotic fluid; often called the "bag of waters."

Amniotomy   Artificial rupture of the amniotic sac.

Analgesic   An agent that reduces pain.

Anemia   The condition of having less than the normal number of red blood cells or hemoglobin.

Anesthesia   The loss of feeling or sensation resulting from the administration of certain drugs or gases.

Apgar score   A newborn health scoring system developed by Virginia Apgar given at one and five minutes after birth; maximum total score is ten.

Apnea   Cessation of breathing.

Areola   Dark-colored skin surrounding the nipple.

Baby blues   Mild depression that may last a couple of weeks following childbirth, usually characterized by mixed feelings of happiness, sadness, excitement, and letdown.

Betamimetic   Adrenaline-like drugs used to relax the uterus.

Bilirubin   A chemical that results from the breakdown of blood.

Biophysical profile   Prenatal test that combines an ultrasound with a nonstress test.

Birth defect   A congenital (present at birth) abnormality.

Blastocyst   Stage of development of the fertilized egg about four days after fertilization.

Bloody show   Vaginal discharge that originates in the cervix and consists of blood and mucus; increases as the cervix dilates during labor.

Bradycardia   Low heart rate.

Bonding   Process of attachment between parents and babies.

Braxton-Hicks   Name often used for contractions that occur before the normal time for labor.

Breech   Presentation in which the fetus is positioned with feet or buttocks toward the cervix.

Bronchopulmonary dysplasia   A chronic lung disease with persistent difficulty breathing and abnormal changes seen on chest x-ray; sometimes follows lung diseases in newborn babies.

Carpal tunnel syndrome   A nerve disorder affecting the hand caused by a pinched nerve; often associated with the swelling and weight gain that accompany pregnancy.

Cerclage   A surgical procedure in which a purse-string type stitch in the cervix is used in an attempt to prevent premature birth.

Cervical incompetence   A condition in which the cervix opens before a pregnancy has reached term; can be treated by surgical procedure called cervical cerclage.

Cervix The cone-shaped neck of the uterus that opens for delivery of a baby.

Cesarean delivery Surgical incision through the mother's abdomen into the uterus to deliver the baby; also called C-section.

Chorion The outer maternal membrane surrounding the fetus.

Chorionic villi sampling Procedure in which a small sample of cells is taken from the placenta for testing.

Chorionicity Term used to describe the arrangement of the chorions in a multiple pregnancy. See *dichorionic* and *monochorionic.*

Chromosome A structure in a cell nucleus that consists of genes. Twenty-three pairs of chromosomes, each pair containing one chromosome from each parent, carry the entire genetic code.

Circumcision Removal of the foreskin from the penis.

Cobedding Putting multiple birth babies to sleep in the same bed or incubator.

Colostrum Thin, yellow-colored liquid produced by a mother's breasts in the first days after giving birth.

Concordance Term for similarity in fetal growth of multiples during pregnancy.

Conjoined twins Identical twins who share body parts or organs.

Continuous positive airway pressure (CPAP) Treatment with a breathing machine to blow a continuous stream of air into the airway and lungs.

Contraction Tightening and shortening of the uterine muscles causing dilatation and thinning of the cervix and the descent of the baby into the birth canal.

Corticosteroid Synthetic hormones given to the mother to help mature fetal lungs.

Crowning The appearance of the top of the baby's head at the vaginal opening during labor.

Dietitian   A professional who plans diet programs for people with special health needs to ensure proper nutrition. A registered dietitian (RD) has special qualifications.

Diamniotic   Refers to two separate amniotic sacs.

Dichorionic   Placental structure with two chorions.

Dilatation   The amount that the cervix opens during labor, from 0 to 10 centimeters.

Discordance   Unequal fetal growth of multiples during pregnancy.

Doppler flow   Technique used to visualize blood flow in blood vessels using ultrasound waves to reflect off blood cells as they move.

Doula   A woman experienced in childbirth who provides support to the mother before, during, and after childbirth.

Ductus arteriosus   Blood vessel in the fetus that joins the aorta with the pulmonary artery; normally closes off at birth.

Edema   Puffiness or swelling that is caused by fluid retention in the body tissue.

Effacement   Thinning and shortening of the cervix during labor, from 0 to 100 percent.

Electronic fetal monitoring   Recording of the fetal heartbeat using an electronic instrument.

Engagement   Occurs when the fetus descends into the pelvic cavity.

Embryo   Term for a developing baby until eight weeks after conception.

Engorgement   Breast swelling and tightness that occurs when a mother's milk comes in.

Entanglement   Tangling or knotting of twins' umbilical cords.

Epidural anesthesia   Injection of local anesthetic in the epidural space of the spinal canal to numb the nerves of the uterus and birth canal.

Episiotomy   An incision into the perineum (area between the vagina and the anus) to enlarge the vaginal opening.

External cephalic version Procedure performed using a doctor's hands on the mother's abdomen to turn a fetus to a vertex presentation.

Fetal distress Change in fetal activity or heartbeat, or meconium-stained amniotic fluid, indicating the fetus is in possible danger.

Fetal fibronectin A protein produced within the tissues of the plancental membranes; present in the cervix and vagina in early pregnancy and before delivery.

Fetal heart rate The number of beats of the fetal heart during pregnancy. Normal fetal heart rate is 120 to 160 beats per minute.

Fetal oxygen saturation monitoring Measuring fetal oxygen levels using a transducer placed against the fetus' skin during labor.

Fetus A baby growing in the mother's uterus; term used after eight weeks gestation.

Folic acid A B vitamin important in cell development. Inadequate folic acid intake before—and in—early pregnancy is related to neural tube defects in the fetus.

Forceps Tong-like instruments used at delivery to help move a baby down through the birth canal.

Fraternal twins Two babies in one pregnancy developing from two separate, fertilized eggs.

Fundus The upper, rounded portion of the uterus.

Funneling Widening of the cervix at the end connected to the uterus; appears Y-, or funnel-shaped, on ultrasound.

Gestation Length of a pregnancy counted in weeks, from the first day of the mother's last menstrual cycle before conception until the baby is delivered.

Gestational diabetes Carbohydrate intolerance diagnosed during pregnancy in which the blood sugar levels are elevated.

Gamete intrafallopian transfer (GIFT) An infertility treatment that involves removing eggs from a woman's ovaries, inserting them into the fallopian tube with sperm, and allowing fertilization to occur in the woman's body.

Group B streptococcus (GBS)   Bacteria present in the reproductive tract of some pregnant women that can be passed to the fetus during pregnancy, delivery, or after birth.

HELLP syndrome   A group of symptoms that occur in pregnant women who have hemolytic anemia (H), elevated liver enzymes (EL), and low platelet (LP) count.

Higher-order multiples   Triplets, quadruplets, quintuplets, and more.

High-risk pregnancy   A pregnancy with a higher than normal chance of developing complications.

Home uterine activity monitoring (HUAM)   Monitoring of uterine contractions using a portable device to transmit a recording of the contractions via a telephone to health care providers; often used for women with preterm labor.

Human chorionic gonadotropin (hCG)   A hormone produced during pregnancy that is present in a woman's blood and urine.

Hyaline membrane disease   Respiratory distress in a premature baby that is caused by a lack of surfactant.

Hydramnios   An excess of amniotic fluid. See *polyhydramnios.*

Incompetent cervix   A defect of the cervix that makes it unable to withstand the pressure and weight of pregnancy resulting in early, gradual, and painless dilatation and effacement.

Infertility   The inability to conceive or carry a baby to term.

Intrauterine growth restriction   Inadequate growth of a fetus compared to the gestational age.

Intravenous (IV)   A small needle or tube inserted into a vein to allow fluids into the blood stream.

Intraventricular hemorrhage (IVH)   Bleeding into or around the fluid-filled cavities (ventricles) of the brain.

In vitro fertilization (IVF)   A procedure to help infertile couples conceive in which eggs and sperm are fertilized in a laboratory and later transferred to a woman's uterus.

Isolette   A clear plastic box used as a bed for premature babies.

Jaundice Yellow discoloration of the skin and eyes due to high levels of bilirubin, a chemical that results from the breakdown of blood.

Kangaroo Care Holding an NICU baby skin-to-skin to provide close human contact and to facilitate parent-infant attachment.

Kegel exercises Exercises to strengthen the pelvic floor done by contracting the perineal muscles.

Kick counting Counting the number of times a fetus moves during a certain period.

Lactation Function of secreting milk or period during which milk is secreted.

Lactation consultant Professional with special training and skills to help women with breastfeeding. Certified lactation consultants (IBCLC) must pass an examination.

LDR Labor/delivery/recovery room.

LDRP Labor/delivery/recovery room/postpartum room.

Lochia Vaginal discharge of mucus, blood, and tissue that occurs after delivery.

Low birth weight Weighing less than 2,500 grams or 5½ pounds at birth.

Magnesium sulfate Medication used to treat high blood pressure in pregnancy; also used for preterm labor.

Marginal cord insertion Connection of the umbilical cord on or near the edge of the placenta.

Mastitis Painful infection of the breast.

Maternal-fetal specialist Obstetrician who has additional training and specializes in the care of both mother and fetus in high-risk pregnancies; also called a perinatologist.

Meconium The greenish black, sticky substance passed as a baby's first bowel movements.

Miscarriage Loss of a pregnancy before the fetus can survive outside the uterus.

Monoamniotic Refers to multiple fetuses sharing one single amniotic sac.

Monochorionic Refers to multiple fetuses sharing one chorion/placenta.

Monozygotic Arising from a single fertilized egg.

Morning sickness Nausea and vomiting that usually occurs in the first trimester of pregnancy; often accompanied by aversions to foods and odors.

Mucus plug A plug of mucus that is present in the cervix during pregnancy.

Multifetal pregnancy reduction Termination of one or more fetuses in a multiple pregnancy.

Multiple birth Delivery of more than one baby in a pregnancy.

Neonatal Concerning the first twenty-eight days after birth.

Neonatal intensive care Unit (NICU) Specialized nursery with trained staff and equipment for the care of sick and premature babies.

Neonatologist Pediatrician with additional training in the care of high-risk newborns.

Necrotizing enterocolitis (NEC) A serious intestinal problem in premature babies.

Neural tube defect Abnormality of the brain or spinal cord, or the coverings that occurs during fetal development.

Nonstress test Monitoring the fetal heart rate to assess the fetal response to its own movements.

Oligohydramnios Too little amniotic fluid.

Oxytocin Pituitary hormone that causes uterine contractions and stimulates the breasts to release milk.

Palpation Hands-on technique used to detect the presence of uterine contractions.

Perinatal Referring to the time before, during, and after birth.

Perinatologist Obstetrician who has additional training and specializes in the care of both mother and fetus in high-risk pregnancies; also called a maternal-fetal specialist.

Periventricular leukomalacia (PVL) Softening of the white matter of the brain near the ventricles due to damage and death of brain tissue.

Pitocin   Brand name for the synthetic form of the hormone oxytocin used to induce labor.

Placenta   Vascular disc-shaped organ with the purpose of maternal-fetal gas and nutrient exchange; also called afterbirth.

Placenta previa   Condition in which the placenta is attached too low on the uterine wall, fully or partially covering the cervix.

Pneumothorax   Collapse of lungs as air accumulates outside them.

Polyhydramnios   Excessive amounts of amniotic fluid around the fetus.

Postpartum   The period of time after delivery, sometimes called the fourth trimester.

Postpartum depression   Strong feelings of sadness, anxiety, or despair after childbirth that interfere with a mother's ability to function and do not go away after a few weeks; onset may be delayed for several weeks or may develop out of unresolved baby blues.

Preeclampsia   See *pregnancy induced hypertension*.

Pregnancy induced hypertension (PIH)   A complication of pregnancy characterized by swelling, high blood pressure, and protein in the urine; also called toxemia and preeclampsia.

Premature   Refers to a baby born before thirty-seven weeks gestation.

Premature rupture of membranes (PROM)   Rupture of the amniotic sac before labor begins.

Presentation   Refers to the part of the fetus that is presenting at the cervical opening.

Preterm   Before thirty-seven weeks gestation.

Prolapsed umbilical cord   When the umbilical cord slips out through the cervix ahead of the baby; can be life threatening if the cord is compressed by the cervix, cutting off blood flow to the placenta and fetus.

Prostaglandin   Substances in the body that can stimulate uterine contractions of labor and birth.

Pulmonary edema   A condition in which fluid accumulates in the lungs.

Quickening   The first fetal movements felt by a pregnant woman.

Respiratory distress syndrome (RDS)   Respiratory distress that is caused by a lack of surfactant; also called hyaline membrane disease.

Retinopathy of prematurity (ROP)   Condition in which there is scarring and abnormal growth of the blood vessels in the retina of a baby's eye.

Rooming-in   When a newborn stays in the same room as the mother after birth.

Rupture of membranes   Breaking of the amniotic sac.

Salivary estriol   Maternal hormone of pregnancy that appears with labor and can be detected in saliva.

Scalp electrode   A small wire attached to the skin of the fetal head that is connected to a fetal heart rate monitor.

Selective reduction   Termination of a specific fetus in a multiple pregnancy.

Singleton   Refers to a single baby in a pregnancy.

Small for gestational age (SGA)   Infant size and weight that are smaller than normal for the length of gestation.

Spina bifida   A birth defect resulting from the abnormal development of the spinal cord.

Station   A number representing the relationship between the presenting part of the fetus and parts of the maternal pelvis called the ischial spines.

Supertwins   Same as higher-order multiples.

Surfactant   Substance produced in the lungs that allows lung tissues to expand and contract easily when breathing; may be absent or decreased in infants born preterm.

Teratogenic   Causing abnormalities in a developing fetus.

Tocolytic   Medication used to slow or stop preterm labor.

Toxemia   See *pregnancy-induced hypertension.*

Triplets   Three babies in the same pregnancy.

Twins   Two babies in the same pregnancy.

Twin-to-twin transfusion syndrome (TTTS)   A condition that affects identical twins with a shared placenta. Blood passes disproportionately from one baby to the other through connecting blood vessels within their shared placenta.

Ultrasound   A test to view internal organs using high-frequency sound waves that echo off the body and create a picture.

Umbilical cord   The connection between the placenta of the mother and the fetus through which blood, oxygen, and nutrients are transported to the fetus and waste products are removed.

Uterine activity   Contracting and relaxing of the uterine muscle.

Uterine irritability   Low-strength, frequent tensing and muscular activity in the uterus.

Vacuum-assisted delivery   A method of delivery using a suction cup on the head of the fetus to help move the baby down the birth canal.

Vagina   Female organ that extends from the outside of the body to the cervix; the passageway for delivery of a baby.

Vanishing twin   Death and disappearance of a multiple in the first three months of pregnancy.

VBAC   Vaginal birth after a prior cesarean birth.

Velamentous cord insertion   Abnormal attachment of the umbilical cord to the placenta.

Version   A maneuver designed to turn the fetus from an undesirable position to a more acceptable one to facilitate delivery.

Vertex   Refers to the fetal head.

Very high multiples   More than three babies in the same pregnancy.

Very low birth weight   Weighing less than 1,500 grams or 3¼ pounds at birth.

Zygote   The fertilized egg before it begins to divide and grow.

Selected Bibliography

Alexander, G. R., Kogan, M., Martin J., Papiernik, E. "What Are the Fetal Growth Patterns of Singletons, Twins, and Triplets in the United States?" *Clinical Obstetrics and Gynecology* 41, no. 1 (1998): 114–125.

American Academy of Pediatrics and American College of Obstetricians and Gynecologists. Perinatal Guidelines. Guidelines for Perinatal Care, 1997.

Benirschke, K. "The Biology of the Twinning Process. How Placentation Influences Outcome." *Seminars in Perinatology* 19, no. 5 (1995): 342–350.

Buekens, P., Wilcox, A. "Why Do Twins Have a Lower Mortality Rate Than Small Singletons?" *American Journal of Obstetrics and Gynecology* 168 (1993):937–941.

Callahan, T. L., Hall, J. E., Ettner, S. L., Christiansen, C. L., Greene, M. F., & Crowley, W. F. "The Economic Impact of Multiple-Gestation Pregnancies and the Contribution of Assisted-Reproduction Techniques to Their Incidence." *New England Journal of Medicine* 331, no. 4 (1994):244–249.

Cohen, L. M., Capeless, E. L., Krusinski, P. A., Maloney, M. E. "Pruritic Urticarial Papules and Plaques of Pregnancy and Its Relationship to Maternal-Fetal Weight Gain and Twin Pregnancy." *Archives of Dermatology* 125, no. 11 (1989):1534–1536.

Coonrod, D. V., Hickok, D. E., Zhu, K., Easterling, T. R., Daling, J. R. "Risk Factors for Preeclampsia in Twin Pregnancies: A Population-Based Cohort Study." *Obstetrics and Gynecology* 85, no. 5 pt. 1 (1995):645–650.

Copper, R. L., Goldenberg, R. L., Das, A., Elder, N., Swain, M., Norman, G., Ramsey, R., Cotroneo, P., Collins, B. A., Johnson, F., Jones, P., Meier, A. M. "The Preterm Prediction Study: Maternal Stress Is Associated with Spontaneous Preterm Birth at Less Than Thirty-Five Weeks' Gestation." National Institute of Child Health and Human Development Maternal-Fetal Medicine Units Network. *American Journal of Obstetrics and Gynecology* 17, no. 5 (1996):1286–1292.

Crane, J. M., Van den Hof, M., Armson, B. A. & Liston, R. "Transvaginal Ultrasound in the Prediction of Preterm Delivery: Singleton and Twin Gestations." *Obstetrics and Gynecology* 90, no. 3 (1997): 357–363.

Crowther, C. A. " Hospitalisation and Bed Rest for Multiple Pregnancy" (Cochrane Review). In: The Cochrane Library, Issue 3. Oxford: Update Software, 2000.

De Catte, L., Camus, M., Bonduelle, M., Liebaers, I., Foulon, W. "Prenatal Diagnosis by Chorionic Villus Sampling in Multiple Pregnancies Prior to Fetal Reduction." *American Journal of Perinatology* 15, no. 5 (1998):339–343.

Dhont, M., De Neubourg, F., Van der Elst, J., De Sutter, P. "Perinatal Outcome of Pregnancies After Assisted Reproduction: A Case-Control Study." *Journal of Assisted Reproductive Genetics* 14, no. 10 (1997):575–580

Dommergues, M., Mahieu-Caputo, D., Dumez, Y. "Is the Route of Delivery a Meaningful Issue in Triplets and Higher Order Multiples?" *Clinical Obstetrics and Gynecology* 41, no. 1 (1998): 24–29.

Dyson, D. C., Danbe, K. H., Bamber, J. A. Crites, Y. M., Field D. R., Maier, J. A., Newman, L. A., Ray, D. A., Walton, D. L., Armstrong, M. A. "Monitoring Women at Risk for Preterm Labor." *New England Journal of Medicine,* 338, no. 1 (1998):15–19.

Ellings, J. M., Newman, R. B., Hulsey, T. C., Bivins, H. A., Jr., Keenan, A. "Reduction in Very Low Birth Weight Deliveries and Perinatal Mortality in A Specialized, Multidisciplinary Twin Clinic." *Obstetrics and Gynecology* 81 (1993):387–391.

Elliott, J. P., Radin, T. G. "The Effect of Corticosteroid Administration on Uterine Activity and Preterm Labor in High-Order Multiple Gestations." *Obstetrics and Gynecology,* 85, no. 2 (1995):250–254.

Elliott, J. P., Radin, T. G. "Quadruplet Pregnancy: Contemporary Management and Outcome." *Obstetrics and Gynecology,* 80, no. 3, pt 1 (1992):421–424.

Fitzsimmons, B. P., Bebbington, M. W., Fluker M. R. "Perinatal and Neonatal Outcomes in Multiple Gestations: Assisted Reproduction Versus Spontaneous Conception."*American Journal of Obstetrics and Gynecology* 79, no. 5 (1998):1162–1167.

Gabbe, S. G., Niebyl, J. R., Simpson, J. L. (Eds.). *Obstetrics: Normal and Problem Pregnancies.* New York: Churchill Livingstone, 1996.

Gardner, M. O., Goldenberg, R. L., Cliver, S. P., Tucker, J. M., Nelson, K. G., Copper, R.L. "The Origin and Outcome of Preterm Twin Pregnancies." *Obstetrics and Gynecology* 85, no. 4 (1995):553 556.

Goldenberg, R. L., Iams, J. D., Miodovnik, M., Van Dorsten, J. P., Thurnau, G., Bottoms, S., Mercer, B. M., Meis, P. J., Moawad, A. H., Das, A., Caritis, S. N., McNellis, D. "The Preterm Prediction Study: Risk Factors in Twin Gestations." *American Journal of Obstetrics and Gynecology* 175 (1996):1047–1053.

Gromada, K. K. and Spangler, A. K. "Breastfeeding Twins and Higher-Order Multiples." *Journal of Obstetric, Gynecologic and Neonatal Nursing* 27, no. 4 (1998):441–449.

Haning, R. V. Jr, Seifer, D. B., Wheeler, C. A., Frishman, G. N., Silver, H., Pierce, D. J. "Effects of Fetal Number and Multifetal Reduction on Length of In Vitro Fertilization Pregnancies." *Obstetrics and Gynecology* 87, no. 6 (1996):964–968.

Hardardottir, H., Kelly, K., Bork, M. D., Cusick, W., Campbell, W. A., Rodis, J. F. "Atypical Presentation of Preeclampsia in High-Order Multifetal Gestations." *Obstetrics and Gynecology* 87, no. 3 (1996): 370–374.

Hecht, B. R.and Magoon, M. W. "Can the Epidemic of Iatrogenic Multiples Be Conquered?" *Clinical Obstetrics and Gynecology* 41, no. 1 (1998):126–137.

Imseis, H. M., Albert, T. A., Iams, J. D. "Identifying Twin Gestations at Low Risk for Preterm Birth with a Transvaginal Ultrasonographic Cervical Measurement at 24 to 26 Weeks' Gestation." *American Journal of Obstetrics and Gynecology* 177, no. 5 (1997):1149–1155.

Janke, J. "The Effect of Relaxation Therapy on Preterm Labor Outcomes." *Journal of Obstetric, Gynecologic and Neonatal Nursing* 28, no. 3 (1999):255–263.

Keith, L., Papiernik, E., Oleszczuk, J. J. "How Should the Efficacy of Prenatal Care Be Tested in Twin Gestations?" *Clinical Obstetrics and Gynecology* 41, no. 1 (1998):84–93.

Keith, L. G., Papiernik, E., Keith, D. M., Luke, B. (Eds.). *Multiple Pregnancy—Epidemiology, Gestations and Perinatal Outcome.* New York: The Parthenon Publishing Group, 1995.

Keys, S. L., Elliott, J. P. "Vaginal Lever Pessary in Patients with Multiple Gestation, Preterm Labor and Low Fetal Station. A Report of Three Cases." *Journal of Reproductive Medicine* 42, no. 11 (1997): 751–755.

Kiely, J. L. "What Is the Population-Based Risk of Preterm Birth Among Twins and Other Multiples?" *Clinical Obstetrics and Gynecology* 41, no. 1 (1998):3–11.

Knuppel, R. A., Lake, M. F., Watson, D. L., Welch, R. A., Hill, W. C., Fleming, A. D., Martin, R. W., Bentley, D. L. "Preventing Preterm Birth in Twin Gestation: Home Uterine Activity Monitoring and Perinatal Nursing Support." *Obstetrics and Gynecology* 76 no. 1 (1990):24S–27S.

Kramer, M. S. "Balanced Protein/Energy Supplementation in Pregnancy (Cochrane Review). In: The Cochrane Library, Issue 2. Oxford: Update Software, 1999.

Lantz, M. E., Chez, R. A., Rodrigues, A., Porter, K. B. "Maternal Weight Gain Patterns and Birth Outcome in Twin Gestation." *Obstetrics and Gynecology* 87 no. 4 (1996):551–555.

Leonard, L. G. "Depression and Anxiety Disorders During Multiple Pregnancy and Parenthood." *Journal of Obstetric, Gynecologic and Neonatal Nursing* 27 no. 3, (1998):329–337.

Luke, B. "The Changing Pattern of Multiple Births in the U.S. Maternal and Infant Characteristics, 1973 and 1990." *Obstetrics and Gynecology* 84, (1994):101–106.

Luke, B., Gillespie, B., Sung-Joon, M., Avni, M., Witter, F., O'Sullivan, M. J. "Critical Periods of Maternal Weight Gain: Effect on Twin Birth Weight." *American Journal of Obstetrics and Gynecology* 177 (1997):1055–1062.

Luke, B., and Keith, L. "The Contribution of Singletons, Twins, and Triplets to Low Birth Weight, Infant Mortality, and Handicap in the United States." *Journal of Reproductive Medicine* 37 (1992):661–666.

Luke, B., Keith, L., Witter, F. R. "Theoretical Model for Reducing Neonatal Morbidity and Mortality and Associated Costs Among Twins." *The Journal of Maternal Fetal Medicine* 1 (1992):14–19.

Luke, B. Minogue, J. "Contribution of Gestational Age, and Birth Weight to Perinatal Viability in Singletons Versus Twins." *The Journal of Maternal Fetal Medicine* 3 (1994):263–264.

Lynch, L., Berkowitz, R. L. "Maternal Serum Alpha-Fetoprotein and Coagulation Profiles After Multifetal Pregnancy Reduction." *American Journal of Obstetrics and Gynecology* 169, no. 4 (1993): 987–990.

Makhseed, M., Al-Sharhan, M., Egbase, P., Al-Essa, M., Grudzinskas, J. G. "Maternal and Perinatal Outcomes of Multiple Pregnancy Following IVF-ET." *International Journal of Gynaecology and Obstetrics* 61, no. 2 (1998):155–163.

Malmstrom, P., Biale, R. "An Agenda for Meeting the Special Needs of Multiple Birth Families." *Acta Geneticae Medicae Et Gemellogiae* 39 (1990):507–514.

Maloni, J. "Averting the Bed Rest Controversy. Preventive Counseling Can Help Avoid the Issue." *AWHONN Lifelines* 2, no. 4 (1998):64, 61–63.

Maloni, J. A., Chance, B., Zhang, C., Cohen, A. W., Betts, D., Gange, S. J. "Physical and Psychosocial Side Effects of Antepartum Hospital Bed Rest." *Nursing Research* 42, no. 4 (1993):197–203.

Martin, J. A., MacDorman, M. F., Mathews, T. J. "Triplet births: Trends and Outcomes, 1971–94." National Center for Health Statistics. *Vital Health Statistics* 21, no. 55 (1997):1–20.

Mastrobattista, J. M., Skupski, D. W., Monga, M., Blanco, J. D., August, P. "The Rate of Severe Preeclampsia is Increased in Triplet as Compared to Twin Gestations." *American Journal of Perinatology* 14, no. 5 (1997):263–265.

McGrath, J. M., Conliffe-Torres, S. "Integrating Family-Centered Developmental Assessment and Intervention into Routine Care in the Neonatal Intensive Care Unit." *Nursing Clinics of North America* 31, no. 2 (1996):367–386.

Morales, W. J., O'Brien, W. F., Knuppel, R. A., Gaylord, S., Hayes, P. "The Effect of Mode of Delivery on the Risk of Intraventricular Hemorrhage in Nondiscordant Twins Under 1500g." *Obstetrics and Gynecology* 73 (1989):107–110.

Newman, R. B. "Obstetric Management of High-Order Multiple Pregnancies." *Bailliere's Clinical Obstetrics and Gynecology* 12, no. 1 (1998):109–129.

Newman, R. B., Ellings, J. M., O'Reilly, M. M., Brost, B. C., Miller, M. C., Gates, D., Jr. "Correlation of Antepartum Uterine Activity and Cervical Change in Twin Gestation." *Acta Geneticae Medicae Et Gemellologiae* 46, no. 1 (1997):1–7.

Newman, R. B., Ellings, J. M. "Specialized Care for the Multiple Gestation." *Seminars in Perinatology* 19 (1995):387–403.

Newman, R. B., Godsey, R. K., Ellings, J. M., Campbell, B. A., Eller, D. P., Miller, M. C. "Quantification of Cervical Change: Relationship to Preterm Delivery in the Multiple Pregnancy." *American Journal of Obstetrics and Gynecology* 165 (1991):264–269.

Newman, R. B., Hamer, C., Miller, M. C. "Outpatient Triplet Management: A Contemporary Review." *American Journal of Obstetrics and Gynecology* 161 (1989):547–555.

Newman, R. B., Luke, B. *Multifetal Pregnancy: A Handbook for Care of the Pregnant Patient.* Philadelphia: Lippincott Williams and Wilkins, 2000.

NIH Consensus Development Panel. "Effect of Corticosteriods for Fetal Maturation on Perinatal Outcome." *Journal of the American Medical Association* 273 (1995):413–418.

Nyqvist, K. H., and Lutes, L. M. "Co-bedding Twins: A Developmentally Supportive Care Strategy." *Journal of Obstetric, Gynecologic and Neonatal Nursing* 27, no. 4 (1998):450–456.

Papiernik, E., Keith, L., Oleszczuk, J. J., Cervantes, A. "What Interventions Are Useful in Reducing the Rate of Preterm Delivery in Twins?" *Clinical Obstetrics and Gynecology* 41, no. 1 (1998): 12–23.

Powers, W. F., Kiely, J. L. "The Risks Confronting Twins: A National Perspective." *American Journal of Obstetrics and Gynecology* 170 (1994):456–461.

Powers, W. F., and Wampler, N. S. "Further Defining the Risks Confronting Twins." *American Journal of Obstetrics and Gynecology* 175 (1996):1522–1528.

Roberts, W. E., Morrison, J. C. "Has the Use of Home Monitors, Fetal Fibronectin, and Measurement of Cervical Length Helped Predict Labor and/or Prevent Preterm Delivery in Twins?" *Clinical Obstetrics and Gynecology* 41, no. 1 (1998):94–102.

Rodis, J. F., McIlveen, P. F., Egan, J. F., Borgida, A. F., Turner, G. W., Campbell, W. A. "Monoamniotic Twins: Improved Perinatal Survival with Accurate Prenatal Diagnosis and Antenatal Fetal Surveillance." *American Journal of Obstetrics and Gynecology* 177, no. 5 (1997): 1046–1049.

Sassoon, D. A., Castro, L. C, Davis, J. L., Hobel, C. J. "Perinatal Outcome in Triplet Versus Twin Gestations." *Obstetrics and Gynecology* 75 (1990):817–820.

Schiff, E., Cohen, S. B., Dulitzky, M., Novikov, I., Friedman, S. A., Mashiach, S., Lipitz, S. "Progression of Labor in Twin Versus Singleton Gestations." *American Journal of Obstetrics and Gynecology* 179, no. 5 (1998):1181–1185.

Spellacy, W. N., Handler, A., Ferre, C. D. "A Case-Control Study of 1253 Twin Pregnancies from a 1982–1987 Perinatal Data Base." *Obstetrics and Gynecology* 75, no. 2 (1990):168–171.

Subcommittee on Nutritional Status and Weight Gain During Pregnancy, "Weight Gain in Twin Pregnancies." In *Nutrition During Pregnancy,* 212–221. Washington, DC: National Academy Press, 1990.

Templeton, A. and Morris, J. K. "Reducing the Risk of Multiple Births by Transfer of Two Embryos After In Vitro Fertilization." *New England Journal of Medicine* 339, no. 9 (1998):573–577.

Wein, P., Warwick, M. M. , Beischer, N. A. "Gestational Diabetes in Twin Pregnancy: Prevalence and Long-Term Implications." *Australian and New Zealand Journal of Obstetrics and Gynaecology* 32 (1992): 322–327.

Wenstrom, K. D., Syrop, C. H., Hammitt, D. G., Van Voorhis, B. J. "Increased Risk of Monochorionic Twinning Associated with Assisted Reproduction." *Fertility and Sterility* 60, no. 3 (1993): 510–514.

Wilcox, L. S., Kiely, J. L., Melvin, C. L., Martin, M. C. "Assisted Reproductive Technologies: Estimates of Their Contribution to Multiple Births and Newborn Hospital Days in the United States." *Fertility and Sterility* 65, no. 2 (1996):361–366.

Resources

Chapter Two

Books

The Long Awaited Stork: A Guide to Parenting After Infertility, by Ellen Sarasohn Glazer, 1998, Jossey-Bass Publishers.

Organizations

American Society of Reproductive Medicine
1209 Montgomery Highway
Birmingham, AL 35216-2809
Phone: (205) 978-5000
Fax: (205) 978-5005
E-mail: asrm@asrm.org
http://www.asrm.org

A voluntary nonprofit organization devoted to advancing knowledge and expertise in reproductive medicine and biology. Members must demonstrate the high ethical principles of the medical profession, evidence an interest in reproductive medicine and biology, and adhere to the objectives of the society.

InterNational Council on Infertility
    Information Dissemination, Inc.
P.O. Box 6836
Arlington, VA 22206
Phone: (703) 379-9178

E-mail: inciidinfo@inciid.org
http://www.inciid.org

INCIID (pronounced "inside") is a nonprofit organization dedicated to educating infertile couples about the latest methods to
diagnose, treat, and prevent infertility and pregnancy loss.

RESOLVE, Inc.
1310 Broadway
Somerville, MA 02144-1779
Business office phone: (617) 623-1156
National help line: (617) 623-0744
Fax: 617-623-0252
E-mail: resolveinc@aol.com
http://www.resolve.org

A national non-profit organization that, for more than twenty
years, has assisted people in resolving their infertility by providing
information, support, and advocacy.

Web Sites

Infertility drugs
http://www.ihr.com/infertility/drugs.html

Infertility glossaries
http://www.inciid.org/glossary.html

Success Rates for Assisted Reproductive Technology, National
Summary and Fertility Clinic Reports
http://www.cdc.gov/nccdphp/drh/arts/index.htm

Chapter Three

Organizations

The Center for Study of Multiple Birth
333 E. Superior Street, Suite 463-5
Chicago, IL 60601
Phone: (312) 908-7532
Fax: (312) 908-8500
http://www.multiplebirth.com

Purpose is to stimulate and foster medical and social research in
the area of multiple birth and help parents with the special problems they and their offspring may encounter.

International Twins Association
6898 Channel Road NE
Minneapolis, MN 55432
Phone: (612) 571-3022
E-mail: ITAConvention@aol.com
http://www.intltwins.org

Marvelous Multiples, Inc.
Multiple Birth Prenatal Education
P.O. Box 381164
Birmingham, AL 35238
Phone: (205) 437-3575
Fax: (205) 437-3574
E-mail: marvmult@aol.com
http://www.marvelousmultiples.com

Mothers of Supertwins (MOST)
P.O. Box 951
Brentwood, NY 11717
Phone: (631) 859-1110
E-mail: maureen@mostonline.org
http://www.mostonline.org

National Online Fathers of Twins Club (NOFOTC)
c/o Jeff Maxwell
2804 NW 163rd
Edmond, OK 73013
E-mail: general.info@nofotc.org
http://www.nofotc.org

National Organization of Mothers of Twins Clubs, Inc.
(NOMOTC)
P.O. Box 438
Thompson Station, TN 37179-0438
Phone: (615) 595-0936, 1-877-540-2200
E-mail: NOMOTC@aol.com
http://www.nomotc.org

Multiples Birth Canada (formerly Parents of Multiple Births
    Association of Canada—POMBA)
P.O. Box 234
Gormley, Ontario, Canada L0H 1G0
Phone : (905) 888-0725
E-mail: office@pomba.org
http://www.pomba.org/index.html

The Triplet Connection
P.O. Box 99571
Stockton, CA 95209
Phone: (209) 474-0885
E-mail: tc@tripletconnection.org
http://www.tripletconnection.org

Triplets, Quads & Quints Association
2968 Nipiwin Drive
Mississauga, Ontario, Canada, L5N 1X9
Phone: (905) 826-0734
E-mail: DianeMyers@aol.com
http://www.tqq.com

Twin Services Consulting
E-mail: twinservices@juno.com
http://www.twinservices.org

The Twins Foundation
P.O. Box 6043
Providence RI 02940
Phone: (401) 729-1000
Fax: (401) 751-4642
E-mail:Twins@twinsfoundation.com
http://www.twinsfoundation.com

TWINS Magazine
5350 S. Roslyn, Suite 400
Englewood, CO 80111-2125
Phone: 1-888-55-TWINS (558-9467)
http://www.twinsmagazine.com

Twins and Multiple Births Association (TAMBA)
Harnott House
309 Chester Road Little Sutton
Ellesmere Port CH66 1QQ England
Phone: 151 348 0020
E-mail: enquiries@tambahq.org.uk
http://www.tamba.org.uk

Twin to Twin Transfusion Syndrome Foundation
411 Longbeach Parkway
Bay Village, OH 44140
Phone : (440) 899-TTTS (8887)
Fax : (440) 899-1184
E-mail: info@tttsfoundation.org
http://www.tttsfoundation.org

High Risk Pregnancy Support

Sidelines National Support Network
P.O. Box 1808
Laguna Beach, CA 92652
Phone: (949) 497-2265
E-mail: sidelines@sidelines.org
http://www.sidelines.org

Loss

Center for Loss in Multiple Birth (CLIMB), Inc.
c/o Jean Kollantai
P.O. Box 91377
Anchorage, AK 99509
Phone : (907) 222-5321
E-mail: climb@pobox.alaska.net
http://www.climb-support.org

Twinless Twins Support Group International
9311 Poplar Creek Place
Leo, IN 46765
Phone: (219) 627-5414
E-mail: Twinworld1@aol.com
http://fwi.com/twinless

Web Sites

Twins and Supertwins List
http://www.twinslist.org

Chapter Six

Organizations

Family Medical Leave
U.S. Department of Labor
1-800-959-FMLA (3652)
http://www.dol.gov/dol/esa/fmla.htm

Mother's Access to Careers at Home, Inc.
P.O. Box 123
Annandale, VA 22003
Phone: (703) 205-9664
http://www.freestate.net/match

Home-Based Working Moms
P.O. Box 500164
Austin, TX 78750
Phone: (512) 266-0900
http://www.hbwm.com
E-mail: hbwm@hbwm.com

Working Woman Network
135 W. 50th Street
New York, NY 10020
Phone: (212) 445-6100
www.workingwoman.com

Chapter Seven

Organizations

American Board of Medical Specialties (ABMS)
1007 Church Street, Suite 404
Evanston, IL 60201-5913
Phone: (847) 491-9091
Fax: (847) 328-3596
http://www.abms.org

The ABMS Public Education Program's physician locator and information service allows the public to verify free of charge the board certification status, location by city and state, and specialty of any physician certified by one or more of the twenty-four member boards of the ABMS. You may need the correct spelling of the physician's name.

American College of Obstetricians and Gynecologists
409 12th Street, SW
Washington, D.C. 20024
Phone: (202) 863-2518
Fax: (202) 484-1595
E-mail: resources@acog.org
http://www.acog.org

The ACOG Resource Center offers a list of members in your area, as well as subspecialists in maternal-fetal medicine, reproductive endocrinology, and gynecologic oncology.

Marvelous Multiples, Inc.
P.O. Box 381164
Birmingham, AL 35238
Phone: (205) 437-3575
Fax: (205) 437-3574
E-mail: marvmult@aol.com
http://www.marvelousmultiples.com

Links to multiple birth education classes nationwide.

Society for Maternal-Fetal Medicine
409 12th Street, SW
Washington, D.C. 20024-2188
Phone: (202) 863-2476
Fax: (202) 554-1132
http://www.smfm.org

Boot Camp for New Dads
www.bcnd.org
E-mail: http://www.susan@newdads.com
Phone: (949) 786-3146

Web Sites

Administrators in Medicine (AIM)
http://www.docboard.org

This association of state medical board executive directors provides links to physician profiles in many states, and should have all
states accessible by the year 2000.

Chapter Eight

Book

A Child Is Born, by Lennart Nilsson, 1990, Bantam Doubleday
Dell.

Web Sites

http://www.pregnancycalendar.com/first9months
http://www.pregnancyguideonline.com
http://www.visembryo.com

Chapter Nine

Organizations

American College of Obstetricians and Gynecologists (ACOG)
Resource Center
Phone: (202) 863-2518
Fax: (202) 484-1595
E-mail: resources@acog.org
http://www.acog.org

The ACOG Resource Center will send you up to five different
ACOG Patient Education Pamphlets. Include your full name, e-
mail address, affiliation, mailing address, and the titles and codes
of the pamphlets you want:

- Amniocentesis and chorionic villus sampling (AP107)
- Genetic disorders (AP094)
- Later childbearing (AP060)

GeneClinics
University of Washington School of Medicine
9725 Third Avenue NE, Suite 610
Seattle, WA 98115
Phone: (206) 221-4674
FAX (206) 221-4679
http://www.geneclinics.com
E-mail: geneclinics@geneclinics.org

GeneClinics is a clinical information resource relating genetic
testing to the diagnosis, management, and genetic counseling of
individuals and families with specific inherited disorders.

GeneTests, CH-94
Children's Hospital and Regional Medical Center
P.O. Box 5371
Seattle, WA 98105-0371
Phone: (206) 527-5742

Fax: (206) 527-5743
http://www.genetests.org
E-mail: genetests@genetests.org

GeneTests is a genetic testing resource, funded by the National
Library of Medicine of the NIH and Maternal & Child Health
Bureau of the HRSA. It includes a medical genetics laboratory directory, genetics clinic directory, and an introduction to genetic
counseling and testing concepts.

Web Sites

Ultrasound websites with ultrasound photos and movies
http://www.ob-ultrasound.net
http://pregnancy.about.com/library/ultrasounds/
bltwinusindex.htm

Prevention of spina bifida and other NTDs
http://vm.cfsan.fda.gov
http://www.cdc.gov/ncch/cddh/folic

Chapter Ten

Books

The High-Risk Pregnancy Sourcebook, by Denise M. Chism, 1998,
Lowell House.

*When Pregnancy Isn't Perfect: A Layperson's Guide to Compli-
cations in Pregnancy*, by Laurie A. Rich, 1996, Larata Press.

Organizations

Group B Strep Association
P.O. Box 16515
Chapel Hill, NC 27516
http://www.groupbstrep.org

The Coalition for Positive Outcomes in Pregnancy
507 Capital Court, NE
Washington, DC 20002
Phone: (202) 544-7499
Fax: (202) 546-7105
http://www.storknet.org/CPOP

Chapter Eleven

Organizations

Center for Loss in Multiple Birth, Inc. (CLIMB, Inc.)
c/o Jean Kollantai
P.O. Box 91377
Anchorage AK 99509
Phone: (907) 222-5321
E-mail: climb@pobox.alaska.net
http://www.climb-support.org

Compassionate Friends
Phone: (708) 990-0010
Self-help group for parents, grandparents, and siblings of children.
who have died.

Conjoined Twins International
P.O. Box 10895
Prescott, AZ 86304-0895
http://www.familyvillage.wisc.edu/lib_conjoined.htm

European Research Group on Fetoscopy
E-mail: eurofoetus@eurofoetus.org
http://www.eurofoetus.org

The Florida Institute for Fetal Diagnosis and Therapy
13601 Bruce B. Downs Boulevard, Suite 160
Tampa, FL 33613
Phone: (813) 872-2951

Fax: (813) 971-6985; 1-888-FETAL-77 (888-338-2577)
E-mail: Quintero@fetalmd.com
http://www.fetalmd.com

The HELLP Syndrome Society, Inc.
P.O. Box 44
Bethany, WV 26032
E-mail: j.pyle@mail.bethanywv.edu
http://member.aol.com/hellp1995/hellp.html

Resolve Through Sharing
1910 South Avenue
LaCrosse, WI 54601
Phone: (608) 791-4747; 1-800-362-9567, x4747
Contact: Fran Rybarik
International perinatal bereavement program offering training, seminars, and support materials.

Twin Hope, Inc.
2592 West 14th Street
Cleveland, OH 44113
Phone: (440) 353-1933
E-mail: twinhope@twinhope.com
http://www.twinhope.com

The Twin to Twin Transfusion Syndrome Foundation
National Office
411 Longbeach Parkway
Bay Village, OH 44140
Phone: (440) 899-TTTS (8887)
Fax: (440) 899-1184
E-mail: info@tttsfoundation.org
http://www.tttsfoundation.org

Web Sites

LIMBO (Loss In Multiple Births Outreach) Internet List
To subscribe to the list, send an email message to
listguru@fatcity.com
In the body of the message write: SUB LIMBO-L

Monoamniotic Monochorionic Support Site
E-mail: momo@monoamniotic.org
http://www.monoamniotic.org/

On-line Support for Loss of Multiples
http://boards2.parentsplace.com/cgi-bin/boards/losttwin

Chapter Twelve

Books

The Bed Rest Survival Guide, by Barbara Edelston Peterson and Hallie Beachum, 1998, Avon Books.

Days in Waiting: A Guide to Surviving Pregnancy Bed Rest, by Mary Ann McCann, 1999, A Place to Remember.

Organizations

Sidelines National Support Network
National Office
P. O. Box 1808
Laguna Beach, CA 92652
Phone: (949) 497-2265; (760) 598-5331; (949) 581-5266
E-mail: sidelines@sidelines.org
http://www.sidelines.org

Offers, among other services, a bed rest checklist

Web Sites

Pregnancy Bed Rest
Information and support for families and caregivers
http://www.son.wisc.edu/~son/bedrest

Twins and Supertwins Mailing List
Bed Rest in Multiple Pregnancy
http://www.owc.net/~twins/bedrest.htm

Chapter Thirteen

Web Sites

American Society for Reproductive Medicine
Fact Sheet: Multiple Gestation and
    Multifetal Pregnancy Reduction
http://www.asrm.org/Patients/FactSheets/
Multiple_Gestation_Fact.pdf

FIGO
http://www.figo.org

An international organization of obstetricians and gynecologists
whose mission is to promote the well-being of women and to
raise the standard of practice in obstetrics and gynecology

FIGO Committee for the Study of Ethical Aspects of
    Human Reproduction
http://www.md.huji.ac.il/figo/INDEX.HTM

MEDLINE searches through PUBMED
http://www.ncbi.nlm.nih.gov/PubMed/PubMed

Provides access to a library of medical research

Part III

Organizations

Coalition for Improving Maternity Service (CIMS)
National Office
P.O. Box 2346
Ponte Verde Beach, FL 32004
Phone: (888) 282-CIMS (2467); (904) 285-1613
Fax: (904) 285-2120
E-mail: info@motherfriendly.org
http://www.motherfriendly.org

Chapter Fourteen

Organizations

The American Academy of Pediatrics
141 Northwest Point Blvd.
Elk Grove Village, IL 60007-1098
Phone: (847) 434-4000
Fax: (847) 434-8000
E-mail: http://kidsdocs@aap.org
http://www.aap.org

American College of Obstetricians and Gynecologists
409 12th St., S.W.
Washington, D.C. 20090-6920
Phone: (202) 863-2518
Fax: (202) 484-1595
E-mail: resources@acog.org
http://www.acog.org

The ACOG Resource Center can provide a list of members in your area, as well as subspecialists in maternal-fetal medicine, reproductive endocrinology, and gynecologic oncology.

American Society of Anesthesiologists
520 N. Northwest Highway
Park Ridge, IL 60068-2573
Phone: (847) 825-5586
E-mail: mail@ASAhq.org
http://www.asahq.org/PublicEducation/Childbirth.html

Doulas of North America (DONA)
13513 North Grove Drive
Alpine, UT 84004
Phone: (801) 756-7331
Fax: (801) 763-1847
E-mail: AskDONA@aol.com
http://www.dona.com

Chapter Fifteen

Organizations

National Marrow Donor Program
List of cord blood registries
Phone: 1-800-526-7809
http://www.marrow.org/FAQS/cord_blood_faqs.html

Chapter 16

Organizations

American College of Obstetricians and Gynecologists
Resource Center
Phone: (202) 863-2518
Fax: (202) 484-1595
E-mail: resources@acog.org
http://www.acog.org

The ACOG Resource Center will send you up to five different
ACOG Patient Education Pamphlets. Include your full name,
e-mail address, affiliation, mailing address, and the titles and
codes of the pamphlets you want:

- Birth control AP005
- Cesarean birth AP006
- Having twins AP092
- Vaginal birth after cesarean delivery AP070

Chapter Seventeen

Books

Depression After Childbirth : How to Recognize, Treat, and Prevent Postnatal Depression, by Katharina Dalton and Wendy
Holton, 1996, Oxford University Press.

Overcoming Postpartum Depression & Anxiety, by Linda Sebastian, 1998, Addicus Books.

Postpartum Survival Guide, by Ann Dunnewold and Diane G.
Sanford, 1994, New Harbinger Publishing.

This Isn't What I Expected: Overcoming Postpartum Depression, by Karen R. Kleiman and Valerie D. Raskin, 1994, Bantam Doubleday Dell.

Organizations

Depression After Delivery (DAD)
P.O. Box 278
Belle Mead, NJ 08502
Phone: (908) 575-9121; 1-800-944-4773 (Voice-mail information)
http://www.behavenet.com/dadinc

Depression Awareness, Recognition, and Treatment Program
National Institute of Mental Health
5600 Fishers Lane, Rm. 15C-05
Rockville, MD 20857
Phone: 1-800-421-4211
http://www.nimh.nih.gov

Postpartum Stress Center
1062 Lancaster Avenue, Suite 8
Rosemont, PA 19010
Phone: (610) 525-7527
E-mail: Kkleinman@aol.com
http://www.postpartumstress.com

Postpartum Support International
927 North Kellog Avenue
Santa Barbara, CA 93111
Phone: (805) 967-7636
E-mail: postpartum@aol.com
http://www.chss.iup.edu/postpartum

Chapter Eighteen

Organizations

American Academy of Pediatrics
141 Northwest Point Boulevard
Elk Grove Village, IL 60007-1098
http://www.aap.org

On-line pediatrician referral service is currently under development.

Chapter 20

Books

Born Too Soon, by Elizabeth Mehren, 1998, Kensington Publishing Corporation.

Breast Feeding Your Premature Baby, by Gwen Gotsch, 1999, La Leche League International.

Caring for Your Premature Baby: A Complete Resource for Parents, by Alan H. Klein and Jill Alison Ganon, 1998, Harper Reference.

Preemie Parents' Companion: The Essential Guide to Caring for Your Premature Baby in the Hospital, at Home, and Through the First Years, by Susan L. Madden M.S., 1999, Harvard Common Press.

You Are Not Alone: The NICU Experience, September 1998, Children's Medical Ventures, Inc.

Your Premature Baby : Everything You Need to Know About the Childbirth, Treatment, and Parenting of Premature Infants, by Frank P. Manginello and Theresa Foy Digeronimo, 1991, John Wiley & Sons.

Your Premature Baby and Child: Helpful Answers and Advice for Parents, by Amy E. Tracy and Dianne I. Maroney, edited by Judy C. Bernbaum and Jessie Groothuis, 1999, Berkley Pub Group.

Organizations

American Association for Premature Infants (AAPI)
P.O. Box 46371
Cincinnati, OH 45246-0371
http://www.aapi-online.org

A national advocacy organization dedicated to improving the quality of health of premature infants and providing developmental and educational services for their families

Children's Medical Ventures, Inc.
Hospital ordering: 1-800-377-3449
Parent ordering: Use on-line catalog or
call (888) SOOTHIE (766-8443)
http://www.childmed.com

Developmental care products and parent support for premature babies.

Lutes & Lutes Consulting, Inc.
Linda M. Lutes, M.Ed.
Infant Development Specialist/Educator/Consultant
106 Lakehoma Parkway
Mustang, OK 73064
Phone: (405) 818-2625
Fax: (405) 376-5051
E-mail: lindamlutes@aol.com

National Institute on Deafness and Other
   Communication Disorders
National Institutes of Health
31 Center Drive, MSC 2320
Bethesda, MD 20892-2320
http://www.nidcd.nih.gov/health/parents/index.htm

Parent Care, Inc.
101½ South Union Street
Alexandria, VA 22314-3323

Web Sites

Database of Neonatology Research
http://www.cochrane.org/revabstr.mainindex.htm

Emory University Developmental Continuity Program
http://www.emory.edu/PEDS/NEONATOLOGY/DCP
Information on prematurity and developmental outcomes with
milestones for corrected age.

Internet Discussion Forums and E-mail List
http://home.vicnet.net.au/~garyh/preemie.htm
http://www.preemie.org

List of Neonatology Websites
http://members.home.net/cotton/neoweb.html

National Association of Neonatal Nurses
http://www.nann.org/

Neonatology on the Web
http://www.neonatology.org/

Parent Support
http://www2.medsch.wisc.edu/childrenshosp/
parents_of_preemies/overview.html

Recommended Standards for Newborn ICU Design
http://www.nd.edu/~kkolberg/DesignStandards.htm

Chapter 22

Books

Breastfeeding: A Parent's Guide, 7th ed., by Amy Spangler, 1999, self-published.

Breastfeeding Your Premature Baby, by Gwen Gotch, 1999, La Leche League International.

Mothering Multiples, by Karen Kerkhoff Gromada, 1999, La Leche League International.

Organizations

The International Board of Lactation Consultant Examiners
   (IBLCE)
7309 Arlington Boulevard, Suite 300
Falls Church, VA 22042-3215
Phone: (703) 560-7330
Fax: (703) 560-7332
E-mail: iblce@erols.com
http://www.iblce.org

International Lactation Consultant Association (ILCA)
4101 Lake Boone Trail, Suite 201
Raleigh, NC 27607
Phone: (919) 787-5181
Fax: (919) 787-4916
E-mail: ilca@erols.com
http://www.ilca.org/

La Leche League International
1400 N. Meacham Road
Schaumburg, IL 60173-4048
Phone: (847) 519-7730
Fax : (847) 519-0035
http://www.lalecheleague.org

Web Sites

Breastfeeding More Than One
http://www.parentingweb.com/lounge/multiples.htm

Breastfeeding Twins
http://www.nursingmother.com/helpme/
helpme_images_twins.html

La Leche League International
http://www.lalecheleague.org/bfmultiple.html

Breast Pumps and Breastfeeding Accessories

Hollister/Ameda
Phone: 1-800-323-4060 (US); 1-800-263-7400 (Canada)
http://www.hollister.com/products/breast.htm

Kisses From Heaven
P. O. Box 6742
Lees Summit, MO 64064
Phone: 1-800-459-0461
http://www.kissesfromheaven.com

Medela, Inc.
P.O. Box 660
McHenry, IL 60051-0660
Phone: 1-800-435-8316
Fax: (815)363-9941
http://www.medela.com

Nurse EZ Twin Nursing Pillow
Basic Comfort, Inc.
445 Lincoln Street
Denver, Colorado 80203

Phone: (303) 778-7535; 1-800-456-8687
Fax (303) 778-0143
E-mail: sales@basiccomfort.com
http://www.basiccomfort.com

White River Concepts
925 C Calle Negocio
San Clemente, CA 92673
Phone: (949) 366-8960; 1 800-342-3906
Email: custsvc@whiteriver.com
http//www.whiteriver.com

Chapter 23

Books

The Art of Parenting Twins: The Unique Joys and Challenges of Raising Twins and Other Multiples, by Patricia Maxwell Malmstrom and Janet Poland, 1999, Ballantine Books.

Raising Multiple Birth Children: A Parents' Survival Guide, by William Laut, Kristin Benit, and Sheila Laut, 1999, Chandler House Press.

Twins, Triplets and More, by Elizabeth M. Bryan, 1998, St Martins Press.

When You're Expecting Twins, Triplets, or Quads: A Complete Resource, by Barbara Luke and Tamara Eberlein, 1999, Harper Perennial.

Car Seats

American Academy of Pediatrics
Division of Publications
P.O. Box 747
Elk Grove Village, IL 60009-0747

- 2000 Family Shopping Guide to Car Seats
  Safety and Product Information
  http://www.aap.org/family/famshop.htm
- Car Seat Shopping Guide for Children with Special Needs
  http://www.aap.org/family/99cars.htm

U.S. Department of Transportation Auto Safety Hotline
1-888-327-4236

Nursery Equipment

Arms Reach
Phone: 1-800-954-9353
Fax: (818) 991-5999
http://www.armsreach.com

More Than One (equipment)
Mainly Multiples (announcements, cards, invitations)
1727-8A Sardis Road N., Suite 276
Charlotte, NC 28270
Phone: 1-800-388-TWIN (8946)
http://www.morethan1.com

Nursery Product Safety

Office of Information and Public Affairs
Washington, D.C., 20207
http://www.cpsc.gov/cpscpub/pubs/pub_idx.html
Write or go online for free copies of these brochures:

- Consumer Product Safety Commission
- Nursery Equipment Safety Checklist
- The Safe Nursery, A Buyer's Guide

The Danny Foundation—Nursery Safety
P.O. Box 680
Alamo, CA 94507
1-800-83-DANNY (3-2669)
http://www.dannyfoundation.org

National Sudden Infant Death Syndrome Resource Center
2070 Chain Bridge Road, Suite 450
Vienna, VA 22182
Phone: (703) 821-8955
Fax: (703) 821-2098
E-mail: sids@circsol.com
http://www.circsol.com/sids

Sudden Infant Death Syndrome Alliance
1314 Bedford Avenue, Suite 210
Baltimore, MD 21208
Phone: 1-800-221-7437; (410) 653-8226
Fax: (410) 653-8709
http://www.sidsalliance.org

On-Line Baby Gift Registries

eTOYS
Phone: 1-800-GO-ETOYS (463-8697)
http://www.etoys.com

Babies R Us/Toys R Us
Phone: 1-888-Toys-Web (869-7932)
http://www.babiesrus.com

Target
Phone: 1-800-888-9333
http://www.target.com

Premature Clothing

Le Petite Baby
1915 SE 34th Avenue
Portland, OR 97214-5709
Phone: 1-800-767-9374
Fax: (413) 473-2005
http://www.snuggletown.com/preemie

The Preemie Store . . . and More!
17195 Newhope Street, Suite 105
Fountain Valley, CA 92708
Phone: (714) 434-3740; 1-800-O-SO-TINY (676-8469)
Fax: (714) 434-7510
http://www.preemie.com

Tiny Bundles
11468 Ballybunion Square
San Diego, CA 92128
Phone: (858) 451-9907
http://www.tinybundles.com

Index

A

A&B (apnea and bradycardia)
episodes, 277
abdomen
dark line down (linea nigra),
75
itching, 73
shooting pain, 70
stretch marks, 75
abortion, 192
Accutane, 90
aches and pains, 70–72
addiction of babies, 89–90
additives in food, 54–55
AFI (amniotic fluid index), 167
AFP (alpha-fetoprotein) testing,
117–118
after-pains, 250–251
age and multiple pregnancy, 9
alcohol use, 88
alpha-fetoprotein (AFP) testing,
117–118
amniocentesis, 119–120
for treating TTTS, 172–173
amnioInfusion, 168
amniotic fluid, 14
low volume of and IUGR,
164

oligohydramnios, 164, 169
polyhydramnios, 167
premature rupture of mem-
branes (PROM), 139–141
problems with, 166–168
water breaks, 220
amniotic fluid index (AFI), 167
amniotic sac, 14
amniotomy, 236
analgesics, 207
anemia
mothers and, 74
premature babies and, 279
antacids during labor, 223
anxiety during pregnancy, 34
Apgar score, 265
apnea, 277
apnea and bradycardia (A&B)
episodes, 277
ART (assisted reproductive
technologies), 21–22
artificial sweeteners, 55
assisted reproductive technologies (ART), 21–22

B

baby blues, 255

baby showers for multiples, 337–338

back labor, 229–230

backaches, 70–71

bassinets, 331–332

bathing of newborns, 267

bed rest, 181–188
    coping with, 184–188
    at home, 185–187
    in the hospital, 187–188
    problems with, 182–184

bedding for cribs, 332

betamethazone, 148–149

betamimetics, 145–147

bilirubin, premature babies and, 280

biophysical profile (BPP), 121, 172

birth. *See* cesarean birth; vaginal birth

birth control after delivery, 257

birth defects data, 113–114

birth plan, 197
    sample, 353–356

birth rate data, multiples, 7–8

birth weight
    factors contributing to lower weight, 108–109
    ideal weight for multiples, 109
    low birth weight, 133
    and mother's weight gain, 39, 57
    preterm birth and, 133
    very low birth weight, 133
    See also intrauterine growth restriction (IUGR); small for gestational age (SGA)

birthing centers, 212

blastocyst stage, 23

bleeding after giving birth, 251

blood clotting complication, after IUFD, 177

blood glucose testing of newborns, 269

blood vessel changes, 72

bloody discharge, 136

bonding with babies, 300–306
    in the hospital, 304–306
    multiple babies and, 302–303
    truths about bonding, 301–302

Boot Camp for Dads, 103

bottle feeding multiples, 326–327

BPD (bronchopulmonary dysplasia), 276

BPP (biophysical profile), 121, 172

bra support, 63

Braxton-Hicks contractions, 136

breaking water, 220

breast milk for premature newborns, 278

breast pumping, 323–325

breastfeeding, 307–326
    benefits to baby, 311–312
    benefits to mother, 309–310
    disadvantages of, 313
    feeding rotation, 317
    feeding scenario, 318
    higher-order multiples and, 317–318
    lactation consultant, 100–101, 273, 319
    milk production, 314–315
    mother's health and energy, 325–326

premature or sick babies, 322
during recovery, 246–247
simultaneous nursing,
319–322
starting, 315–317
troubleshooting, 319
breasts, condition of after birth,
251–252
breech delivery, 233–234
Brethine, 145–147
bronchopulmonary dysplasia
(BPD), 276

C
caffeine, 54–55
calcium, recommended amounts
of, 44–45
calories, needs per baby, 40–41
car bed, 335–336
car seatbelts, positioning during
pregnancy, 87–88
car seats, 334–336
carpal tunnel syndrome (CTS),
72
case manager, 95, 272–273
castor oil, 90
cat litter, 56
Celestone, 148–149
cerebral palsy, 133, 282
cervical cerclage, 150–151
cervix, changes in and preterm
labor, 141–142
changes in and labor,
228–230
cesarean birth, 239–244
incisions, 242–243
operating room environment,
241–242
preparing for, 240–241
the procedure, 242–244

special situations, 216–217
See also recovery and post-par-
tum care
changing table, 334
cheeses to avoid, 56
children, caring for during
pregnancy, 80–83
chloasma, 75
cholestasis, 73–74
chorioamnionitis, 140
chorion, 14
chorionic villus sampling (CVS),
118–119
chorionicity, 14
chronic abruption, 170
chronic lung disease (CLD), 276
circulation
after giving birth, 253
during pregnancy, 74
circumcision, 269–270
classes, prenatal 102–104
CLD (chronic lung disease), 276
clomiphene citrate (Clomid), 20
clothing, maternity, 62–63
clothing for babies, 332–333
co-bedding of multiples,
110–111, 291–294
in NICU, 293
cocaine, 89–90
cohosh, 90
colostrum, 246
combined vaginal/cesarean
delivery, 216
complications in multiple
pregnancy
amniotic fluid problems,
166–168
fetal loss, 175–179
gestational diabetes, 165–166
high blood pressure, 157–162

intrauterine growth restriction (IUGR), 162–165
placental problems, 169–174
preterm labor and birth, 131–155
umbilical cord problems, 174–175
compresses for engorged breasts, 252
conjoined twins, 15
constipation, 66
continuous positive airway pressure (CPAP), 276
contraction stress test (CST), 121
contractions
detecting, 136–137
after giving birth, 250–251
organized contractions, 136
preterm labor, 137
types of, 135–136
uterine activity monitoring at home, 144
uterine irritability, 135–136
conversion table (pounds/grams), 268
cord blood banking, 237–238
corticosteroids
high blood pressure treatment, 162
preterm labor treatment, 148–149
Coumadin, 90
CPAP (continuous positive airway pressure), 276
cradles, 331–332
cribs, 331–332
CST (contraction stress test), 121

CVS (chorionic villus sampling), 118–119

D
dads. See fathers
death of fetus. See fetal loss
delayed interval birth, 152
delivery
fetal loss and, 178
fetal position and, 214–215
with high blood pressure, 162
planning for, 211–217
timing of, 212
where should multiples be born, 212–214
See also cesarean birth; vaginal birth
depression, 35
postpartum depression, 256–257
developmental care for babies, 283–289
benefits of, 284
co-bedding of multiples, 291–294
Kangaroo Care, 289–291
requesting, 294
dexamethazone, 148–149
diabetes. See gestational diabetes mellitus (GDM)
diagnosis of multiple pregnancy, 16–18
diapers, 333–334
diastasis recti, 72–73, 253–254
DIC (disseminated intravascular coagulation), 177
dichorionic-diamniotic chorionicity, 14
diet. See nutrition

digestion
 early pregnancy, 64–65
 later in pregnancy, 66
dilation, cervical,
 in labor, 227–230
 preterm, 141
disability plans and high-risk
 pregnancy, 79
disseminated intravascular
 coagulation (DIC), 177
dizygotic, 12
DNA testing, 16
Doppler flow ultrasound, 122,
 172
doulas, 202–203, 339
drug addiction, 89–90
drugs and pregnancy, 89–90
Dubowitz/Ballard Exam for
 Gestational Age, 265–266
due date, 96

E
E. coli, 55
eating disorders and nutrition,
 54
eclampsia, 158
 See also high blood pressure
EDC (estimated date of
 confinement), 96
edema, 74
 high blood pressure and, 159
effacement, 227
emotional issues, 31–38
 about babies in NICU,
  295–298
 balancing your concerns,
  35–37
 common concerns, 32–33
 fathers and, 33–34

postpartum coping tips,
 257–258
support resources, 37–38
worries that are out of
 control, 34–35
employment issues for working
 mothers, 77–80
endometritis, 251
endotracheal tube, 276
enema, 222
engorged breasts, 252
epidural anesthesia, 205,
 210–211
episiotomy, 226
estimated date of confinement
 (EDC), 96
ET tube, 276
evening primrose oil, 90
exercise
 during pregnancy, 82–85
 after giving birth, 254
 pelvic rock exercise, 71
external cephalic version,
 233–234
eye prophylaxis for newborns,
 266

F
Family Medical Leave Act, 80
FAS (fetal acoustic stimulation),
 120–121
FAS (fetal alcohol syndrome),
 88
fathers
 Boot Camp for Dads, 103
 emotions during pregnancy,
  33–34
 support during labor and
  delivery, 201–202

fatigue, 67–68
fats, 47
fertility drugs, and incidence of
    multiples, 20–21
Fertinex, 21
fetal acoustic stimulation (FAS),
    120–121
fetal alcohol syndrome (FAS),
    88
fetal fibronectin (fFN) test,
    142–144
fetal growth and development,
    105–111
    beginning of pregnancy,
        105–106
    intrauterine behavior,
        109–111
    multiple fetal development,
        108–109
    single fetal development,
        106–107
fetal heart monitor during labor,
    223–224
fetal loss, 175–179
    early pregnancy loss, 175–176
    grieving process, 177–179
    later pregnancy loss, 176–177
fetal movement
    reporting, 99–100
    what to expect, 122–123
fetal oxygen saturation
    (FSaO*sub*2) monitor,
    224–225
fFN (fetal fibronectin) test,
    142–144
fish to avoid, 47
fluid intake, 52–53
flushing, and blood vessel
    changes, 72

folic acid, 43
    for preventing neural tube
        defects (NTDs), 118
    supplement, 51
Follistim, 21
food. See nutrition
food-borne illnesses, 55–56
food pyramid, 41–42
forceps during delivery, 142
fraternal multiples, 12–13
    chorionicity, 14
    determining, 15–16
FSaO*sub*2 monitor, 224–225
full rooming-in, 300
funneling of the cervix, 141

G
gamete intrafallopian transfer
    (GIFT), 21
gastrointestinal discomforts after
    birth, 249
GDM. See gestational diabetes
    mellitus (GDM)
general anesthesia, 209
genital herpes, cesarean delivery
    and, 216–217
gestational assessment of
    newborns, 265–266
gestational diabetes mellitus
    (GDM), 165–166
    detection of, 166
    and nutrition, 53
gestational sac, 17
gingivitis, 72
Gonal F, 21
grieving process, fetal loss,
    177–179

H

hand problems, carpal tunnel
  syndrome (CTS), 72
handling of premature babies,
  286
hCG (human chorionic
  gonadotropin) levels, 64
HDN (hemorrhagic disease of
  the newborn), 266
hearing tests for newborns, 270
heartburn, 66
HELLP syndrome, 159
  See also high blood pressure
help after returning home,
  338–339
hemorrhage, postpartum
  complication, 246
hemorrhagic disease of the
  newborn (HDN), 266
hemorrhoids, 72
Hepatitis B vaccine, for
  newborns, 269
herbal preparations and
  pregnancy, 90
herpes (genital), cesarean
  delivery and, 216–217
high blood pressure, 157–162
  frequency of, 157–158
  prevention, 160
  signs and symptoms, 159
  treatment, 160–162
high-impact exercise, 84
higher-order multiples, 13
  breastfeeding, 317–318
  defined, 4
  delivery methods, 216
  ideal weight for, 109
  pregnancy risks, 127
  preventing, 22–23
  See also triplets

home births, 212
home uterine activity
  monitoring (HUAM), 144
homemakers and caring for
  other children, 80–83
hospital staff, during labor and
  delivery, 203–204
hospitalization
  admission during labor,
    221–222
  for bed rest, 187–188
  for high blood pressure, 161
  for preterm labor, 149–150
  See also neonatal intensive care
    unit (NICU)
HUAM (home uterine activity
  monitoring), 144
human chorionic gonadotropin
  (hCG) levels, 64
Humegon, 21
hyaline membrane disease,
  132–133
hydralazine, 162
hydramnios, 167
hyperbilirubinemia, premature
  babies and, 280
hyperemesis gravidarum, 65
hypertension. *See* high blood
  pressure
hypothyroidism, testing
  newborns for, 267

I

identical multiples, 10–12
  chorionicity, 14
  determining, 15–16
illegal drugs and pregnancy,
  89–90
immature oocyte retrieval, 23

in vitro fertilization (IVF), 21
  preventing higher-order
    multiples, 23
incompetent cervix, 150–151
incubators, 275
indomethacin, 147–148
inducing labor, 235–236
infection
  premature babies and, 279
  and premature rupture of
    membranes (PROM), 140
  and vaginal discharge,
    137–138
infertility treatments
  assisted reproductive tech-
    nologies (ART), 21–22
  conception timing, 105–106
  concerns with pregnancy
    after, 24–29
  difficulties after, 26–28
  incidence of multiples, 20–21
  and multiple pregnancy, 9
  ovulation-stimulating drugs,
    20–21
  prenatal care after, 25–26
  preventing higher-order
    multiples, 22–23
insomnia, 68–70
interdelivery time, 234
intimacy and sexual relations
  during pregnancy, 86–87
intracytoplasmic sperm injection
  (ICSI), 21
intrauterine fetal demise
  (IUFD), 176–177
intrauterine growth restriction
  (IUGR), 108–109,
    162–165
  See also birth weight

intrauterine pressure catheter
  (IUPC), 224
intravenous line/fluids, 223
intraventricular hemorrhage
  (IVH), 133
  premature babies and, 281
iron supplements, 51
  anemia and, 74
isolettes, 275
itching, 73–74
IUFD (intrauterine fetal
  demise), 176–177
IUGR. See intrauterine growth
  restriction (IUGR)
IUPC (intrauterine pressure
  catheter), 224
IVF. See in vitro fertilization
  (IVF)
IVH. See intraventricular
  hemorrhage
IVs during labor and delivery,
  223

J
jaundice
  mothers and, 73
  premature babies and, 280

K
Kangaroo Care, 289–291
kicks. See fetal movement
kidney function, after giving
  birth, 253

L
labetolol, 162
labor, 227–235
  evaluating progress of,
    227–228

hospital admission, 221–222
inducing, 235–236
pain relief during, 205–211
signs of, 219–221
Stage 1, 228–230
Stage 2, 230–235
Stage 3, 235
labor augmentation, 236
labor curve, 227
labor/delivery/recovery (LDR) room, 213
labor/delivery/recovery/post-partum (LDRP) room, 213
lactation consultant, 100–101, 273, 319
Lamaze classes, 103
laser surgery, for treating TTTS, 173
LDR room, 213
LDRP room, 213
leg cramps, 71
Level II ultrasound, 115
lifting, 84
linea nigra, 75
Listeriosis, 55–56
local anesthetic, 207
lochia, 251
loss of fetus. See fetal loss
low birth weight, 133
    risk for with twins, 126
    risk for with triplets, 127
low-impact exercise, 84

M
magnesium sulfate
    high blood pressure treatment, 161
    preterm labor treatment, 147
magnesium supplements, 51–52
marginal cord insertion, 174

marijuana, 89
Marvelous Multiples® Course, 103
massage, 85
mastitis, 252–253
maternal-fetal specialist. See peri-natologist
maternity insurance, 79
maternity supporter, for backaches, 71
meconium,
    bathing and, 267
    in amniotic fluid, 220
    use of IUPC with, 224
medicated pain relief, 207–209
menu samples, 49–50, 350–351
Metrodin, 21
mineral supplements, 51–52
monoamniotic, 12
    cord entanglement and, 174
monochorionic-monoamniotic chorionicity, 14–15
monozygotic, 10
morning sickness, 64–65
mother-friendly care, 197–198
movement of babies. See fetal movement
multifetal pregnancy reduction, 191–196
    decision making, 194–196
    the procedure, 193
    risks and complications, 194
multiple pregnancy, defined, 4
multiples
    birth rate data, 7–8
    defined, 4

N
naming babies, 202–204
nausea, 64–65

necrotizing enterocolitis (NEC), 133, 281
neonatal intensive care unit (NICU), 104, 271–273
  co-bedding guidelines, 293
  emotional issue for parents, 295–298
  light and sound in, 287–288
  reducing environmental stress in, 288–289
neonatal nurse, 272
neonatal nurse practitioner, 272
neonatologist, 100, 272
neural tube defect (NTD), 117–118
newborns
  appearance and characteristics, 262–264
  developmental care for, 283–289
  initial care and testing, 266–270
  in intensive care, 271–282
  procedures and treatments, 265–266
  well-baby care in hospital, 261–270
  See also premature newborns
NICU. *See* neonatal intensive care unit
nifedipine
  high blood pressure treatment, 162
  preterm labor treatment, 148
nonimpact conditioning, 84–85
nonmedicated pain relief, 206
nonnutritive sucking, 286–287
nonstress test (NST), 120–121, 172

nonvertex positions, 216
nourishment of premature newborns, 277–278
NST (nonstress test), 120–121, 172
NTD (neural tube defect), 117–118
nursery for the babies, 329–331
nursing. *See* breastfeeding
nutrition, 39–60
  additives in food, 54–55
  breads, grains, cereal, rice, and pasta, 42–43
  calorie increases per baby, 40–41
  cheeses to avoid, 56
  dairy products, 44–45
  diabetes and, 53
  eating disorders and, 54
  fats, 47
  fluid intake, 52–53
  fruits, 43
  meat, poultry, fish, dry beans, eggs, and nuts, 46–47
  menu samples, 49–50, 350–351
  recommendations, 40–50
  snacks, 48–49
  supplementing your diet, 50–52
  vegetables, 44
  vegetarians and, 53
nutritional supplements, 52

O
obstetric nurses, 94
obstetrician
  choosing, 92–93
  questions to ask, 198

occupational therapist, 273
OHSS (ovarian hyperstimulation syndrome), 21
oligohydramnios, 164, 169
organized contractions, 136
ovarian hyperstimulation syndrome (OHSS), 21
over-the-counter medications, 90
ovulation-stimulating drugs, 20
    preventing higher-order multiples, 22–23
    side effects, 21
oxygen for premature newborns, 275–277

P
pain management
    labor and birth, 205–211
    recovery and postpartum care, 248–249
parenting multiples
    after infertility, 28–29
    See also bonding with babies
partial rooming-in, 300
patent ductus arteriosus (PDA), 280
pediatrician, choosing, 100
pelvic rock exercise, 71
Pergonal, 21
"peri-care," 248
perinatal case manager, 95
perinatal nurse practitioners, 94
perinatologist, choosing, 93–94
perineum care, 248
periventricular leukomalacia (PVL), 281–282
phenylketonuria (PKU) testing, 267

photography during labor and delivery, hospital policy on, 200
PIH (pregnancy-induced hypertension). *See* high blood pressure
Pitocin, 229, 236
PKU (phenylketonuria) testing, 267
placenta previa, 89, 138, 169–170
placental abruption, 89, 138, 140–141, 170–171
placentas
    delivery of, 235
    in multiple pregnancy, 13–15
planning for birth, 199–217
    delivery decisions, 211–217
    items to bring to the hospital, 199–201
    pain relief in labor and birth, 205–211
    support in labor and delivery, 201–203
pneumothorax in premature babies, 277
positioning of babies, 284–285
positions of babies, delivery methods and, 214–216
postpartum blues, 254–256
postpartum care. *See* recovery and postpartum care
postpartum contractions, 250–251
postpartum depression, 256–257
preeclampsia. *See* high blood pressure

Pregnancy Discrimination Act, 80

pregnancy-induced hypertension (PIH). *See* high blood pressure

pregnancy massage, 85

pregnancy yoga, 85

premature newborns
appearance and characteristics, 263–264
breast milk for, 278
breastfeeding, 322
developmental care for, 283–289
health problems of, 279–282
in intensive care, 271–282
needs of, 275–278
survival statistics, 274–275
See also neonatal intensive care unit (NICU); preterm labor and birth

premature rupture of membranes (PROM), 139–141

prenatal care, 91–104
choosing a care provider, 91–95
first appointment, 95–97
after infertility treatments, 25–26
schedule for visits and tests, 97–102

prenatal diagnosis and testing, 113–123
alpha-fetoprotein (AFP) testing, 117–118
amniocentesis, 119–120
biophysical profile (BPP), 121
chorionic villus sampling (CVS), 118–119
Doppler flow ultrasound, 122

fetal movement, 122–123
nonstress test (NST), 120–121
ultrasound, 114–117

prenatal education, 102–104

prenatal vitamins, 50–51

prescription medications, 90

preterm labor and birth, 131–155
causes of, 134–135
cervical cerclage, 150–151
complications of, 132–134
defining preterm, 131–132
delayed interval birth, 152
home uterine activity monitoring, 144
hospitalization, 149–150
medications for treatment, 145–149
predicting, 141–144
progressive muscle relaxation, 153, 154
reducing chances of, 153, 155
relaxation therapy, 152–153
signs of, 135–139
test for predicting, 142–144
vaginal pessary, 151

Procardia, 148

progressive muscle relaxation, 153, 154

PROM (premature rupture of membranes), 139–141

prostaglandin, 236

protein supplement caution, 47

pruritic urticarial papules and plaques of pregnancy (PUPPP), 73

pubic hair shave prep, 222–223

pudendal block, 207

PUPPP (pruritic urticarial
      papules and plaques of
      pregnancy), 73
Puregon, 21
PVL (periventricular leukomala-
      cia), premature babies and,
      281–282

Q
quadruplets. *See* higher-order
      multiples
questions to ask your doctor,
      198
quickening, reporting, 99–100

R
race
   lower birth weights in multi-
      ples and, 108
   and multiple pregnancy, 9
RDA for multiple pregnancy, 40
RDS (respiratory distress
      syndrome), 132–133, 276
recommended dietary allow-
      ances (RDA) for multiple
      pregnancy, 40
recovery and postpartum care,
      245–258
   coping tips, 257–258
   first hours of recovery,
      246–247
   hospital care during, 247–248
   other discomforts, 249–250
   pain management, 248–249
reduction. *See* multifetal
      pregnancy reduction
reflux, 66
relaxation therapy, for preterm
      labor, 152–153
Repronex, 21

rescue cerclage, 152
respiratory distress syndrome
      (RDS), 132–133, 276
respiratory therapist, 273
retinopathy of prematurity
      (ROP), premature babies
      and, 280
risks of multiple pregnancy
   dealing with the risks,
      127–129
   overview, 125–126
   twin pregnancy, 126 127
   triplet pregnancy, 127
   quadruplet pregnancy, 127
ritodrine, 145–147
rooming-in with babies in the
      hospital, 299–300
ROP (retinopathy of prematu-
      rity), premature babies
      and, 280
round ligament pain, 70
rupture of membranes. *See*
      premature rupture of
      membranes (PROM)

S
salivary estriol test, 142–144
sample birth plan, 353–356
sample menus, 49–50, 350–351
screening tests for newborns,
      267, 269
seatbelts, positioning during
      pregnancy, 87–88
secondhand smoke hazards, 89
sedatives, 207
selective reduction, 192
Serophene, 20
sexual relations during
      pregnancy, 86–87

SGA (small for gestational age), 163, 265
shave prep, 222–223
shoes, 63
shortness of breath, 67
Siamese twins. *See* conjoined twins
SIDS. *See* sudden infant death syndrome (SIDS)
singleton, defined, 4
skin
    changes during pregnancy, 75
    itching problems, 73–74
sleep problems, 68–70
small for gestational age (SGA), 163, 265
    See also birth weight
smoking during pregnancy, 89
snacks, 48–49
social activities during pregnancy, 85–86
social worker, 273
spina bifida, AFP testing for, 117
spinal block, 209
steroids. *See* corticosteroids
stress and stability in newborns, signs of, 284, 285
stress during pregnancy, 34
stretch marks, 75
strollers, 336–337
sucking, nonnutritive, 286–287
sudden infant death syndrome (SIDS)
    smoking and, 89
    soft bedding and, 332
sugar substitutes, 55
superovulation, 20
supplementing your diet, 50–52
support groups, *See* Resources
surfactant, 133

swelling, 74
    after birth, 249–250
    high blood pressure and, 159
swimming, 84

T
targeted imaging for fetal anomalies (TIFFA) study, 115
teratogen, 78
terbutaline sulfate, 145–147
term newborns
    appearance and characteristics, 263–264
    See also newborns
termination of fetus. *See* multifetal pregnancy reduction
tetracycline, 90
time between births, *See* interdelivery time
TIFFA study (Level II ultrasound), 115
tocotransducer, 224
total parenteral nutrition (TPN), 65
toxemia. *See* high blood pressure
toxoplasmosis, 56
TPN (total parenteral nutrition), 65
tranquilizers, 207
travel during pregnancy, 87–88
trichorionic-triamniotic chorionicity, 14
triplets
    defined, 4
    ideal weight for, 109
    pregnancy risks, 127
    weight gain guidelines, 58
    See also higher-order multiples

trizygotic, 12
TTTS. *See* twin-to-twin transfusion syndrome (TTTS)
"twin skin," 253
twin-to-twin transfusion
 syndrome (TTTS)
 detection of, 172
 Doppler flow ultrasound,
  122, 172
 IUGR and, 164
 nonstress testing for, 121
 oligohydramnios, 169
 overview, 171
 polyhydramnios, 167
 shared placenta and, 15, 171
 slower weight gain, 108–109
 treatment, 172–174
 ultrasound for identifying,
  116
twinning, defined, 4
twins
 defined, 4
 fetal positions, 215
 food pyramid servings for, 42
 ideal weight for, 109
 pregnancy risks, 126–127
 weight gain distribution, 59
 weight gain guidelines, 58
twins clubs, *See* Resources

U
ultrasound, 114–117
 biophysical profile (BPP), 121
 for determining identical or
  fraternal twins, 15–16
 for diagnosis of multiple
  pregnancy, 16–18
 Doppler flow ultrasound,
  122, 172

funneling of the cervix
 detection, 142
IUGR detection, 164
during labor and delivery, 225
Level II ultrasound, 115
umbilical cord problem
 detection, 173–174
umbilical cord
 cord care for newborns, 267
 problems, 174–175
urinary catheter, 226
urinary tract infections, 67
urination, 66–67
uterine irritability contractions,
 135–136
uterus
 after giving birth, 250–251
 in labor, 229
 growth of during pregnancy,
  62

V
vacuum-assisted delivery,
 225–226
vaginal birth
 the birth, 231–232
 after cesarean, 236–237, 242
 delivery of babies, 230–231
 procedures, 222–226
 the second baby, 233–234
 time between births, 234–235
 See also delivery; recovery and
  postpartum care
vaginal discharge
 after giving birth, 251
 preterm labor and, 137–138
vaginal pessary, 151
"vanishing twin" theory,
 175–176, 192–193

vasa previa, 174

VBAC. *See* vaginal birth, after cesarean

vegetables, 44

vegetarians and nutrition, 53

velamentous cord insertion, 174

vertex/nonvertex position, 214–215

vertex/vertex position, 214

very high multiples
   defined, 4
   weight gain guidelines, 58

very low birth weight, p.133
   risk for with twins, p. 126
   risk for with triplets, p. 127

vitamin K, for newborns, 266

vitamins, prenatal, 50–51

W

walking, 84

walking epidural, 208

warmth for premature newborns, 275

water breaks, 220

weighing of newborns, 266–267
   conversion table (pounds/grams), 268

weight gain in pregnancy, 57–60
   and birth weight, 39, 57
   distribution of weight, 59–60
   guidelines for, 58–59

weight loss and muscle tone, after giving birth, 253–254

working mothers, special issues for, 77–80

worries that are out of control, 34–35

Y

yoga, 85

Z

zygote
   and fraternal multiples, 12
   and identical multiples, 10